T0146226

Deliver Me from Pain

Deliver Me from Pain

Anesthesia and Birth in America

JACQUELINE H. WOLF

The Johns Hopkins University Press
Baltimore

Printed in the United States of America on acid-free paper

2 4 6 8 9 7 5 3 1

The Johns Hopkins University Press

2715 North Charles Street

Baltimore, Maryland 21218-4363

www.press.jhu.edu

Library of Congress Cataloging-in-Publication Data

Wolf, Jacqueline H.

Deliver me from pain : anesthesia and birth in America / Jacqueline H. Wolf.

p. ; cm.

Includes bibliographical references and index.

ISBN-13: 978-0-8018-9110-6 (hardcover : alk. paper)

ISBN-10: 0-8018-9110-8 (hardcover : alk. paper)

1. Anesthesia in obstetrics—United States—History.   2. Childbirth—United
States—History.   3. Natural childbirth—United States—History.   I. Title.
[DNLM: 1. Delivery, Obstetric—history—United States.   2. Delivery,
Obstetric—psychology—United States.   3. Anesthesia, Obstetrical—
history—United States.   4. History, 19th Century—United States.
5. History, 20th Century—United States.   6. Labor Pain—history—United States.
7. Labor Pain—psychology—United States.   8. Socioeconomic Factors—
United States. WQ 11 AA1 W854d 2009]

RG732.W76 2009

617.9′682—dc22   2008021274

A catalog record for this book is available from the British Library.

*Special discounts are available for bulk purchases of this book. For more information,
please contact Special Sales at 410-516-6936 or specialsales@press.jhu.edu.*

The Johns Hopkins University Press uses environmentally friendly book materials,
including recycled text paper that is composed of at least 30 percent post-consumer
waste, whenever possible. All of our book papers are acid-free, and our jackets and
covers are printed on paper with recycled content.

To my close women friends, the doulas of my life

CONTENTS

*T*his book is the product of personal experience as well as scholarship. I owe a special debt to two of my oldest friends, Mary Ludden DeJong and Estelle Carol, for introducing me to social birth almost thirty years ago. I realize now that in attending the births of three of their six children (two home births for Mary and one low-tech hospital birth for Estelle) and watching Mary and Estelle closely as they labored, I internalized their casual attitudes. "So that's how you behave during birth," I said to myself as I watched first Mary and, several years later, Estelle relax through contractions. By the time I was pregnant, birth held no fear for me. I knew exactly what to expect and what to do, thanks to these wonderful role models. (That is, to a point. Seeing Mary and Estelle give birth without anesthesia and with barely a grimace was a little deceiving. I vividly recall the moment Mary arrived to help me through my labor. I managed to open one eye and with great difficulty gasp in the midst of a contraction, "I can't believe you've done this four times.")

My interest in exploring the topic of this book stemmed from those events. Having so enjoyed my birth experiences as both witness and eventually mother, I looked forward to discussing birth physiology and the history of birth practices with medical students, undergraduates, and graduates via the lectures and classes I offer today through the departments of social medicine and history at Ohio University. I was stunned to find that the young women attending my medical school lectures and history classes met my enthusiasm for birth and birth practices not with keen interest but with wide-eyed horror. This I had not anticipated. What happened to the passion and fearlessness with which women approached childbirth? How had unbridled enthusiasm in the 1970s for women's unique strength and power during labor and birth been replaced in the late 1990s with abject fear and a fervent wish to avoid every sensation of birth? Seeking answers to these questions set me on the path that became this book, and so I am grateful to the students who taught me at least as much as I taught them.

I also owe special thanks to Sam Wilen, the kind of attentive partner for whom "husband-coached" childbirth was invented. If he had left my side even momentarily during my labor with our daughter, Cora, I would have lost control. His voice carried me through. He also nurtured this book in many small ways, most notably giving me hours of valuable writing time as the project neared completion by transcribing several of the oral history interview tapes with mothers and physicians, translating mysterious words and acronyms like "parous" and "VBAC" as "Paris??" and "V-Back??"

I could not have even begun researching and writing this book without the aid of several granting agencies. I was the fortunate recipient of a multiyear National Institutes of Health–National Library of Medicine Publication Grant, two Ohio University Research Challenge grants, an Ohio University College of Osteopathic Medicine Office of Research Direct Grant Award, and an Ohio University Research Committee Award.

In the course of my research for this book, I interviewed several dozen mothers and physicians who generously shared with me their varied and fascinating birth experiences. I wish I could thank them each by name, but, alas, in the era of HIPAA they must remain anonymous. As I prepared for these oral history interviews, Amanda Konradi, a sociologist formerly of Ohio University and now at Loyola College of Maryland, helped me (a historian accustomed to studying yellowing documents rather than interviewing living people) to construct the questionnaires I used to probe the experiences of mothers and doctors.

As I worked on this project, I met often with Katherine Jellison and Steven Merritt Miner as the RRC (Ruthless Readers' Club). We were each writing a book—Katherine on the history of the American infatuation with the white wedding, Steve on the experience of the Soviet people during World War II—and our weekly critiques of each other's work proved essential to our progress. Katherine and Steve are colleagues in the best sense of that word; I am grateful for their support, friendship, and unremitting constructive criticism. Steve Rubenstein was also a valued member of the RRC, until he left Ohio University for the University of Liverpool.

Norman Gevitz, Janet Golden, Barbara Katz Rothman, my brother Robert V. Wolf, and an anonymous reviewer for the Johns Hopkins University Press read one version or another of this book (in Rob's case several versions) and offered many suggestions for improvement, almost all of which I gratefully incorporated. This book is far sounder thanks to their generous help.

I am also grateful to Donald Caton, Timothy R. B. Johnson, and Wanda Ronner; each of these physicians gave this book an invaluable medical scan. Their work and interest in the history of women's health and medicine made their input particularly helpful. Any errors that remain are, of course, mine alone.

My brother Kevin Wolf, an actuary specializing in health care costs, was unstinting with his knowledge of the history of the health insurance industry and maternity coverage. An Excel master, he also maintained the bar graph tracking the annual rise of the cesarean section rate that appears in Chapter 6. My parents, Herbert and Nancy Wolf, and my brother Glenn Wolf provided meals and a touch of home during my numerous research visits to Chicago and Boston.

Jacqueline Wehmueller at the Johns Hopkins University Press has been a dream editor, gently offering suggestions throughout the research, writing, and production processes. Lois Crum, a freelance copy editor for Johns Hopkins, provided elegant wordsmithing and a sharp eye.

Thanks, too, to Linda Ross and Angela Cross for helping me find photographs and to Jeff Brown for his assistance with the book's illustrations.

I owe many a "eureka!" moment to archivists. Special thanks to Debra Scarbrough, Mary Hyde, and Pamela Van Hine of the American College of Obstetricians and Gynecologists; Stacey Peeples of the Pennsylvania Hospital Historic Collections; Susan Sacharski of the Northwestern Memorial Hospital archives; Patrick Sim, Judy Robins, and Karen Bieterman of the Wood Library–Museum of Anesthesiology; Russell Johnson and Marcia Meldrum of the UCLA Louise M. Darling Biomedical Library History and Special Collections Division; Monica Ralston of the Minnesota Historical Society; the late Archie Motley of the Chicago Historical Society; Susan Rishworth of the American College of Surgeons; Heidi Butler, formerly of the Rush University Medical Center Archives; Jack Eckert of the Countway Medical Library at Harvard University; Stephen Greenberg of the National Library of Medicine, History of Medicine Division; Kathy Jacob of the Schlesinger Library; and Marian Taliaferro of the Association of American Medical Colleges.

My daughter, Cora Wilen, was three when I began to write my dissertation, seven when I began to write my first book, and ten when my first book was published. She is now a stunning seventeen and long accustomed to a mother who spends every daylight hour of every weekend working in her study. Cora: Thanks for being my occasional companion in that study, curled up on the floor reading while I was writing. However you choose to give birth, I hope the births of your children will be as wondrous an event in your life as your birth was for me. And if your children are half as magnificent as you are, your life will indeed be blessed.

Deliver Me from Pain

"Terrible Torture" or "The Nicest Sensation I've Ever Had"?

Conflicting Perceptions of Labor in U.S. History

Of all the bitterly contested obstetric treatments of the past 160 years, the administration of anesthesia for labor pain has prompted the longest-lasting disagreement. William T. G. Morton inadvertently sparked this discussion when he demonstrated the miraculous use of ether during surgery before an enthralled audience at Massachusetts General Hospital in Boston in 1846. Within a year, James Young Simpson exhibited the anesthetic properties of chloroform to similarly enthusiastic colleagues in Edinburgh, Scotland. In the wake of these two exciting discoveries, doctors almost immediately began using ether and chloroform during childbirth as well as surgery. Controversy generated by that move has been a hallmark of obstetrics ever since.[1]

Like other public debates about women's reproductive health and medicine, the century-and-a-half-long discussion of the necessity and efficacy of obstetric anesthesia has been characterized by hyperbole. Voices of moderation have been drowned out by the proponents of two extreme and contradictory views of labor. The words of two nineteenth-century physicians exemplify these views. One argued that birthing chambers were principally scenes of "cheerfulness and gayety." The other portrayed labor as "terrible torture, hopeless of relief." These diametrically opposed views have persisted. The statements of two mothers in the twentieth and twenty-first centuries paint the same irreconcilable pictures. One described her unmedicated labor as "the most ecstatic, interesting, adventurous, exciting, enjoyable and personally triumphant accomplishment I have yet known." The other condemned unanesthetized childbirth as "a barbaric ritual." No matter the century, proponents of the "cheerful" and "ecstatic" view of labor contend that obstetric anesthesia is wholly unnecessary and extremely dangerous; proponents of the "terrible" and "barbaric" view declare anesthesia to be an unequivocal necessity for all women who care about dignity, comfort, and health.[2]

These contradictory positions have their origins in two rival obstetric philosophies, personified by the arguments between obstetricians Charles Meigs and James Young Simpson in the mid-nineteenth century and J. Whitridge Williams and Joseph DeLee in the early twentieth. Meigs and Williams argued that birth is primarily a physiological event requiring skilled and attentive but largely hands-off medical care. Simpson and DeLee contended that birth is primarily a potentially pathological event requiring skilled, attentive, and largely hands-on medical care.

Disagreement about the use of obstetric anesthesia has been an integral component of this long-running dispute. Today, those who view birth as chiefly a physiological occurrence observe, "Obstetric anesthesia is unique in medicine in that we use an invasive and potentially hazardous procedure to provide a humanitarian service to healthy women undergoing a physiological process." Those who emphasize the potential for pathology during birth contend, "There is no other circumstance where it is considered acceptable for a person to experience severe pain, amenable to safe intervention, while under a physician's care." The two positions continue to be argued among obstetricians, among women, and between women and their obstetricians.[3]

For most mothers, birth is a deeply personal experience, central to their lives; their feelings about it are heartfelt and often immutable. Even if women were able to anticipate birth objectively or reexamine it dispassionately after the fact, consensus would remain unlikely. Wide variations in how women experience labor pain make rational discussion about this topic unusually difficult. The experience of pain is peculiar to the individual, even given identical medical conditions. Innate personality traits, ability to tolerate discomfort, religious beliefs, access to social and emotional support, social status, immediate environment, past experience, learned expectations, and cultural nuances all contribute to how an individual anticipates and reacts to pain. Recent studies about labor pain in particular indicate that women's prior anxiety about pain, expectation of severe pain during labor, and belief that labor pain is a negative phenomenon are factors associated with the most painful labors. Given these and other variables, individuals experience pain through many lenses. A woman might perceive labor as a terrifying task, as an opportunity to display strength and heroism, as well-deserved or wholly undeserved punishment, as the normal consequence of a specific and self-limiting condition, as utterly unbearable, or as easily dismissed suffering preceding great reward.[4]

Culture and experience also dictate how pain should be expressed, and that

expression—stoic silence, occasional wincing, low moaning, constant complaining, or uncontrolled hysteria, to name only a few examples—can further shape
the nature of the physical feeling. Behavior while giving birth is a particularly
good example of this phenomenon; in cultures where the custom is to remain
silent, women experience the sensations of labor differently than in cultures
where screaming is the expected reaction. Asking and answering the important
cultural question "How am I supposed to behave in this situation?" dictates not
only outward behavior but often physical and emotional sensation as well.[5]

Thus, while the physiology of birth is fundamentally the same for all women,
the experience of birth is not. Even in countries with similar standards of living,
cultures dictate differing practices that shape women's knowledge and perception
of birth before and after the fact, for various cultures offer dramatically different
"right" answers to a host of questions: Who should be present to sustain a laboring woman? Does a woman even need emotional support during labor? Who is
qualified to offer the expertise that keeps both mother and baby safe throughout
labor and birth? What is the definition of "normal" labor? Where is an appropriate place to labor and give birth? What positions should women assume during
labor? What treatments are beneficial during labor? Under what conditions are
these treatments given? Who is qualified to administer them? What treatments
should be avoided? How should a mother behave during labor? How should the
baby be handled in the immediate aftermath of birth? The answers to these questions mold women's anticipation of and reactions to labor and their overall experience of giving birth.[6]

Even women from the same culture, class, and era—that is, women undergoing essentially the same set of cultural and medical rituals during birth—can
experience labor very differently. This difference in perception and proclivity became acutely clear to me while participating on a panel of women invited to share
their birth experiences with third-year medical students at Ohio University. Over
two hours, we took turns describing the births of our children and answering students' questions. At one point in my narrative, I described the stretching of the
perineum at the end of second-stage labor as "a burning sensation." Another
woman, who spoke after I did, described the same stretching—without recalling
or alluding to my earlier description—as feeling like she was "on fire." These
two descriptions of the same bodily occurrence, though both employed a fire
metaphor, differed markedly in tone and emphasis. I experienced the sensation
as interesting and mild; my colleague could not sufficiently emphasize how "terrible" it was. If our birth-experience panel had been listed in the course syllabus

as simply "women discuss a personal health incident" and we had avoided mention of body parts and only described physical sensations, students might have assumed most of us were talking about different events. Each of us clearly experienced what is customarily referred to as "the pain of childbirth" differently, and each chose to highlight different aspects of the event.

Contemporary obstetric textbooks, in contrast, describe labor uniformly and dispassionately. They explain that first-stage labor has two phases: a latent phase when cervical effacement and early dilation occur, usually over many hours and sometimes days, and a shorter, active phase when the cervix rapidly finishes dilating. The very end of this active phase is known as "transition" because it signifies the culmination of first-stage labor and the beginning of the second stage. The terms *latent* and *active* imply what women often describe when they discuss the entire first stage of labor: a slow, relatively lengthy, more easily handled (latent) portion of the first stage that gradually increases in intensity, followed eventually by a brief but far more intense (active) later segment during which it is difficult to stay in control. The same textbooks describe the second stage of labor as the mother's uncontrollable urge to bear down, an urge prompted by the piston-like movement of the uterus expelling the fetus.[7]

The vast majority of women report that transition is the most painful part of labor. During transition the cervix dilates rapidly (in ten to twenty minutes or so) from about eight to ten centimeters; that is, it fully opens. Contractions intensify at this time, coming one after another with little time for relief or rest between contractions. After the cervix is fully dilated, first-stage contractions cease and women can start pushing when they have the urge to do so. Whereas hard-to-handle pain is the salient characteristic of transition, the urge to push is the salient characteristic of second-stage labor.

Women who experienced childbirth without any medication during the mid-to-late twentieth century attest to the sensations of labor as they are hinted at in modern obstetric texts. These women describe early first-stage labor as "easily handled." In contrast, they describe transition as "the part of labor that many of us felt was painful." Just as the segments of first-stage labor feel different from one another, second-stage labor is unlike any portion of first-stage labor, according to these women's reports. One described second-stage contractions as "no pain at all, only very hard work." Another considered the pushing stage "joyful, not painful." Some women have even described second-stage labor as "the fun part" of birth.[8]

Many sources corroborate these descriptions. Robert Bradley, a Colorado obstetrician who had delivered more than four thousand babies by 1962, pointedly asked his "experienced unmedicated patients," If you could receive gas anesthesia for only ten minutes during labor, which ten minutes would you choose? In essence Bradley was asking, What part of labor hurts most? His patients chose transition. Not one woman in Bradley's informal survey chose early first-stage labor, any portion of second-stage labor, or the moment of birth for this imaginary respite.[9]

Witnesses to labor, however, have traditionally misinterpreted women's experience. Although transition causes the vast majority of women by far the most discomfort, second-stage labor looks and sounds to observers like the most painful portion. Watching women strain with the force of their uterine muscle as it pushes the fetus out of the womb is a powerfully disquieting sight. Yet the sight is deceptive. One physician and mother of four, who was a lay midwife for ten years before starting medical school in 1986, described second-stage labor in the same way so many other women do: as painless, or more accurately as better than painless. She explained, "It actually feels good to push." She admitted, though, that unschooled observers often think they are witnessing indescribable agony as women push, and she understands why. She recalled, "We [lay midwives] used to call it 'animaling out.'" The medical sociologist Barbara Katz Rothman also vividly described the probable reason why witnesses misunderstand women's experience. In writing of her own first birth, Rothman termed second-stage labor "the strangest, and in some ways the nicest, sensation I've ever had." Yet as she pushed, she "heard noises coming out of my throat that I couldn't believe—like the soundtrack of a horror movie."[10]

The unsettling sights and sounds of second-stage labor are likely why doctors, beginning with the introduction of anesthesia in the mid-nineteenth century and continuing well into the 1960s, customarily administered general or regional anesthesia only at the end of second-stage labor, as the baby's head crowned. In other words, women often weathered the first stage, transition, and most of the second stage without any anesthesia, only to be rendered unconscious as their babies were born. The experience of the physician-witness trumped the experience of the patient, highlighting the importance of physicians'—as opposed to patients'—perceptions when formulating medical treatment. The traditional timing of the administration of obstetric anesthesia is a classic example of medical authority usurping patient need when defining "necessary" medical protocol.[11]

Because obstetricians' medical writings in the nineteenth and early twentieth centuries were more subjective than current obstetric texts, those writings illustrate why physicians wanted to ensure that anesthesia rendered women unconscious at the moment of birth. James Young Simpson said of second-stage labor:

"the extremity of suffering seems to be beyond endurance." Joseph DeLee, in his 1925 edition of *The Principles and Practice of Obstetrics*, explained that a woman feels "the greatest anguish" as her baby's head emerges from her body—"as if she were torn open." He warned ominously, "The pain may be so great that the patient faints or is temporarily insane."[12]

DeLee's 1925 text also demonstrates the influence of culture and society on medical and lay views of labor pain. Like many of his contemporaries, he contended that the severity of labor pain depended on a woman's race and class: women of "uncivilized races" had easy labors, whereas "highly cultured women" had "hard, painful labors." DeLee also argued that women's personality quirks shaped their labors: women of "quiet, even temperament" weathered labor easily, whereas "nervous, hysteric" women tended to turn "an otherwise normal labor [into] a pathologic trend."[13]

These many varied discussions and observations about labor pain and its treatment over the past century and a half are worth special study, for the medical and lay communities have always differentiated between labor pain and other types of pain. While labor pain has received unremitting attention and a kaleidoscopic array of proposed antidotes, Western medicine has exhibited considerably less interest in other types of pain. Western healers have paid so little attention historically to pain in general that defining pain as a medical problem is a relatively new concept for Western medicine. Only in the past few decades, with pain medicine now a specialty, has pain itself come to be viewed as a physical abnormality worthy of its own attention and treatment. Yet even in light of this new specialty, most physicians continue to respond with indifference to patients' complaints of pain at office visits. These doctors view pain only as a messenger, and once it has delivered its message, they dismiss its relevance.[14]

Some scholars attribute doctors' dismissal of pain to the scientific explanation for pain—that it is a complex signal traveling from the site of an injury over nerve cells to the brain. In focusing on the physiology of pain rather than on the meaning of pain to the sufferer, physicians strip pain of personal significance and transform it into a meaningless, if troublesome, sensation, of interest only because of the clinical message it conveys to the physician.[15]

In dismissing the personal context of pain, though, physicians overlook a vital opportunity, since context delineates an individual's experience of pain and predicts reaction to its treatment. As one pain scholar points out, for example, the automatic trust and confidence accorded physicians in the United States gives emergency room doctors (who are almost always strangers to the patients they treat) the otherwise inexplicable ability to calm patients' anxiety, subdue their pain, and improve their breathing simply by uttering soothing assurances. Cultural expectations prompt patients' reactions to pain and its treatment as surely as these expectations prompt patients' reactions to ER physicians.[16]

Thus, depending on the cultural milieu, offers of comfort from physicians and loved ones can subdue pain, including labor pain. One retired obstetrician recalled that as a first-year resident in 1951, his training included sitting with women for lengthy periods while they labored. Again and again, he would find a woman screaming in agony and fear, sit next to her bed, take her hand, talk to her quietly, and find that the distraught woman calmed down and remained in control as long as he remained by her bedside. These experiences taught him a valuable lesson: "The doctor in the room . . . [is] worth 100 milligrams of Demerol."[17]

The corollary to this doctor's observation is that medical personnel can also exacerbate patients' anxiety and discomfort. Many mothers charged in the 1950s, for example, that callous treatment by nurses and doctors in maternity wards worsened the mothers' painful ordeals. This cavalier treatment also likely made women more amenable to receiving drugs during labor; in the 1950s and 1960s physicians and nurses commonly gave women multiple injections of opioid analgesics (often coupled with scopolamine) throughout first-stage labor, followed eventually by nitrous oxide, cyclopropane, ether, or regional anesthesia in the delivery room. How a sufferer anticipates pain often dictates the amount and type of medication required to subdue the pain. Thus, the vast obstetric anesthesia arsenal of the mid-twentieth century could have been a self-fulfilling prophecy of sorts: hearing from other women about their exceedingly unpleasant ordeals in the hospital, women anticipated labor pain as unbearable and accepted heavily drugged labors and deliveries with gratitude and relief.[18]

The Western notion of pain as a purely physiological occurrence unaffected by a cultural lens or personal history has had enormous impact on Western birthing practices. Labor pain has long been viewed as such assuredly overwhelming torment—indeed birth has become the quintessential example of excruciating pain—that pain has come to eclipse giving birth as an experience with inherent meaning, deserving of distinct treatment. This phenomenon is not unheard of in the history of American women's health and medicine. Menarche, rather than occasioning discussions between mothers and daughters about maturity, fertility, and sexuality, instead prompts explanations of hygiene management. Just as the treatment of labor pain sidetracks the meaning of the experience of birth, lessons in how to dispose of menstrual blood overshadow the meaning of menarche. Menstruation has become principally a problem of sanitation management while birth has become principally a problem of pain management.[19]

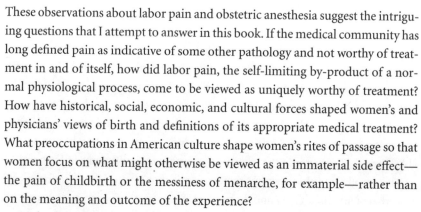

These observations about labor pain and obstetric anesthesia suggest the intriguing questions that I attempt to answer in this book. If the medical community has long defined pain as indicative of some other pathology and not worthy of treatment in and of itself, how did labor pain, the self-limiting by-product of a normal physiological process, come to be viewed as uniquely worthy of treatment? How have historical, social, economic, and cultural forces shaped women's and physicians' views of birth and definitions of its appropriate medical treatment? What preoccupations in American culture shape women's rites of passage so that women focus on what might otherwise be viewed as an immaterial side effect— the pain of childbirth or the messiness of menarche, for example—rather than on the meaning and outcome of the experience?

In this book I argue that cultural and social change rather than medical innovation have shaped mothers' and physicians' attitudes toward obstetric anesthesia and their representation and use of it. In the 1850s, when society idealized physically fragile women, physicians and mothers were unusually susceptible to the argument that obstetric anesthesia was necessary. By the decade beginning in 1910, when the bicycle-riding Gibson girl was in vogue, the lay press helped popularize twilight sleep by contending that it enabled mothers to resume normal activity shortly after giving birth. After World War II, as mothers and their doctors struggled to cope with the demands of the baby boom, medical journals and women's magazines depicted the systemization of birth, represented especially by labor induction and heavily drugged deliveries, as convenient for all participants. In the 1970s, when activists in the women's movement proclaimed that natural childbirth empowered women, mothers eschewed anesthesia. Today, when so many women have dual roles as full-time mothers and full-time employees, the lay press portrays natural childbirth as a foolish choice rather than an empowering one. Epidural anesthesia seems to assure busy, working mothers a pain-free, even relaxing, way to give birth. Women's and physicians' views and use of obstetric anesthesia have been so closely allied with contemporary cultural perceptions of the ideal woman and her appropriate role in society that rational formulation of obstetric practices, particularly the use of anesthesia, has been problematic throughout the time period examined in this book.

Because this is a history of one obstetric treatment, several of the conclusions in this book differ from those found in more general historical works on American birth practices. Although historians have long argued, for example, that women controlled birth practices until birth moved from home to hospital (and the majority of births in the United States did not occur in the hospital until the early 1940s), I found that women's desire for obstetric anesthesia allowed physicians to shape birth practices long before hospital birth became the norm. As early as the mid-nineteenth century, physicians could dictate when obstetric anesthesia would be administered in the birthing chamber. As described above, physicians customarily based the timing of anesthetic administration on the disturbing way women looked and sounded at the end of second-stage labor rather than on what women felt throughout labor. Women tended to accept this practice unquestioningly. Because most of the women who summoned physicians to their births had ceased attending other women's births (and so lacked experience with the rhythms of labor), they trusted doctors' more learned authority. Thus, well before hospitalized birth became the norm, women relied on (male) physicians to determine one of the most elementary aspects of treatment during labor, estimating when the most painful moment in childbirth occurred, something only women were in a logical position to determine.[20]

This is also the first historical examination of U.S. childbirth practices to study contemporary childbirth. In particular, I examine the dramatic change in attitudes toward obstetric anesthesia in the past thirty-five years. During that time the lay press has gone from idealizing natural childbirth and urging women to eschew pain relief to idealizing surgical childbirth and advising that women insist on epidural anesthesia throughout most of labor. Ironically, the feminist movement, which sparked birth reform and widespread interest in natural childbirth in the early 1970s, is also the progenitor of the heavily medicalized births popular today. The cultural concepts of "control" and "choice," first coined in the context of birth by the feminists active in the natural childbirth movement, are the concepts physicians and mothers use today to justify elective cesarean section and heavy use of epidural anesthesia. This preference for strikingly different birth practices reflects the divergent concerns and needs of two generations of American women. Social change thus continues to shape women's vision of the ideal birth and physicians' treatments.

The book is organized roughly chronologically. Because the history of obstetric anesthesia has few defining moments (at least in the sense that a war or the passage of key legislation prompts a sudden tidal wave of cultural, social, and economic change), chapters overlap in time and are demarcated not by specific incidents but by what I term questions. The questions represent changes in the nature of the ongoing debate about obstetric anesthesia and variations in its formulation and use.

Chapter 1 (1840s through 1890s) examines the question of necessity, as physicians argue about the precise nature of labor and birth and hence the need for any administration of ether or chloroform. This era, when the predominant culture characterized women as unavoidably prone to weakness and debility, proved uniquely amenable to fostering both medical discussion about women's need for obstetric anesthesia and lay interest in the treatment.

Chapter 2 (1890s through 1930s) discusses the question of professional respect. In this period women lobbied for painless childbirth in the form of twilight sleep. As the nationwide crusade for twilight sleep revealed the power of consumers to effect change in medical practice, the initially affronted obstetric community ultimately used the intricate protocol demanded by twilight sleep to elevate the status of obstetricians and obstetrics, a specialty disregarded by colleagues and laity alike.

Chapter 3 (1900 through 1960s) focuses on the question of safety, as the medical and lay communities express concern that obstetric pain relief—which now includes injectable, intravenous, rectal, inhalation, and regional analgesia and anesthesia—might jeopardize the health of mothers and their babies. Paradoxically, even as the public health community warns that the inherent side effects of anesthesia contribute to the high maternal death rate, mothers made anxious by the bustle of hospital maternity wards and the medicalization of birth increasingly choose to be drugged during such a frightening event.

Chapter 4 (1940s through 1960s) examines how the pressures of the baby boom altered physicians' use, and the public's perception, of obstetric anesthesia. In this era, the question of convenience became a paramount concern of obstetricians and mothers. Obstetricians struggled to make birth more predictable and systematic in their effort to contend with their growing patient load, and mothers faced the difficulties of managing households full of small children and living in suburbs far from big-city hospitals. Labor induction, injectable analgesia, and inhalation and regional anesthesia became particularly popular because these treatments, taken together, seemed to make labor and birth predictable, systematic, and "convenient."

Chapter 5 (1950s through 1980s) explores the question of authority as mothers protested what they termed the "dehumanizing" aspects of the systemization of obstetric practice and called for a measure of control over their own medical treatment in general and, specifically, a less technological approach to childbirth.

Women began to eschew anesthesia, natural childbirth became popular, and physicians and hospitals responded to women's complaints with myriad efforts to reform obstetric protocol and maternity-ward routine. The women's movement was instrumental in this reformation. As women gained the right to participate in American economic, political, and social life on a par with men, the image of women unwillingly strapped to delivery room tables, unconscious or groggy from unnecessary and unwanted drugs, became abhorrent.

Chapter 6 (1970s to the present) examines the question of choice as women and physicians increasingly define labor induction, epidural anesthesia, and even cesarean section as a matter not of medical need but of personal preference. As women find themselves increasingly overwhelmed by both full-time motherhood and full-time employment after the successes of the women's movement, they no longer perceive natural childbirth as empowering. Instead, planned induction, epidural anesthesia, and even cesarean section are portrayed as the smarter, easier, and less risky "choices" for the working women about to experience childbirth.

Each chapter begins with the description of a birth. These initial stories immediately offer readers details of the unique medical customs of the period under examination, demonstrate how women viewed physicians and vice versa, indicate how women customarily anticipated birth and reflected on it after the fact, and suggest the questions that are asked and answered in the chapter.

This book also exhibits two peculiarities worth mentioning. I use medical terms throughout. Rather than define the terms as I use them and risk turning a social history into a clinical treatise, I provide a comprehensive glossary at the end of the book. The book also includes numerous anecdotes from oral history interviews I conducted with several dozen mothers and physicians. I have withheld the names of these individuals and describe them only in general terms (gender, first year of medical school or residency, and location of medical education and practice in the case of doctors, and location and dates of children's births in the case of mothers). On the rare occasions when I assign names to the physicians and mothers I interviewed, I use pseudonyms. In the age of HIPAA it is, unfortunately for historians of medicine, necessary to mask identities.

Ultimately, this history of obstetric anesthesia and changing views of labor pain is an examination of the American propensity to characterize labor and birth primarily in terms of pain caused and pain treated. Even today, an era of low maternal and infant mortality, when the traditional anxieties associated with birth have been assuaged, labor evokes great fear. How did a potentially dangerous treatment such as anesthesia, which posed serious risk to mothers and infants throughout most of the history discussed in this book, come to alleviate this fear? And how did this treatment eventually come to be defined by the lay and medical communities as beneficial and necessary—in fact, the more anesthesia the better? Today, as we celebrate the age of evidence-based medicine, we think of medicine as a dispassionate science. Yet the history of obstetric anesthesia reveals the many ingredients in addition to scientific evidence that have contributed to the formulation and sale of medical treatment, particularly in conjunction with a specialty like obstetrics that speaks daily to so many individual and societal hopes and concerns.

CHAPTER ONE

Ether and Chloroform

The Question of Necessity, 1840s through 1890s

On April 7, 1847, Fanny Appleton Longfellow of Cambridge, Massachusetts, pregnant with her third child, became the first woman in the United States to inhale anesthesia while giving birth. Longfellow's decision to use ether was not precipitous; indeed, finding a physician willing to administer the substance took considerable time and effort. Before the birth, her husband, the poet Henry Wadsworth Longfellow, consulted a host of doctors, all of whom denied his request. Each denounced obstetric anesthesia as unnecessary and dangerous. Undeterred, Henry persisted in his search for an amenable doctor.[1]

Ultimately he found Nathan Cooley Keep, a Boston physician specializing in dentistry, who agreed to dispense the desired ether. Keep later reported that Fanny's labor was short and unproblematic. Five and a half hours after labor commenced, Keep began to administer ether, and Fanny sporadically inhaled it. She gave birth a brief thirty minutes later. At one point in this half-hour span, acutely aware of the experimental nature of his venture, Keep withheld the ether, despite Fanny's protest, to ensure that the gas was not interfering with her labor. The action allayed his fears, for he saw no change in the frequency, duration, or strength of Fanny's contractions. He noted, however, that in the absence of ether, "the distress of the patient was great."[2]

In retrospect, both physician and patient were pleased with the experiment. In a letter to the editor of the *Boston Medical and Surgical Journal,* Keep termed the endeavor "highly satisfactory." Fanny was elated: she said the birth was far superior to her two previous, unanesthetized ones and that under the influence of ether, she had never felt better or labored more comfortably. She pronounced ether "certainly the greatest blessing of this age" and declared herself "proud to be the pioneer to less suffering for poor weak womankind." Henry's brother joined the celebration by joking, "If you had asked your wife which she preferred, a boy or a girl, she would have replied, 'I will take ether.'"[3]

Social Change Hastens the Acceptance of Obstetric Anesthesia

Notwithstanding the jubilation, it remains unclear why the Longfellows persisted in seeking a medical treatment that the vast majority of doctors considered reckless. Fanny's previous births offer no clues, since Henry described those two labors as "pretty easy."[4] Perhaps Fanny's pride in her ability to offer hope to "poor weak womankind" suggests the reason for the Longfellows' dogged pursuit of ether.

By the mid-nineteenth century, being a woman and being weak and unhealthy seemed to go hand in hand. The tendency of middle- and upper-class urban women to exhibit infirmity was so widespread that when Catherine Esther Beecher, a pioneer in women's hygiene, asked women around the country to describe the health of the ten women they knew best, one Milwaukee woman provided the prototypical response: "Do not know one healthy woman in the place."[5]

Characterizing birth as unbearable was a logical by-product of this cultural milieu. The development of ether in 1846 and the discovery one year later of the anesthetic properties of chloroform strengthened the tendency. News of the potential of obstetric anesthesia amplified the descriptions of agonizing labors as the possibility of painless childbirth was increasingly dangled before a susceptible audience of seemingly frail women and their concerned doctors.[6]

In the late nineteenth century, Cyrus Edson, commissioner of health of New York, exemplified the American tendency to describe birth in harsh terms by likening the suffering of laboring women to the agony of martyrs tortured during the Middle Ages. He contended that giving birth transformed vulnerable women into lifelong invalids and blamed girls' increased access to formal education for the tragedy. Sitting in a classroom during puberty, he argued, drained girls' strength, leaving little in reserve for childbirth in coming years.[7]

Other physicians elaborated on this argument, explaining that educational demands interfered with the proper growth of girls' bodies. Frequent diagnoses of "structural disease of the ovaries" and "juvenile cervix" appeared in the medical record. Physicians theorized that boys were immune to underdeveloped reproductive systems because boys' bodies developed slowly and evenly throughout adolescence. In contrast, girls' bodies allegedly developed in a brief burst that could result in disaster if at that particular moment their overtaxed brains were monopolizing the energy their bodies needed for proper maturation. One physician proposed solving the problem by removing girls from school during puberty. He advised that during the break girls engage in exercise: walking, gardening, or anything else that did not require "mental labor."[8]

Physicians began to identify new diseases that affected mostly women, thus reinforcing the image of inherently weak women susceptible to maladies customarily avoided by men. One of those illnesses was neurasthenia, a medical condition diagnosed usually in women and known more generically as nervous exhaustion. Neurasthenia was so complex and all-encompassing that New York neurologist George M. Beard needed two full pages in his 1881 book *American Nervousness* to list its symptoms. These symptoms included, among many others, irritability, fear of responsibility, exhaustion after defecation and urination, dry hair, and sensitivity to weather changes. Beard declared neurasthenia most prevalent in the northern United States owing to rapid urbanization; the condition was so well-known there that he needed to offer no proof of its epidemic nature. Other physicians echoed Beard, explaining that genteel urban women, the very women who exhibited weakness and lethargy and had difficulty giving birth, now lived artificial lives. The unnaturalness of cities had turned them into "hot-house product[s]" unable to withstand the rigors of "natural" activities such as birth.[9]

Associating sensitive, genteel urban women with difficult births had a corollary. Working-class women, rural women, Native Americans, and slaves—women who were thought to live "natural" lives—presumably birthed with great ease. One doctor described the typical "squaw" birth: "She performs the usual drudgery of her life up to the very hour of her labor . . . [then] enters her cabin or betakes herself to some stream . . . , gives birth, washes the young 'Injun' in the cold water, straps it upon her back, and before she has been scarcely missed, has returned a full-fledged mother, and resumes her labors unconscious of having undergone any very wonderful ordeal." If her "band" was "on a march" when her time came, she responded similarly, leaving the trail, hastily giving birth, washing the newborn in a stream, strapping the baby to her back, mounting her pony, and then galloping to catch up with her cohorts. "If they experience any of the annoyances of pregnancy that afflict the daughters of artificial life," this doctor contended, "they pay so little attention to them as to attract no notice whatever." Physicians and white laypeople viewed slaves similarly; one planter, for example, observed that slaves never suffered during birth. Midwives who attended female slaves did not share this opinion, however: some placed an ax under the mattress to metaphorically "cut" the pain.[10]

Although connecting more intense suffering during childbirth to urbanization was an attribute of this era, American women's fear of birth was an old story. Fear of dying in childbirth was so culturally ingrained that American women had long marked giving birth in their letters and diaries with some variation of the grateful observation "I am the living mother of a living child" and often nothing

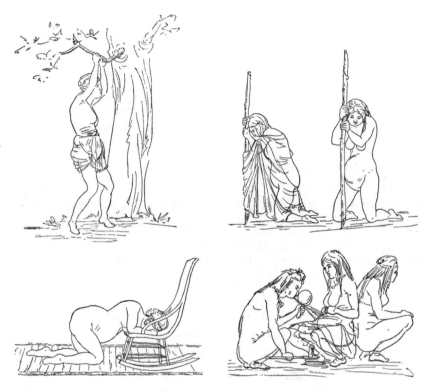

A few of George J. Engelmann's depictions of "primitive peoples" in the United States giving birth. *Upper left:* "a negress" in Louisiana giving birth "while hanging on to the limb of a tree." *Lower left:* "southern Negress" in a kneeling position. *Upper right:* Blackfoot "squaws" leaning on a staff during a contraction. *Lower right:* according to Engelmann, this is the labor position assumed by the Pawnees: squatting, with an assistant supporting the parturient's back and a "medicine man" kneeling before her "with a gourd in one hand, which he rattles constantly, and a pipe in his mouth which he smokes, blowing the smoke under the clothes . . . Evidently a warm vapor bath to soften the parts." *Source:* George J. Engelmann, *Labor among Primitive Peoples* (J. H. Chambers, 1882), 19, 24, 29, 32.

more. Yet even in the eighteenth century, women's apprehension was probably unwarranted.[11]

Historical demographers believe the maternal death rate observed by Maine midwife Martha Ballard between 1785 and 1812 had long been typical. In almost one thousand births, Ballard lost five mothers in the postnatal period and none during delivery. This maternal death rate of 0.5 percent of births, though extremely high by today's standard, was minuscule in comparison to eighteenth- and nineteenth-century perceptions. Historians attribute this exaggerated fear of dying during childbirth to the belief that labor pain was just punishment meted out by God, a principle conveyed and reinforced by the predominant religion. The sheer number of births experienced by many eighteenth-century women likely exacerbated the culturally ingrained fears. Particularly in small towns and rural areas, when the details of just one mother's death in childbirth became well known, the oft-repeated story served to heighten anxiety levels.[12]

Worries about the likelihood of death during childbirth persisted in the nineteenth century. Chicago mother Nettie Fowler McCormick wrote in her diary shortly before the birth of her sixth child in 1872: "O God preserve my life to my husband & children."[13]

Yet the woman who wrote to the *Boston Medical and Surgical Journal* in 1866 to describe birth as "agony which is akin to nothing else on earth" emphasized what had become a far more common concern, for mid-nineteenth-century women exhibited greater apprehension about the pain of childbirth than the possibility of dying during childbirth. The two fears occasionally converged, however, since women often likened labor pain to a near-death experience. Mary Putnam Jacobi described the birth of her first grandchild in 1902 as watching her daughter "plunge . . . down in to a fiery furnace of peril and pain. . . . You cannot forgive that child for what it has cost your child." Another woman described birth as an event that "bursts your brain, and tears out your heart, and crashes your nerves to bits." The specter of women's torment horrified husbands as well, and they tended to echo their wives' gruesome descriptions. One man said of his wife's labor: "I have seen the greatest suffering this day that I have ever known or ever imagined."[14]

Political and social concerns shaped these depictions. Between 1800 and 1900 the fertility rate of white women of childbearing age dropped from 7.04 children to a worrisome 3.56. Mary Virginia Terhune, a novelist, author of domestic manuals, and syndicated columnist for the *Chicago Tribune,* who wrote under the pen name Marion Harland, warned in one of her advice books that for the United States to remain strong, the birthrate had to increase. Observing in 1882 that the "cry for women's suffrage is waxing loud," she scolded, "Is it not that women want to vote, but are not willing to make voters?" The editor of the *Medical Record* accused American women of preferring pets to children. The French had responded to their similarly declining birthrate by offering prizes to large families, but, he lamented, "Anglo-Saxon prudery" would thwart similar action in the United States.[15]

The anxiety over the plummeting fertility rate fomented praise for obstetric anesthesia. While historians argue that the diminished birthrate resulted from in-

creased negotiation and cooperation between marital partners and from wom-
en's active search for contraceptive devices, many nineteenth-century physicians
assumed that women's fear of labor sparked their unprecedented unwillingness to
bear large numbers of children. Obstetric anesthesia, which, in the words of one
physician, "robbed [childbirth] of its chief terror," thus seemed the ideal antidote
to women's new, seemingly antisocial preference for fewer children.[16]

Yet for much of the nineteenth century, when most women still had no access
to anesthesia despite what was becoming a lively discussion about the treatment
among physicians, women sought comfort during birth from other women, just
as they had in prior centuries. During these "social births," female relatives and
neighbors gathered in a laboring woman's home, usually but not always under
the auspices of a midwife, to help with a variety of tasks before, during, and after
childbirth. Birth attendants looked forward to these events, not only as opportunities to see another woman safely and comfortably through labor and its aftermath, but also as occasions to enjoy each other's company. Eventually, the laboring woman repaid her helpers by attending their births. Birth was part of the
social fabric, a quasi-public social event for women only.[17]

Although social birth was less common in isolated rural communities, where
women often found themselves alone or with only a midwife or their husband for
companionship and assistance, even women living in these sparsely populated
areas occasionally enjoyed social birth and certainly looked forward to the possibility of its occurrence. Nellie Brown, who lived in Saint Anthony, Minnesota, in
the late 1850s, informed her sister-in-law that her second birth had been a good
one: she had benefited from "the best of attendance." After she went into labor,
her husband notified a Native American woman who lived nearby with a white
man. That woman summoned two friends, and Brown said of her three helpers,
"The Indian women are very kind and affectionate . . . and they are nearly all
Doctresses and are very skilfull." Brown's only disappointment was that, though
the women stayed with her throughout labor and remained for several hours
after the baby was born, after departing they did not come to see her again. Social birth was also the convention in the South among and between white and
black women. White women often provided aid in the slaves' quarters and slaves
aided white women in their homes.[18]

Over the course of the nineteenth century, as physicians replaced midwives,
women attended each other's births less frequently. But the transition from social
birth under the supervision of a midwife to physician-attended birth without
supporting players was exceedingly slow. Physicians continued to acknowledge
the importance of social birth even in the late nineteenth century by advising that

birth attendants be intimates of a laboring woman and that these close friends and relatives avoid all serious conversation and display a cheerful, encouraging disposition. And even into the early twentieth century in the urban north, midwives remained valued birth attendants in certain circles. Dr. S. Josephine Baker, the first director of the New York City Bureau of Child Hygiene, observed, "If deprived of midwives, [immigrant] women would rather have amateur assistance from the janitor's wife or the woman across the hall than to submit to this outlandish American custom of having a male doctor for confinement." During the unhurried transition from home birth with a midwife and assorted friends and relatives to home birth attended by a doctor with few, if any, others present, when a woman did choose a physician as her primary birth attendant, the doctor's behavior was not radically different from that of a midwife anyway. Like a midwife, the doctor spent long hours with a woman simply waiting for her baby to be born. Thus, doctors provided at least a modicum of companionship in the absence of what had long been a supportive entourage of close women friends and relatives.[19]

A physician's company proved to be qualitatively different than the camaraderie offered by women, however. Some scholars argue that male physicians so altered the atmosphere of the birthing chamber that there was a causal link between women's increased complaints of unbearable labor pain and the growing number of physician-attended home births throughout the nineteenth century. The presence of a male physician, and the corresponding lack of female cohorts, might have prompted women to experience birth as a more formal, anxiety-producing activity. Current studies showing that the presence of female companions during birth shortens labor and reduces the need for anesthesia support this view.[20]

In the absence of social birth, women searched for other comforts. Anita McCormick Blaine, the daughter of industrialist Cyrus McCormick, found solace in returning to her childhood home for the birth of her first child. She wrote to her mother, "From the minute we walked in two weeks ago we have been *at home* & so happy here. . . . You would not see the frightened child I expected to be—but your own child the same as ever waiting for her little one with absolute calmness & happiness."[21]

Not only loneliness in the absence of other women but also sheer ignorance intensified women's fear of birth, for the move from social birth to physician-attended birth coincided with a growing unwillingness on the part of mothers to discuss any aspect of reproduction with their daughters. As girls menstruated earlier and married later, mothers hoped that maintaining their daughters' ignorance would protect them from the sexual dangers they now faced for longer spans of time starting at younger ages. Many girls thus experienced menarche in complete ignorance, terrified that they were bleeding to death. A popular advice book of the era condemned the "false delicacy or cowardice" that now prevented daughters from learning from their mothers, driving them instead to "the prurient whisperings of the schoolfellow . . . or the vulgar gossiping of servant girls." Mothers' reluctance to share information could, of course, result in tragedy. One woman, with tears streaming down her face, brought her pregnant fourteen-year-old to the Minneapolis Maternity Hospital in the 1880s and confessed, "I am more to blame than she is, for I never told her about these things."[22]

Middle- and upper-class women came to rely not on their mothers for information, but on magazines, an inadequate replacement for the now-vanished multigenerational support and advice network. Lottie Tubbs, an Ohio woman who moved to Mexico to do missionary work with her husband, looked forward to monthly issues of the *Ladies' Home Journal* and the *Delineator*, especially during pregnancy. Yet these magazines, on the rare occasion when they contained articles about reproduction, were as unforthcoming as society at large. One article in the *Ladies' Home Journal,* promisingly titled "When a Child First Awakens to Manhood or Womanhood," dismissed any discussion of menstruation or other bodily transformations with the statement, "The physical changes in the period of youthful reaction are well known, and somewhat definitely limited in time, and it is not upon these that I intend to dwell."[23]

Reluctance to discuss reproduction crossed class and racial lines; daughters of slaves also testified to ignorance of conception and birth, even after marriage and during a first pregnancy.[24] With so many women uninformed about even the most fundamental aspects of reproduction, deprived of the support and companionship of cohorts during birth, and prevented from observing other women giving birth, birth became shrouded in mystery. Increasingly, women anticipated the event with incapacitating trepidation. In this environment, the promise of obstetric anesthesia offered much-needed comfort.

The Status of Obstetrics in Nineteenth-Century America

Even as physicians attended more births and midwives fewer, formal medical interest in birth remained sparse. Most physicians considered obstetrics a trivial sideline, unworthy of professional training, attention, and respect. The public exhibited similar disdain. Joseph DeLee, a longtime professor of obstetrics at Northwestern University Medical School who eventually became known as "the father of modern obstetrics," complained that women had long believed that childbirth was so ordinary an event that it required no more solicitous supervision than respiration or digestion.[25]

Given the scanty professional and public interest, medical schools felt no pressure to offer significant training in obstetrics. The training was so meager that DeLee complained of new doctors serving as the sole attendant at a birth without ever having examined a pregnant woman or witnessed a labor. One physician recalled that after graduation from medical school, his ignorance was so profound that at the first birth he attended as a licensed physician, he determined that the patient had a massive tumor blocking the birth canal. He panicked, sure that the baby could not be born and the woman would die. He soon discovered, however, that the suspected tumor was the baby, who arrived quite safely without aid from the terrified doctor.[26]

Medical students had so little exposure to birth that in the 1850s when James P. White of the University of Buffalo became the first instructor in the country to allow medical students to attend births, students passed resolutions thanking him. Local physicians and the surrounding community were considerably less appreciative. An editorial in the *Buffalo Courier* termed White's method of teaching midwifery "*gross outrage.*" Assurances by University of Buffalo officials that the best European teachers used similar techniques did not quell the furor. Neither did a letter from medical students published in the *Buffalo Medical Journal* testifying that their training had been in accordance with every standard of decency. Nothing appeased the offended. The Committee on Education of the Medical Association termed White's approach "utterly incompetent" and admonished, "No practitioner ever had any desire to see the presenting part emerge under the arch of the pubis for any additional knowledge that might be gained by such an exposure." Published evaluations of White's teaching methods became so strident that White sued one Buffalo newspaper for libel. He lost the case. [27]

Recalling the brouhaha fifty-four years later, J. Whitridge Williams, professor and director of obstetrics at Johns Hopkins University and later dean of the medical school there, observed that the Medical Association's indignation over White's allowing medical students to view a birth effectively reinforced the prevailing notion among physicians that practicing obstetrics was demeaning. Even as Williams penned that rebuke in 1904, however, obstetric training had not changed much since White's day. Physicians still received medical degrees attesting to their competence to provide medical care at a birth without ever having witnessed a birth.[28]

Such inadequate training took its toll on maternal health. DeLee blamed general practitioners and midwives in equal measure for the country's high maternal morbidity and mortality rates. While he deplored the "careless and ignorant midwives" who cared for 43 percent of the women who gave birth in Chicago in 1895, he just as vehemently denounced the physicians in general practice who persisted in attending the occasional birth despite having little or no obstetric training. Other obstetricians echoed DeLee's complaint. One Boston physician had grown so weary of being summoned to emergencies by colleagues "who have absolutely no appreciation of what they are doing" that he noted obstetrics was the only medical field in which doctors without special training could claim competence even though there was no branch of medicine that offered the unskilled doctor more opportunity to harm the patient.[29]

Individuals like DeLee stepped in to fill the void in medical education. In 1895 he opened the Chicago Lying-in Dispensary (also referred to informally by neighborhood women as the Maxwell Street Dispensary) in a heavily populated immigrant neighborhood west of Chicago's downtown. The dispensary had three purposes: to provide skilled obstetricians free of charge to poor women in their homes, to prevent maternal death, and to train medical students. Medical students from around the country paid to apprentice there, and one or more students always accompanied a dispensary doctor to births. DeLee touted this training as the dispensary's most important service: "It is a fact that midwifery has been and still is the most neglected branch of medical teaching and the mortality records of the Board of Health bring melancholy proof of this fact." The dispensary board boasted in its first annual report that the free service provided aid not just to working-class women but also to "the wives of our important citizens [because]. . . .The doctors taught by the Dispensary are destined to practice among the affluent as well as the poor and both thus receive the benefits of the institution." Chicago's wealthiest families were cognizant of this aspect of the service, and the dispensary, which relied heavily on donations to provide its free service, quickly became a popular charity, counting among its benefactors such prominent Chicago families as the McCormicks, the Loebs, and the Schaffners.[30]

The Maxwell Street Dispensary proved an unqualified success. Dispensary physicians and their apprentices, "under adverse conditions with a group of patients physically below par," maintained a maternal mortality rate of .14 percent, less than one-fourth of the nationwide rate, .59 percent. European physicians termed DeLee's venture the best of its kind in the world.[31]

DeLee was not alone in this type of work. In 1910 the American Gynecological Society Committee on Medical Education paid homage to every home birth dispensary in the country when the committee concluded that urban medical charities like DeLee's, not medical schools, had been instrumental in training future physicians in the science and art of obstetrics. Clinical experience in obstetrics did not become an integral part of medical school curricula until the 1920s. Only then did the isolated efforts of medical charities to dispense obstetric training become unnecessary.[32]

In the nineteenth century, with medical schools neglecting obstetric training, the task of improving and standardizing obstetric practice was nearly impossible. This situation did not bode well for the reasoned implementation of any obstetric treatment, especially the use of anesthesia.

Obstetric Anesthesia and the Question of Necessity

As physicians began to examine the relative drawbacks and benefits of obstetric anesthesia, they conducted their discussion in this atmosphere. Hobbled and splintered by institutional and public disdain for their work, the physicians who practiced primarily obstetrics could not even agree on whether obstetric anesthesia was beneficial, let alone necessary.

Discussion among physicians about obstetric anesthesia in the United States and Europe was so uncompromising that one side championed the treatment as "a benefaction beyond all computation" while the other side denounced it as "insane ethereal furor." Assessment of the nature of labor was equally unbending; views were so rigid that doctors with conflicting opinions seemed to be describing wholly different biological events. Opponents of anesthesia portrayed childbirth benevolently, as "a scene of cheerfulness," while advocates portrayed it malevolently, as "terrible torture, hopeless of relief."[33]

In some cases, personal experience shaped doctors' impassioned views. Although the vast majority of labors in these years were uncomplicated, most physicians encountered troubling complications like hemorrhage or postpartum infection in the course of their medical practice. In fact, doctors likely saw a significant percentage of difficult births because midwives customarily summoned a doctor for help when they encountered a problem. These births were at times so traumatic that just one particularly difficult labor could permanently alter a physician's perspective of birth, especially if the negative experience occurred early in a doctor's career. One doctor, responding to a plea for help from a midwife, found a woman bleeding to death with "two blankets and the mattress under her . . . saturated, and the blood dripping through on to the floor." This doctor was unlikely to ever again anticipate birth as a "cheerful" event.[34]

Walter Channing, professor of midwifery and eventually the first dean of the faculty at Harvard Medical College, was the best-known proponent of obstetric anesthesia in the United States, and deeply personal experience likely contributed to his strong advocacy. Channing was married twice, and both his wives had harrowing births. His first wife died of tuberculosis shortly after the birth of their fourth child. His second wife bled to death after the stillbirth of their first child, while Channing was the sole attendant. These incidents probably contributed to Channing's view that labor was the product of "imperfect harmony" among cervix, vagina, and perineum. He postulated that these "unyielding organs," coupled with severe pressure from the baby's head, gave "rise to the agony of childbirth."[35]

By the end of November 1847, only thirteen months after William T. G. Morton first demonstrated the use of ether at the Massachusetts General Hospital, Channing had attended over forty etherized births, more than any other physician in Boston and likely more than any other in the United States. In his classic study on the use of ether during childbirth, he explained that ether suspended pain without affecting contractions. He attempted to assuage the trepidation of dubious colleagues by assuring them that ether did not leave women convulsed, paralyzed, or mentally deranged and that the children born of anesthetized births did not demonstrate mental or physical abnormalities; these were all common fears at the time.[36]

James Young Simpson, an avid promoter of obstetric anesthesia in Scotland, was Channing's philosophical counterpart in Europe. A professor of medicine and midwifery in Edinburgh, he was the first physician (in January 1847, three months before Nathan Cooley Keep's adventure with Fanny Longfellow) to administer ether during a birth. When he first observed its effects, Simpson vowed to find an equally fast-acting anesthetic with none of the disadvantages of ether, drawbacks that included hysteria, vomiting, and lethargy. Over the next two years, this quest drove Simpson to inhale numerous substances: "chloride of hydro-carbon, acetone, nitrate of oxïde of ethyle, ... benzin, the vapour of iodoform, &c." Upon inhaling chloroform, he knew instantly that he had discovered the substance he was searching for. He exulted, "Future generations shall be born in Elysian dreams on beds of asphodel."[37]

In an assessment similar to Channing's, Simpson dubbed labor a series of "fearful sufferings and agonies." He believed that education, tradition, and the inability to avoid childbirth had long prevented physicians from discussing this horrific reality. He credited ether and chloroform with finally allowing the long-deferred discussion about the terrible nature of labor to take place and charged that doctors who refused to administer anesthesia during birth practiced "professional cruelty."[38]

Simpson, who had an affinity for bluster and self-promotion, was instrumental in publicizing obstetric anesthesia throughout the United States and Europe, though his manner occasionally detracted from his mission. After he discovered the anesthetic properties of chloroform, the *Lancet* printed a letter from a doctor denouncing Simpson for traveling around Europe exhibiting chloroform's effects "somewhat after the fashion of a showman . . . at dinner parties, and in drawing-rooms."[39]

In 1853 chloroform received its biggest boost yet when the British physician John Snow famously administered it to Queen Victoria during her eighth birth. The queen described the birth in a letter to her uncle, conveying a sentiment similar to Fanny Appleton Longfellow's six years earlier: "I can report most favourably of it myself, for I have never been better or stronger." Four years later, after Snow attended the birth of Victoria's ninth child, he noted in his casebook: "The Queen . . . kept asking for more chloroform, and complaining that it did not remove the pain. She slept, however, sometimes between the pains. . . . The chloroform was left off for 3 or 4 pains and the royal patient made an effort which expelled the head, a little chloroform being given just as the head passed."[40]

The physicians who considered labor a tolerable and positive force reviled both ether and chloroform. Charles Meigs, a Philadelphia physician and the author of *Obstetrics: The Science and the Art*, was typical. He estimated that cervical contractions in the early part of first-stage labor lasted from fifteen to thirty or forty seconds. Yet sizable intervals of twelve to thirty minutes separated the contractions. Only toward the end of the first stage did the pain-free interludes shorten appreciably, to five, three, and then two minutes, as contractions increased "in violence and duration until the organ is freed from its load."

Meigs determined that the average woman experienced approximately forty-seven contractions during the four hours or so of late first-stage labor and estimated that those intensified contractions lasted a cumulative twenty-five minutes. Those twenty-five minutes, however, were dispersed among more than three and a half hours of relief. Of ether he wrote, "I should find the objection to it less and the inducement greater, were the twenty-five minutes of pain to be always twenty-five consecutive minutes. . . . when they are distributed through two hundred and forty minutes . . . , I look upon the exhibition as unnecessary and uncalled for." Although he conceded that some women exhibited distress even between contractions, Meigs contended that most women were comfortable except when experiencing a contraction. He thus argued that the birthing chamber was more often a happy scene "instead of the shrieks and anguish and despair that have been so forcibly portrayed."[41]

Simpson's and Meigs's contrasting views of labor are clearest in their descriptions of second-stage labor. Meigs differentiated between first-stage contractions (he called these "sharp, agonizing, and dispiriting pains") and the pistonlike contractions of labor's second stage, when the uterus pushes the baby out (a sensation he characterized as indescribable, incomparable to any other feeling). He noticed that women seemed calmer, less fearful, and more focused during the second stage, "like one who has a task set for her." Henry N. Guernsey, professor of obstetrics and diseases of women and children at the Homeopathic Medical College of Pennsylvania, echoed this general description in the 1860s. Guernsey told medical students that while first-stage labor made women "unusually peevish and despondent," their irritation and hopelessness disappeared during the second stage as they went "to work manfully."[42]

Simpson's view contrasted with Meigs's and Guernsey's, in that he deemed first-stage labor relatively benign and second-stage labor excruciating. He repeated a colleague's description of second-stage labor as proof of this assessment: "The pulse gradually increases in quickness and force; the skin grows hot; the face becomes intensely red; drops of sweat stand upon the forehead; and a perspiration, sometimes profuse, breaks out all over the body; frequently violent tremblings accompany the last pain, and at the moment that the head passes into the world, *the extremity of suffering seems to be beyond endurance.*" Another physician offered an equally dramatic portrayal focusing on the baby's head rather than the mother's body: "pushing along, crushing along against . . . that sensitive channel, and caught by a resistant perinaeum . . . hurled back time after time." He wondered, "What heart is so hard as to withhold chloroform in that hour of bitterness and despair!"[43]

The doctors offering this negative assessment of labor readily acknowledged that anesthesia relieved not only women's pain but also physicians' obligation to witness the unsettling sights and sounds of labor. Thus, Simpson termed anesthesia not only a "great blessing" to women but also a "great boon" to the practitioner. A Virginia physician similarly recalled in 1895 that before he began to routinely employ anesthesia, he often sat anguished by women's bedsides, forced to listen to "moanings from almost insufferable agony." He too found chloroform "not only a blessing to the patient but to the physician also."[44]

Physicians communicated directly and passionately with one another about their views of obstetric anesthesia. In an 1848 letter, Meigs advised Simpson that anesthesia was unnecessary; doctors could free laboring women from fear and pain simply by offering reassurance. This particular discussion did not remain private, as Meigs publicly condemned Simpson's advocacy of anesthesia in the *Philadelphia Medical Examiner*. Simpson responded to the rebuke by comparing childbirth with walking, noting that both could be arduous physiological functions mitigated by human ingenuity. Using the very same phrase Meigs had employed in his writings to describe labor, Simpson asked, Did Meigs walk from Boston to New York, because walking was a "desirable, salutary, and conservative manifestation of life-force?" Or did he take the railway?[45]

Simpson engaged in similar correspondence with Francis Henry Ramsbotham, a well-known London obstetrician who eschewed anesthesia throughout his career. Before the advent of anesthesia, the two shared an interest in placenta previa; after the introduction of ether, their primary topic of conversation changed, and the two began arguing about the necessity and safety of obstetric anesthesia. Their exchange indicates that Simpson's enthusiasm for ether was immediate: soon after its introduction, he wrote to Ramsbotham excitedly, asking if he had tried it yet. Simpson assured Ramsbotham that all doctors would soon be using ether even during uneventful births, and he chastised Ramsbotham for his hesitancy, contrasting the quick acceptance of ether in Edinburgh with the foolish reluctance of London physicians to embrace the treatment.[46]

The Simpson-Ramsbotham correspondence demonstrates that entire medical communities reacted very differently to obstetric anesthesia. In 1851 most London physicians were apparently still reluctant to embrace it. Simpson admonished Ramsbotham for "the opposition to it in *your* houses—whilst every *village* in Scotland has it—even those as far north of Newcastle." Simpson attributed Ramsbotham's objections to anesthesia to ignorance and prejudice. He never did convince Ramsbotham of his point of view, however. In one fourteen-page response, Ramsbotham told Simpson he had no interest in learning "how much poison I can administer without causing death." Simpson responded by assuring him that "the ladies themselves will keep medical men right about the proper quantity in parturition," simply by falling asleep when they had enough. Throughout their years-long exchange of views, Simpson continued to laud Edinburgh as an enlightened medical bastion and condemn London as a relative backwater.[47]

Despite Simpson's spirited efforts, his skeptical correspondents remained unswayed. Meigs noted that aspiration of ether and chloroform had on occasion caused sudden death, and he wondered how colleagues could justify exposing healthy women and their infants to such unnecessary danger. He admonished, "What sufficient motive have I to risk the life . . . of [even] one in a thousand [laboring women], in a questionable attempt to abrogate one of the general conditions of man?" Channing, ever the ally of Simpson's, countered that the previous 999 cases were reason enough.[48]

Both camps, particularly in the earliest, most rancorous days of the debate, exploited religion to defend their stance. Some doctors insisted that the use of anesthesia in obstetrics violated the Christian mandate that women give birth "in sorrow." Others countered that employing anesthesia did not defy biblical command any more than clearing land challenged the biblical admonition, "Thorns also and thistles shall it bring forth to thee." Anesthesia was a product of human ingenuity, these physicians explained, and therefore a "God-given" gift, just as the plow was. Simpson contended that God overtly sanctioned anesthesia by putting Adam in a dreamlike state while extracting his rib. Another doctor dismissed this reasoning: "Dr. Simpson surely forgets that the deep sleep of Adam took place before the introduction of pain into the world during his state of innocence!"[49]

Two starkly different philosophies nurtured these conflicting views. Physicians who viewed birth foremost as pathological—with pain one of the most troubling features of the pathology—favored the use of ether or chloroform. Physicians who viewed birth primarily as physiological, with the overwhelming likelihood of a good outcome, urged as routine during birth only the presence of a highly skilled, alert doctor. These two ideologies proved so compelling that doctors who practiced obstetrics came to identify with one of two informal philosophical camps: the "operators," to whom birth was primarily pathological, or the "nonoperators," who viewed birth as primarily physiological.[50]

Members of the group that eventually became the operator camp argued that obstetric anesthesia was not only palliative but also therapeutic. Simpson contended that chloroform sped mothers' recovery and produced more viable children. Channing also celebrated the therapeutic properties of ether: he claimed it hastened cervical dilation, lessened resistance of the perineum, prevented maternal exhaustion, and ensured that women would evacuate their bowels by the second day after birth "as if a miracle had been performed." Another doctor described a woman who had suffered such severe headaches after giving birth that she lay in darkness and silence for days. The day after her first birth under chloroform, however, the doctor arrived at her home to find the shutters open and the room bathed in light.[51]

Despite the conflicting claims for efficacy, Walter Channing was alone in his attempt to gather information on how doctors used and assessed obstetric anesthesia. In one of the first efforts in the United States to collect data to test the value of a medical practice, Channing sent a questionnaire to Boston-area colleagues to learn about their experience with ether and chloroform. He elicited responses by pointedly appealing to physicians' civic pride, observing that Boston, as "the birthplace of etherization," was the ideal site for such a study. Forty-six physicians responded to Channing's solicitation, describing 516 anesthetized births. The vast majority assessed ether favorably. One doctor testified to "the happiest results; not one unpleasant symptom having followed its use." Another observed that women did well with ether and seemed to recover from childbirth more quickly than normal. One physician said that in one case, when he used chloroform instead of ether, his patient suffered severe hemorrhage. He was unsure, however, if chloroform had prompted the bleeding. Only one doctor reported that most of his patients "preferred to trust to their powers of endurance" rather than inhale either ether or chloroform.[52]

The entire medical community debated the issues raised by Channing, Simpson, Snow, Ramsbotham, and Meigs, using language as contentious and uncompromising as these better-known physicians. One doctor extolled "the great superiority of allowing Nature to conduct the whole process of the birth." He condemned anesthesia for reducing patients "to a point very little separated from death itself." Another charged that the very nature of labor rendered obstetric anesthesia inherently dangerous and ineffective because the average labor lasted too long to permit the safe use of anesthesia. Other doctors unreservedly praised anesthesia. One told colleagues that in more than one thousand deliveries, he had not experienced a single difficulty with chloroform. He attributed the complaints of detractors to inadequate training or lack of talent.[53]

Through most of the nineteenth century, advice literature for mothers largely avoided this debate, mentioning obstetric anesthesia only cursorily, if at all. When advice manuals did allude to anesthesia, they customarily reiterated the view of the physicians who eschewed it. Marion Harland, not only the writer of domestic manuals but also the mother of six children, tried first to quell women's anxiety whenever she discussed birth. "Do not allow your imagination to wander off into the dreary forebodings of disaster and death. . . . [Look] resolutely away from the gloomy to the bright side . . . you can further a happy consummation of present trials more ably than could the combined medical skill of a continent." Mrs. P. B. Saur, a physician trained at the Philadelphia Women's College and presumably a mother, authored *Maternity: A Book for Every Wife and Mother* in 1889. She described labor as a predictable and measured process with pains increasing in rapidity and severity so gradually that women became accustomed to them with little assistance. She advised that remaining confident and cheerful was the best pain remedy. Saur did recommend using chloroform ("one of the greatest and most valuable discoveries ever conferred on suffering humanity") during particularly long labors but recommended that most births be allowed to run their course unaided by any medicine.[54]

Although the authors of maternal advice books remained wary about obstetric anesthesia through the end of the nineteenth century, the weight of medical opinion came to favor its use during that same time. A conversation among physicians in 1884 exemplified the gist of that medical conversation. Speaking before a group of colleagues, a Virginia physician deplored any remaining reluctance to use anesthesia during birth. He chastised colleagues who allowed women to suffer "an *agony*, from the Greek, a struggle as if in the pangs of death." A doctor from West Virginia rose from the audience to ridicule that depiction of labor, insisting that in fifteen years of practice he had never seen a single instance of such torture. To the contrary, he noted, he had been impressed with how easy birth was for the vast majority of his patients. A Texas physician disagreed. "I do not know, sir, what kind of pains the women in West Virginia have, but I want you all to know that the women in Texas suffer the same old pains during parturition!" The audience laughed as the Texas doctor recalled Meigs's impassioned opposition to obstetric anesthesia several decades before: "Having been taught by Dr. Charles D. Meigs, of Philadelphia, not to use chloroform . . . I was afraid to have a bottle of it in the house." Since then his attitude had changed markedly. Now when a woman asked if he could ease her pain, he "thanked God that, through the science of chemistry and the discovery of Sir James Y. Simpson, whose name is immortal, I am enabled to reply 'Yes!' and to carry her safely through the agonies of her parturition!" The audience applauded. By the end of the nineteenth century, the question of necessity was off the table.[55]

Women's Experience of Birth

Most women were largely unaware of physicians' nineteenth-century debates. Rather than doctors' strong opinions, class, more than any other single factor, arguably shaped the experience of birth for women. A woman's class influenced both her perception of "normal" labor and her physician's decisions about treatment. Regardless of the mother's class, however, births in the United States did have certain commonalities.

The most conspicuous feature of the nineteenth-century birth experience was women's reticence to discuss it. Even when writing to intimates, women did not mention a pregnancy until after giving birth, and then they referred to the event only cursorily. Anna Bentley, who left her Maryland home in the spring of 1826 for a Quaker community on the Ohio frontier, wrote long, intimate letters to her mother and sister for more than three decades. Yet even superficial details of her births failed to appear in those letters. After the birth of her tenth child in 1834, Bentley acknowledged the birth five days after the fact by reporting only, "I got up and dressed without assistance, washed and dressed the babe, went to scouring." In 1836, after the birth of her last child, she did not write to her mother for several weeks, eventually reporting only that her cousin Meg, who had been there to assist, left a day after the birth to care for her own sick child. For a birth attendant to leave so quickly was unusual, and Meg and Bentley parted reluctantly, "with tears of sisterly affection."[56]

Men were equally reluctant to speak of pregnancy and birth. James Peet, an itinerant Methodist minister living in St. Paul, Minnesota, never mentioned his wife's 1856 pregnancy in his diary until the birth of his son: "This a.m. at 7¾ oclock we were presented with a new responsibility—a Son—our first born—O Lord may it become . . . a good Christian Man, or else take it back again to thyself before it should grow up to Sin and wretchedness." Nineteen months later, Peet wrote similarly of another pregnancy and birth: "Mrs. P was taken 'in labor' at about 2½ Oclock this a.m. and at about 4¾ Oclock p.m. presented us with a boy, our 2nd Born, which weighs when dressed 8 lbs. is 20 inches long."[57]

This virtual silence surrounding pregnancy and birth crossed class and regional lines. Gertrude Thomas, a wealthy, educated woman born in 1834, lived on large plantations in Georgia both before and after marriage. Beginning at age fourteen and for the next forty-one years, Thomas kept a journal detailing the events in her life. Yet even in her journal she did not mention the birth of her first child until fifteen months after the fact; and then she did so briefly: "I was confined with a sickness which did not last very long and the advent of the birth of a son was hailed with a degree of rapture mingled with silent yet fervent thanks to God, the giver of all good things."[58]

Only after her sixth child was born in 1863 did Thomas offer significant detail of a birth in her journal, for this birth had been extraordinary: she had received chloroform. She was "pleased with the result," though "not altogether satisfied with its safety." Her mother, who was in charge of dispensing the chloroform despite a doctor's presence, was particularly leery of the experiment. She so feared chloroform would harm her daughter that she did not give it nearly as often as the doctor commanded. Nevertheless, Thomas deemed the ability of chloroform to dull pain "magical." She mused, "Of all the ways to select for committing suicide I should think it preferable."[59]

It is unclear whether women and men wrote so tersely of birth because they

deemed it a vulgar event, a difficult ordeal they did not wish to recall, or a biological function so mundane as to be unworthy of elaborate mention. Some combination of the three is likely. In 1865, weary and depressed about the war, Thomas
expressed anxiety about her seventh pregnancy: "I have thought of my dying
when the hour of trial comes. Mr. Thomas says I always say I expect to die, but I
don't think so. I know I have thought of it this time more than usual and if I do
die, I hope that my baby will die with me." She also noted that at times pregnancy
prevented her from faithfully reporting important events in her journal. "The excessive languor and indisposition I suffer from previous to the birth of my children unfit me entirely for a regular course of writing."[60]

Other women's letters and diaries seemed to indicate that terse descriptions of
birth had less to do with embarrassment, debility, or weariness and more to do
with the notion that birth was a commonplace event. When a woman did give details of a birth, she usually did so because some aspect of the birth had been extraordinary, like Anna Bentley's birth attendant's early departure or Gertrude
Thomas's use of chloroform. Doctors' casebooks indicate that women were blasé
enough about labor that they waited many hours before sending for medical
help, postponing a summons so long in some cases that babies arrived before the
physician. Lottie Tubbs, the Ohio missionary living with her husband in Mexico,
did not even realize she was in labor before she precipitously gave birth to her second baby. She felt sick the day before the birth: "just an ordinary stomachache
like I have had lots of times." Her cook suspected the baby's arrival was imminent,
but Tubbs dismissed the idea. Waking that night to go to the bathroom, she was
stunned to find the baby's head coming. She quickly got into bed, and "two very
easy pains brought the child. I didn't suffer any to speak of." Bertha Van Hoosen,
the first woman head and professor of obstetrics at a coeducational medical
school (the Loyola University School of Medicine in Chicago), described in her
autobiography her own arrival in 1863 in advance of the doctor; it was a story she
probably heard often from her mother. Van Hoosen joked that the doctor entered
her mother's house to find the newborn Bertha "kicking at my placenta, aimlessly
waving my fists and howling, as I have many times since, at the unfitness of the
male midwife."[61]

Virtually all women, including the wealthiest and the poorest, gave birth at
home through the nineteenth century. Josephine Laflin, who lived in Chicago,
traveled often in Europe, and summered with her family in Massachusetts, gave
birth to her third child at home in 1898 with two physicians in attendance. Midwives, as well as nurses, doctors, and medical students working for medical charities, similarly attended births in the homes of impoverished women. In 1888 the

first annual report of the Augusta Memorial Visiting Nurses in Chicago, an organization offering free home health care to the poor, noted that its first obstetric case was an eighteen-year-old mother who gave birth in her kitchen on a cold January day beside a virtually fireless stove. When a nurse arrived the next day to provide the new mother with postpartum care, the nurse discovered the baby had no clothing and the young mother had not eaten since the baby's birth. When the nurse asked why, the mother responded that Tommy had no work. The nurse explained, "Tommy was the husband, but he looked a mere boy."[62]

Until the first decades of the twentieth century, only very desperate women gave birth in hospitals. The New England Hospital, the sole maternity hospital in Boston for many decades, described itself as "the only place where a woman . . . can receive the comfort and care so necessary at the period of childbirth, if she is not so fortunate as to possess a good home and friends." The hospital listed soldiers' wives, women who had been deserted by their husbands, and unmarried women (who sought to "spare their friends the mortification of seeing an illegitimate child among them")—in other words "the respectable needy"—as their clientele.[63]

Single women clearly anticipated and experienced birth far differently than married women. The desire of single women to avoid bringing shame on family and friends could be so strong that a woman who died of childbed fever in 1868 at New England Hospital begged nurses just before her death, "Don't let my parents ever hear what has been my fate." Another single woman who gave birth at the Maternity Hospital in Minneapolis in 1889 died shortly after the birth from, according to nurses, "a sense of shame and disgrace which so preyed upon her mind, that life became a burden too heavy for endurance."[64]

For these women, the physical pain of childbirth was likely inconsequential compared to the humiliation of their circumstance. Or perhaps they believed labor pain was richly deserved punishment. We do not know because, unlike married women of means, they left no record of their experience. In any event, labor pain was not the primary torment for some birthing women in this period, nor was hope for its relief even a fleeting desire.

Even so, wealthy women giving birth at home were not the only women to receive ether or chloroform in the nineteenth century. At some point the medical community made obstetric anesthesia available, on occasion, to the desperate women giving birth in charity hospitals. In 1888 the New England Hospital board took up the question of which anesthetic, ether or chloroform, was better for use during birth and solicited opinions from Boston-area physicians to settle the matter. At the Boston Lying-In Hospital, founded in 1832 to provide maternity care for indigent married women, obstetric records indicate that though the vast majority of women did not receive anesthesia, doctors used ether when a woman seemed to be in unusual distress or when forceps were required. During one particularly long labor in 1886, for example, a twenty-six-year-old first-time mother received "ether to full anesthesia" at 8:50 a.m., 1:00 p.m., and 5:50 p.m., when the doctor finally applied forceps. During another birth that same year, a woman described as "very noisy and unmanageable thro out labor" received "ether to full anesthesia for 5 min." Boston Lying-In Hospital's policy of using ether during births deemed problematic by physicians continued in ensuing years.[65]

The Philadelphia Lying-In Charity Hospital, founded in 1828, followed a similar pattern of anesthesia usage. The hospital offered two services, free medical attendance at home births and hospitalized maternity care for homeless women. In the early 1890s, the charity's medical records indicate that doctors and nurses viewed labor much as the famed Philadelphia obstetrician Charles Meigs had more than forty years before: as a positive force to be encouraged rather than nullified. "Pains very good" was a near-constant descriptive refrain in patients' records.[66]

When records indicated that ether or chloroform was applied, mention of the treatment was usually accompanied by a description of the patient's annoying behavior prior to anesthetic administration, implying that nurses and doctors administered anesthesia less for women's needs than for the needs of harried medical personnel. "Pa. very nervous—excitable. Gave chloroform to quiet patient"; "Kept pa. under influence of chloroform until 6 p.m. Pa. very nervous and unmanageable"; and "Patient was very nervous and excited; rolling about the bed and unmanageable . . . mild etherization begun to assist in controlling the patient" were typical entries. This strategy occasionally backfired, however. An 1891 entry in a patient's chart read, "Patient hysterical. Gave ether but caused patient to be more excitable." Far less frequent were notes indicating that a physician administered anesthesia to relieve the patient: "Pa. very weak owing to long labor. . . . Dr. Hopkinson applied forceps. . . . Pa. kept under ether"; "The perineum was lacerated. Anesthetic was given and three stitches taken"; "Patient complained of headache and dizziness of vision. Gave chloral per rectum."[67]

By the mid-1890s, anesthesia was still only rarely used at this hospital. When a doctor or nurse did administer it that late in the century, however, there is evidence of less hesitant use. In one particularly long labor in 1895, doctors administered chloral rectally to an Irish woman, followed by an opium suppository, followed for more than twelve hours by ether given with each pain.[68] This use of multiple drugs remained exceedingly rare, however.

In January 1906 the Philadelphia Lying-In Charity Hospital began to provide nurses and doctors with preprinted patient charts. Each chart included space for remarks about anesthesia administered during the second stage of labor, specifically, whether anesthesia had been administered to the obstetrical degree (intermittently with each contraction but without loss of consciousness) or to the surgical degree (prompting loss of consciousness). The preprinted notation about anesthesia likely reflected the increased use of anesthesia (as well as its use only during second-stage labor), but the forms also seemed to encourage its use, for with the advent of the charts, anesthetic administration during birth became the norm, in stark contrast to previous years. Of the 34 births recorded at the hospital during July and August of 1907, for example, only 7 women had no anesthesia, 24 had anesthesia to the obstetrical degree, and 3 had anesthesia to the surgical degree.[69]

By the first decade of the twentieth century, doctors clearly administered obstetric anesthesia quite readily to women. They did so, however, only as second-stage labor was ending. In addition to notations on the preprinted hospital charts of impoverished women, well-off women now similarly mentioned this use of anesthesia when they described their home births in diaries and letters. Two women's stories are typical.

At about eleven-thirty on the evening of August 29, 1890, Anita McCormick Blaine, who had been having light contractions all day, told a close family friend that she felt "some little pains as if she had eaten a 'green apple'" and was going to try to sleep. The friend, Missy Hammond, also went to bed. Five hours later Blaine's husband, Emmons, woke Hammond and asked her to bring some cracked ice for Blaine. Hammond entered Blaine's room to find her sitting up in bed, leaning against her husband. The doctor, who had been there for about forty-five minutes, faced Blaine holding both of her hands in his. Hammond later reported to Blaine's mother: "I can never tell you how the . . . sweetness, dignity and strength of her character came out in those trying hours. Emmons was *all in all* to her. I came and went but was not of much use. . . . I must tell you of the patient strength and the touching sweetness that through all, our dear Anita exhibited. At last (when Dr. W. knew the time was at hand, Emmons left the room, and with the nurse holding one hand and I the other, she unconscious from the chloroform, the dear baby boy 'came into this land of ours.' His first cry awakened her. She says it was like calling her from death to life."[70]

Katharine Kerr Moore had a similar experience in June 1921 when she gave birth to her third child at home in Chicago. At about eight o'clock in the evening, she began to feel early labor pains and hurried to finish her ironing before the birth. While she ironed, her husband Max summoned a nurse, who arrived at about ten o'clock. Moore slept fitfully from eleven until two, when she awakened the nurse and instructed her to phone the doctor. The doctor arrived at about three, examined Moore, and assured her that her labor was progressing well. Then he went to sleep in another room. While the doctor slept, Moore's husband and the nurse stayed with her and, according to Moore, "were a great help to me and really worked hard, rubbing my back . . . and listening to my grunts and groans." At 6:35 a.m., Moore announced to her husband and the nurse that the baby's head was coming. The doctor heard the announcement "and came rushing forth (much refreshed & surprised to find that we had let him sleep so long." He immediately administered chloroform, and Moore said afterward, "I didn't know anything for 5 minutes or so, when it was all over."[71]

By the end of the nineteenth century, rendering women unconscious or semiconscious at the moment of birth, and usually only at the moment of birth, was a common practice in homes and hospitals alike. What physicians saw and heard—women forced during second-stage labor to bear down and emit involuntary groans because of the powerful force of the uterine muscle pushing the fetus from the birth canal—as opposed to what mothers felt came to dictate the traditional timing of the administration of obstetric anesthesia. Women likely accepted doctors' assessment of when to administer anesthesia because of women's lack of familiarity with birth. Without the experience enjoyed by previous generations of women, who had so often served as birth attendants, women in the late nineteenth and early twentieth centuries were increasingly content to defer to physicians' judgment in all aspects of childbirth, welcoming ether or chloroform as the moment of birth neared, even though this treatment saved women from little, if any, discomfort.[72]

Physicians' Practice and Experience at Births

Like the women they cared for, nineteenth-century physicians tended to describe births tersely. The pithy notes in doctors' casebooks seemed to imply that births were largely benign, almost incidental events. Visits to patients for other reasons customarily warranted a sizable paragraph of symptoms and therapies, but doctors most often described a birth in few words. "Labor natural and easy," "labor normal," "labor natural and quick," and "very quick, comfortable time" were phrases sprinkled throughout medical logs to wholly describe a birth. John Snow's style of recording a birth was representative in that he devoted only a single line to most births in his casebooks: "Sunday 29 October 1848. Mrs. Buck-ingham. Delivery (Male)" was a typical entry.[73]

This succinct method of marking a birth in the medical record was set aside, however, when a physician used ether or chloroform. The novelty of anesthetics clearly excited physicians; their descriptions of births became considerably longer as they recorded anesthetic effects in some detail. John Snow's expanded note-taking style was typical: "16 Oct. 1848. Mrs. Sutton. Delivery (Fem). Was called at a quarter to four a.m. and found that she had been in labour 3 or 4 hours. Pains had been strong and bearing down, and the os uteri was about half dilated. She inhaled chloroform. . . . she was kept unconscious the greater part of the time, a little more vapour being given whenever consciousness returned. . . . there were all the usual straining and other demonstrations of strong bearing down pains. She rambled in her mind occasionally but was quiet and manageable. Was quite unconscious of the birth, but recovered it in 2 or 3 minutes."[74]

Records kept by William Thornton Parker, a Boston physician, provide an-other example. Beside the description in his casebook of a patient's symptoms, treatment, and prognosis, Parker identified and underlined the diagnosis in the margin. Amid the burns, pneumonias, fevers, sore nipples, mumps, and cholera infantums described in the casebook, only one case had its diagnosis circled in-stead of underlined: an 1848 case of "Chloroform in Labour." The parturient, a Mrs. Kimball, who was giving birth to her fifth child, had "hitherto suffered much more than women in general," owing to a small pelvis. To ease Kimball's "great terror & apprehension," Thornton procured and used chloroform for the first time. Immediately after its administration, Kimball's pulse dropped from 80 to 50. Although she remained conscious throughout the birth, she declared appre-ciatively that the chloroform had reduced her pain to "nothing." Parker described the event as memorable.[75]

By the 1880s and 1890s, the use of anesthesia was apparently common enough that doctors no longer exhibited excitement about its use. Their descriptions of anesthetic administration shortened accordingly. All accounts of births, with or without anesthesia, were once again brief. Physicians with private patients, in particular, now used chloroform or ether so routinely that its administration seemed barely worthy of mention. In one typical notation, a Rochester, Min-nesota, physician wrote: "First child. Used chloroform last hours. labor easy. birth not known to her."[76]

According to the physicians who used anesthesia regularly, women shared their early enthusiasm for the treatment. Channing described one distraught woman who moaned, "I am dying, I am dying," before receiving ether, only to mutter, "How beautiful! How beautiful," after receiving it. Another doctor reported that when he asked a patient what she thought of chloroform, she responded, "It was heaven." In 1850 a Buffalo, New York, doctor reported giving chloroform to a woman who admonished upon her first inhalation, "Why did you not give it to me before!" Another patient, in labor with her fourth child, was so eager to continue receiving chloroform that her physician observed, "It was sometimes rather amusing to see how she clung to the sponge when I directed its removal from her face."[77]

Women did occasionally override the reluctance of some physicians who were unprepared by outlook or training to use obstetric anesthesia. One physician, unschooled in the use of ether, arrived at a woman's home to find a bottle of ether and a sponge on the bedside table. The doctor examined the woman, "found every thing favorable for a safe and speedy termination of the labor," and assured his patient that the baby would be born within two hours without any interference— presumably a pointed reference to the ether on the nightstand. The woman, however, was resolute. She demanded the ether. The physician acquiesced, poured an ounce on the sponge, and the patient held it to her mouth and nose. For the remainder of her labor, she called for the ether whenever she awoke. The baby was born one hour after the initial inhalation.[78]

Women thus played an important role in the increasing acceptance of obstetric anesthesia, to the distress of some physicians. One doctor protested, "Sometimes the patient herself wants *too much*, and will not be denied." Wary doctors often delayed anesthesia administration despite women's requests, fearing that a woman might become so engrossed in her efforts to obtain more anesthetic that she would cease assisting with the birth.[79] Most physicians who employed anesthesia, however, seemed to welcome women's appeals. In an 1848 letter to Meigs, Simpson boasted that in Edinburgh doctors administered chloroform because "the ladies themselves insist in not being doomed to suffer, when suffering is so totally unnecessary." Simpson similarly scolded his London colleague Francis Henry Ramsbotham: "Here all our ladies demand relief—& quite right."[80]

Yet in the absence of patient pressure, most physicians in the thirty or so years after the introduction of obstetric anesthesia administered ether or chloroform only given a clear indication. Since professional standards in obstetrics did not exist, these indications varied depending on the experience and inclination of the physician; they could range from a first birth, to a breech birth, to a prolonged birth, to the need for forceps, to a woman's nervousness. Discernible patterns of anesthesia use did not exist except within individual doctors' obstetric logs.

The policies of the nation's few lying-in hospitals exhibited unique inclinations as well.[81]

Exactly how doctors administered anesthesia also varied widely. Most commonly, they dispensed chloroform with a cotton handkerchief; this method alleviated the burden of carrying a large, ungainly device to patients' homes. The cotton-handkerchief method precluded all attempts at standardization, however, and so rules governing anesthesia administration, like the indications for obstetric anesthesia, came to be based on a vague combination of physician inclination, experimentation, anecdotal evidence, and patient demand.[82]

Accordingly, dosages could be notoriously imprecise. One physician described his recommended protocol: when a woman's cervix was "almost" dilated, pour "about" two drachms of chloroform on a folded handkerchief, hold the handkerchief "5 or 6 inches" from the patient's face, and "slowly approach nearer and nearer until the edges of the handkerchief overlap the upper part of the cheek." When a woman's breathing became "at all loud," this doctor recommended removing the handkerchief, waiting for the effects of the chloroform to subside, and then repeating the process. Another physician described his anesthetic regimen in a series of non sequiturs in 1885: (1) Never use anesthesia in easy normal cases. (2) If the patient is nervous and uncontrollable, administer chloroform at the start of every pain. (3) If total unconsciousness is necessary, use ether instead of chloroform.[83]

Physicians' protocol depended largely on their view of labor pain. John Snow customarily administered chloroform during first-stage labor, "for the suffering caused by the dilating pains in the first stage of labour is often very great, and the chloroform is consequently of the utmost service when employed at this time." Most physicians even in these early years, however, administered anesthesia much later in labor. Joseph DeLee insisted that a physician's cheerful demeanor and offer of encouragement and sympathy would see a woman through first-stage labor. He advised administering anesthesia lightly and intermittently only at the start of second-stage labor. Then, as the baby's head emerged, a moment DeLee described as "the period of greatest anguish" for women, he recommended rendering the mother unconscious.[84]

Physicians considered two factors, their own time and their patient's safety, as they developed their techniques to administer obstetric anesthesia. One physician observed, "Even a doctor of small reputation can hardly be expected to remain immovable beside one patient for a day, or for twenty hours or more." Thus the treatment John Snow had given Queen Victoria, now described as "unremitting care, watching the patient almost continuously through many hours, and

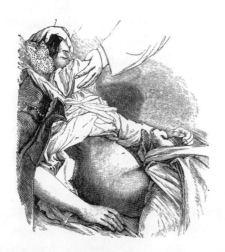 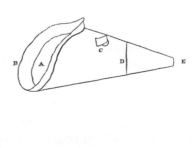

Left: administering chloroform via handkerchief. *Source:* T. Spencer Wells, *Diseases of the Ovaries: Their Diagnosis and Treatment* (D. Appleton, 1872), 144. *Right:* inhaler for the administration of ether or chloroform, made of pasteboard and lined with tinfoil. *A* is the opening for the mouth and nose; *B* is the doeskin leather surrounding the opening to ensure better fit; *C* allows expired air to escape; *D* represents the end of the conical sponge soaked with chloroform or ether; and *E* is the opening that allows air into the inhaler. *Source:* Walter Channing, *A Treatise on Etherization in Childbirth* (William D. Ticknor, 1848), 126.

giving the chloroform drop by drop, just as needed," was deemed out of the question for most doctors.[85] Administration during the relatively brief second stage of labor, however, was feasible. Other doctors limited chloroform or ether to second-stage labor for safety reasons. They found that inducing unconsciousness any earlier weakened contractions, prolonged labor, and endangered mother and baby. Side effects were often so pronounced when anesthesia was administered during first-stage labor that DeLee commented in 1918 that he preferred to have women forgo narcotics during birth altogether, but certainly throughout the first stage.[86]

Yet by the early twentieth century, virtually all physicians had learned to appreciate anesthesia when faced with a difficult birth. A half century after Nathan Cooley Keep celebrated Fanny Longfellow's etherized birth, anesthesia had become such a vital tool during problematic labors that in 1902 one experienced doctor urged younger colleagues to administer chloroform at all births so that they would be adept at its administration when faced with a complicated birth.[87]

As this advice indicates, by the turn of the twentieth century, many if not most doctors used obstetric anesthesia with little reservation. This tendency appeared in even the remotest locales. A physician who practiced in the gold-, silver-, and copper-mining camps of Nevada and Montana for twenty-five years used chloroform in almost exactly half of seven hundred births. He used it "carefully but freely, and without the least hesitation," to induce "a perfectly unconscious birth," even in the absence of indication.[88]

By the early twentieth century, some physicians also clearly recognized that the offer of ether or chloroform attracted patients. For doctors attempting to build a practice in a small town, anesthesia proved a particularly helpful lure. When a doctor in Waukesha, Wisconsin, promised he would no more go to "a case of confinement without my scissors as without my chloroform and mask," women learned of his vow and word quickly spread. "You get that doctor," they told each other; "he gives you chloroform." Another physician, who allowed women to sniff a chloroform-soaked handkerchief at will during labor, assured colleagues that the treatment persuaded mothers both to summon him for subsequent births and to encourage the newly married woman next door to hire him as well. Conversely, a doctor who eschewed anesthesia during birth unless he felt the treatment was clearly warranted complained in 1904 that patients had abandoned him because he refused to "do something" as they labored.[89]

Increasingly, physicians who continued to practice the traditional "watchful waiting" during birth were the exception. By the end of the nineteenth century, medical discussion about the necessity of anesthesia and the nature of labor had largely ended in favor of anesthetic use. With the question of necessity settled, other questions arose, questions that changed the focus of debate and women's and physicians' perception and use of anesthesia.

After Simpson's use of ether at a birth in Edinburgh in January 1847, word of his triumph traveled so fast that within a few months even laypeople living across the Atlantic, like Fanny Appleton Longfellow, savored the potential of obstetric anesthesia. U.S. culture at the time encouraged this interest; earlier, when society had not characterized women as unavoidably weak and sickly and when the female support network seen in social birth had been more reliable, obstetric anesthesia might not have garnered as much attention.

As the incidence of social birth waned during the nineteenth century, doctors replaced midwives and their laywomen assistants. As they did so, physicians contributed significantly to women's perception of birth. Birth has always been a powerful experience for onlookers, and nervous doctors, unaccustomed to seeing others strain as mightily as women do in second-stage labor, exacerbated women's traditional apprehension. Women undergoing unmedicated labors re-port that their behaviors during the second stage are involuntary and they feel little if any pain, especially when compared with the pain of transition, but doc-tors in the nineteenth century were unaware of this fact because they gained al-most no knowledge of childbirth from formal training.[90]

The anxiety doctors displayed as witnesses to birth in the nineteenth century thus likely heightened women's anxiety. Now lacking the acquaintance with so-cial birth enjoyed by previous generations, women increasingly anticipated and experienced birth only through their own fear, loneliness, and pain. As women approached birth in ignorance, physicians' perceptions became the predominant view of the nature of birth. Women's desire for obstetric anesthesia then allowed physicians to exert more control in birth practices, and one manifestation of this new authority accorded to physicians in the birthing chamber was dictating when obstetric anesthesia would be administered.[91]

As the descriptions of birth recounted in this chapter indicate, doctors admin-istered anesthesia most commonly only at the end of second-stage labor. Al-though women have testified over and over that transition, the end of first-stage labor, is the most painful portion of labor, second-stage labor looks and sounds far more painful to those witnessing birth. Simpson, Channing, and DeLee were all typical in that they wrote vividly of the agony they believed women experi-enced as their babies exited their bodies. Thus, in the case of the administration of obstetric anesthesia, the experience of the physician-witness trumped the ex-perience and need of the patient.[92]

Nineteenth-century surgical patients understandably preferred the blessing of ether or chloroform during surgery, but why did so many mothers, after weath-ering all of first-stage labor and most of second-stage labor without pain relief, find oblivion preferable to consciousness at the moment of birth? Unfamiliar with the rhythms of labor because they had not taken part in social birth, women came to rely on physicians to tell them when they needed anesthesia. They be-came convinced that doctors' chosen timing rescued them from the most excru-ciating pain imaginable.

Obstetric anesthesia brought about a fundamental change in birth practices that still reverberates. Decades of bitter disagreement among physicians about the necessity and utility of anesthesia lessened their ability to standardize obstet-ric practice in a deliberate and collaborative manner. Ether and chloroform also prompted the medical community to view laboring women differently than they had in the past: as the helpless victims of a bodily process rather than as the most important participants in that process. One physician typified this attitude, explaining in 1887 that he allowed women to hold a chloroform-soaked handkerchief throughout labor because it made women so "grateful . . . to have something to do" during childbirth.[93]

Doctors' efforts during birth were clearly coming to be valued more than women's. A change in nomenclature reflected the shift: midwives traditionally employed the phrase "catching babies" to describe what they did, but doctors now "delivered" babies. Whereas "catching" a baby acknowledged the central role of the woman who provided the baby to be caught, "deliver" implied that the baby could not appear without the physician to make the delivery.

Anesthesia altered not only the predominant lay and medical perceptions of the nature of childbirth but also the portrayal of the appropriate behavior of doctors and mothers during childbirth. Doctors who used ether or chloroform began to refrain from conversing with laboring women. Snow was one of many who cautioned that conversation with a woman under the influence of chloroform would excite her, rendering her uncontrollable.[94] Learning that external physical stimulus could induce violent response in a lightly anesthetized person portended the ironclad caveat that women under the influence of anesthesia, and particularly twilight sleep, discussed at length in the next chapter, needed absolute silence to ensure the desired effect.

Thus, not only did the incidence of social birth wane through the nineteenth century, but women could not necessarily count on the physicians who replaced social birth networks to provide any companionship. This development reinforced the ostensible need for anesthesia. Only a few decades before, female friends and relatives had surrounded laboring women, sustaining them with camaraderie, encouragement, and advice rather than anesthesia. In contrast, from the mid-nineteenth century onward, women increasingly weathered the vicissitudes of labor alone, with chloroform or ether their only comfort.

CHAPTER TWO

Twilight Sleep

The Question of Professional Respect, 1890s through 1930s

*I*n 1912 Mrs. Cecil Stewart left the United States to give birth to her second child in Freiburg, Germany, under the auspices of physicians Bernhard Krönig and C. J. Gauss. Stewart's sister accompanied her. Word of Krönig's and Gauss's work on Dämmerschlaf, an injectable combination of scopolamine and morphine, motivated the two women to make the long journey. As news of Dämmerschlaf (twilight sleep) crossed the Atlantic, the prospect of painless childbirth had become a topic of conversation in upper-class American social circles, turning Krönig's and Gauss's Frauenklinik (women's clinic) into a mecca for select pregnant Americans.

Before embarking on the trip to Freiburg, Stewart had asked Mrs. C. Temple Emmet, the first American to give birth under Dämmerschlaf, for more information on the Frauenklinik and its novel treatment. Information from Emmet was not forthcoming, however. Instead, she responded to each of Stewart's entreaties with the same terse statement: "The Head Nurse will tell you everything."

Despite the lack of detailed information, Stewart headed to Germany with her sister. Finally arriving in Freiburg after an extended stay in London, Stewart checked into a hotel one "cold, wet, dismal October night," sent her English doctor's letter of introduction to the Frauenklinik, and then settled in, anticipating an imminent visit from Krönig. Days passed and he never came. Eventually, Krönig's head nurse arrived to answer Stewart's questions, just as Emmet had promised. The nurse told Stewart that to see Dr. Krönig she would have to go to the clinic. He would not come to her.

Incredulous at being ordered to go to the doctor rather than being visited by him, Stewart remained at the hotel. A few days later, one of the younger clinic physicians came to see her and immediately put her at ease: "He did not bother me with questions, nor ask me when I thought the baby would come, nor how I felt, nor any of the disagreeable things doctors usually say to one in these circumstances." Instead, the young physician took her hand and assured her, "I have come to comfort you." The next day Stewart went to see Krönig.

Krönig examined her, and because her baby was breech and he did not trust the taxi service to get her to the clinic after dark, he ordered her to sleep each night at the clinic. When Stewart balked, the nurse suggested she continue spending her days at the hotel. Mollified, Stewart went back to the hotel for dinner. Upon returning to the clinic later that evening with her sister, she anticipated "a whole staff to meet us." The two women were stunned to discover that they had to let themselves into the building, find their way to Stewart's room alone, and turn down her bed without assistance.

Three weeks later, when Stewart was asleep in her "big and high-ceilinged [room] with beautiful white tiles," a sharp pain awoke her. She sat up and rang the bell next to the bed. The head nurse rushed in and, learning of Stewart's pain, injected her with scopolamine-morphine, readied the room for the birth, and later administered a second injection. When Dr. Gauss came to examine Stewart, she told him what she had told the nurse earlier: "I have an awfully bad pain." Gauss responded, "Yes, you *have* a very bad pain." Stewart was pleased: "It was the first time a doctor had ever admitted that I had a bad pain when I had one. Before, they had always known better than I had, and they had told me, 'Oh, no, you have not got any pain at all; *that* is *nothing*; you'll have to have much worse pains than that.' Just Dr. Gauss's admitting that my pain *was* pain made me feel comforted and happy."

Under the influence of twilight sleep, Stewart slept. The next morning, three "chambermaids . . . making a fearful racket" woke her. Terribly annoyed at the intrusion, Stewart wondered how clinic doctors could permit such an irritant when she was about to give birth. Just then the door opened and the head nurse came in triumphantly carrying Stewart's baby. Stewart was stunned. "I can't believe it; it is a fairy tale! It isn't *true*!" The head nurse assured her that the baby was indeed hers; she had given birth the night before.

Thrilled, Stewart sat up in bed to eat a "wonderful breakfast" followed by a glass of milk and biscuits at ten o'clock and later that afternoon "a real German lunch, with soup, and an omelet, and boiled beef and cabbage, and potatoes, and roast hare, and carrots and peas, and a salad and dessert." After the scrumptious meals, the staff moved Stewart from the room she had occupied before the birth to a room in the private ward with a view of the mountains—"like a beautiful room in a big hotel"—where her sister joined her. Stewart remained there almost a month, briefly walking around the lovely room and brushing her teeth the day after giving birth and sitting up all afternoon on the fourth day. By her fifth day postpartum, she felt better than she had six long weeks after the birth of her first child and went out for a drive. On the tenth day, she began to take thrice-weekly "beauty baths" designed to bring back her "original figure."

Stewart so enjoyed her time in Freiburg that not until a month after giving birth, when her husband became impatient and cabled her to come home, did she, her sister, and her newborn leave the Frauenklinik for Paris and a boat back to the United States. Stewart spent the weeks on board ship "still marveling that I had really had a painless child."[1]

The Significance of Stewart's Experience

Everything about the birth of Stewart's second child and the surrounding circumstances, including the nurses' and doctors' solicitous attention, her inability to remember the birth, her ability to eat immediately afterward, and her quick resumption of normal activity, contrasted sharply with the birth of her first child in the United States. Stewart recalled that experience bitterly:

> It seemed to me that I had always been sacrificed to that baby. I had to wake up in the middle of the night to feed it; I had to wake up early in the morning and late at night when I was tired. But here in Freiburg, between the hours of ten o'clock at night and ten in the morning, you never saw your baby. It was taken away and put in the nursery with the other babies, and you had a beautiful, long, nice sleep; and if the baby needed to be fed in the middle of the night it was fed by a wet nurse, or by someone else in the hospital, or with a bottle of mother's milk that had been gotten. And then, at ten in the morning, the baby would be brought to you all nicely dressed and washed and clean; but if it cried or annoyed you, it was taken out in the daytime, too, so that you always had your nerves at rest, and were never disturbed by the baby's crying, or anything.[2]

Although Stewart's experience was by no means typical of the era, because twilight sleep, whether administered in Germany or the United States, was most often (but not always) a treatment that only privileged women had access to, her story is nevertheless a telling one. Some of her feelings were representative of other women's, no matter their class. Most notably, Stewart was so apprehensive about giving birth that she traveled to Germany to avoid feeling any labor pain, despite her almost total lack of knowledge about twilight sleep. She pointedly expressed gratitude that the young doctor visiting her at the hotel did not quiz her about her pregnancy or the birth she so dreaded; in other words, he did not draw attention to the source of her anxiety. Rather, he simply offered comfort. Later,

Stewart was exceedingly grateful to Gauss for acknowledging her labor pain, pain her American doctors had apparently dismissed during her first birth as inconsequential. Clearly, she faulted her doctors back home for their lack of empathy and their paternalistic insistence that her pain was trivial.

Stewart's other reactions to her experience were class-based. Although she was annoyed when Krönig did not come to her hotel and the staff failed to greet her when she moved into the clinic, the treatment Stewart ultimately received from physicians and nurses exceeded her expectations. She was especially delighted that she did not have to care for her baby if she did not feel like it. A round-the-clock wet-nursing service was a logical complement to the birth Stewart found so satisfying: having no memory of giving birth, she did not have to be inconvenienced in any way after the birth either. And no one treated Stewart like an invalid after her baby was born; she ate delicious food and resumed her normal activities in short order, reinforcing the sensation that she had never given birth.

Although Stewart's experience was obviously a rarity, her delight with twilight sleep ultimately impacted a great many American women. In 1914 details of her adventure appeared in an article published by *McClure's Magazine.* The article described women who had traveled to Germany from all corners of the world, from India, Russia, South Africa, and South America in addition to the United States, to experience painless childbirth. "The rumor has gone out from mouth to mouth, among women to the ends of the earth," the article's authors announced, "that here, at last, modern science has abolished that primal sentence of the Scriptures upon womankind: 'In sorrow thou shalt bring forth children.'"[3]

Public reaction to the article was unprecedented. So many women wrote to *McClure's* with inquiries that other lay publications around the country vied for similar attention by running related stories. Edified by all the publicity, American women organized to demand twilight sleep from their doctors. The effect of this orchestrated campaign proved to be profound.[4]

With the advent of twilight sleep, not only indigent and single women but also for the first time upper- and middle-class women had compelling reason to give birth in the hospital. Accompanying this shift was a new status accorded obstetrics. Dämmerschlaf demanded such elaborate protocol that the treatment conferred respect to the obstetrician.

Although women's organized crusade for scopolamine-morphine was a brief one, the change in obstetric practice initiated by Dämmerschlaf was dramatic. Relatively few women experienced twilight sleep directly during its heyday, yet the treatment changed everything about how American physicians perceived and treated birth and how American women anticipated and experienced it.

Development of and Initial Reactions to Twilight Sleep

After C. J. Gauss described in a German medical journal the first five hundred Dämmerschlaf births, he and Bernhard Krönig became the acknowledged international experts on the use of scopolamine-morphine in childbirth. Other journals subsequently summarized Gauss's case review; one small article appeared in the *American Journal of Obstetrics and Diseases of Women and Children* in 1906. According to this summation, Gauss admitted to problems with twilight sleep. While Dämmerschlaf produced a desirable painless state somewhere between sound sleep and full consciousness, it also generated unpleasant side effects, including slowed pulse, decreased respiration, reddened face, dilated pupils, dry throat, restlessness, and delirium.[5]

Shortly after a second article by Gauss appeared in 1907, describing one thousand Dämmerschlaf births, William Holt, an American physician living in Freiburg, favorably evaluated Gauss's and Krönig's work in the *American Journal of Clinical Medicine*. According to Holt, the semiconscious state induced by repeated injections of small doses of scopolamine and morphine erased the memories of laboring women. Although they still felt pain, they could not recall their discomfort later. Holt praised twilight sleep for preventing mental disease by sparing women any recollection of the trauma of childbirth.[6]

The assorted articles published in prominent European and American medical journals encouraged other physicians to experiment with twilight sleep. Some doctors consequently confirmed Krönig's and Gauss's optimism. Most did not, focusing instead on Dämmerschlaf's disquieting side effects. Krönig and Gauss dismissed critics by arguing that detractors did not specifically employ the Freiburg method of application, a system Krönig and Gauss deemed safe and an enormous blessing.[7]

The conviction of both European and American physicians that refined women could not withstand labor pain—the same concern that had generated interest in ether and chloroform more than fifty years earlier—fueled the initial, intense interest in twilight sleep. One Freiburg nurse likened genteel women's reaction to pain to a racehorse's "fine nerves." Franklin S. Newell, a Harvard University physician who was among the first in the American medical community to embrace and promote twilight sleep, similarly insisted that "civilized" women required solicitous medical attention during birth.[8]

Bernhard Krönig's theory of labor pain, which was virtually identical to American doctors' claims decades earlier that "squaws" and slaves gave birth with ease, supported the still pervasive view that class and ethnicity determined women's ability to weather childbirth. Krönig often told a story that had become legend in twilight sleep circles: he once saw a Gypsy drop behind the group she was traveling with in order to hastily give birth behind a hedge. After washing her baby in a nearby pond, she raced to catch up with her people. Intrigued by what he had witnessed, Krönig persuaded her to give birth to her second child at his clinic so he could more closely observe her stoicism. He concluded that she was neither healthier nor stronger than "a more highly developed type" of woman. She was simply able to surrender herself completely to the process of birth. Krönig theorized that the mental preoccupations of sophisticated, modern women impeded their ability to submit to labor; their lack of abandon, in turn, exacerbated labor pain.[9]

During the first years of experimentation with scopolamine and morphine, a few American physicians traveled to Freiburg to study with Krönig and Gauss. They returned to the United States with mixed reactions. Joseph DeLee, professor of obstetrics at Northwestern University Medical School and founder of the Chicago Lying-in Hospital and home birth dispensary, was unimpressed. He condemned twilight sleep's side effects: prolonged labor, fetal asphyxia, hemorrhage, delirium, "even violence." Another Chicago physician saw more promise in the treatment but warned that twilight sleep in the hands of untrained doctors might prove dangerous. Barton Cooke Hirst, professor of obstetrics at the University of Pennsylvania, complained that he had crossed the Atlantic only to witness what in later years would be called the placebo effect: "The patients were assured beforehand that there would be no suffering; were delivered in a quiet dark room; were given one moderate dose of morphia and became temporarily under its effect; and, being told afterward they had had no pain, probably left the institution impressed with that belief."[10]

One physician attributed the discrepancies in American doctors' assessments of twilight sleep to the varied class-dependent treatments accorded women at the Freiburg clinic. The Frauenklinik had several wards, the first-class ward for refined "women of nervous temperament" and the third- and fourth-class wards for "women of no great intelligence." Only in Freiburg's first-class ward, where each wealthy patient, like Stewart, had her own room, did German doctors claim significant success. That ward was customarily off limits to observers, however, and so most of the visiting American physicians likely never witnessed the full-blown Gauss-Krönig method, a treatment characterized by absolute quiet, constant monitoring, and dosage geared to the needs and personality of each patient. Instead, they spent their time in the third- and fourth-class free wards, where, in the words of one laywoman, they viewed only "the quick peasant births." In these wards, constant commotion distracted the patients, who underwent the simpler Siegel technique of Dämmerschlaf, a method characterized by standardized doses of scopolamine-morphine administered at predetermined intervals. Krönig experimented freely in these "lower" wards in an attempt to dispense with the exacting protocol demanded by the Gauss-Krönig method, which many physicians denounced as notoriously time-consuming and impractical.[11]

Although in most American hospitals the administration of twilight sleep was limited to wealthy women, some American hospitals provided the treatment to the poor, following methods not unlike that in Freiburg's "lower" wards. There is no record of the protocol used, but the Philadelphia Lying-In Charity Hospital supplied scopolamine-morphine to dozens of patients in 1908, six years before *McClure's Magazine* published its renowned article and the nationwide crusade for twilight sleep began. Of the sixty-six women who gave birth at the Charity Hospital in late winter and early spring of 1908, thirty received twilight sleep. This experimentation prompted an immediate change of habit: for the first time, doctors and nurses at the Philadelphia Lying-In Charity Hospital kept detailed notes describing patients' behavior during labor. These notes revealed the most disquieting side effect of scopolamine, uncontrollable delirium.[12]

Nurses noted on one woman's chart, "So perverse and obstreperous! Kicked, writhed, scratched, and yelled like a caged animal. Took three nurses and two internes to manage her. (and then some!)." Another notation on a chart read, "Flopped around like a fish and kept calling, 'Boy, Boy, Boy.'" More often, however, the notes indicated increased patient submissiveness: "Very quiet after hypo. Such a tractable, obliging little patient. No fuss or outcry whatever." Another chart read, "Very quieting effect. Patient did not yell & groan so much. Better relaxation of parts."[13]

Of all the American physicians administering twilight sleep in those early years, Bertha Van Hoosen claimed the greatest success. When she first observed the use of scopolamine in 1904, she could not contain her excitement: "No novice at a spiritualistic séance could have been more deeply impressed than I was at that first clinic." She subsequently experimented successfully with Dämmerschlaf for a number of years in surgery (calling it a "spectacular anesthetic") but remained wary of using it in obstetrics for fear it would harm babies.[14] To give Van Hoosen the opportunity to finally test the "spectacular" treatment in obstetrics, the Women's and Children's Hospital of Chicago turned its obstetric service over to her for a year. Religiously following Gauss's instructions, she administered twilight sleep to the hospital's obstetric patients. The first fifty cases had inconsistent results. Some women fell asleep after two doses, "cooperat[ing] so that the baby could be born in a natural way." Other women shrieked, bolted from bed, and fought with nurses and doctors. These unpredictable reactions prompted Van Hoosen to design a canvas crib, with heavy material enclosing the sides and top of beds, so women could be safely contained while under the influence of twilight sleep. Using the canvas cages, she deemed the next fifty twilight sleep cases successful, and the Women's and Children's Hospital of Chicago continued to administer scopolamine to laboring women for the next twenty-five years.[15]

Van Hoosen eventually honed her own method of application. Finding Krönig's and Gauss's system of adjusting each dose to the needs of individual women unrealistically demanding, she designed a fixed dosage, not unlike the Siegel method used in the third- and fourth-class wards in Freiburg. "Its claims," she boasted, "compete more with the advertising quack than those of the scientific medical man."[16]

Yet most people in the American medical community failed to share Van Hoosen's enthusiasm. That twilight sleep could be used safely only on women who were caged was enough to dissuade most doctors from employing it. In that sense, doctors and nurses at the Philadelphia Lying-In Charity Hospital appear to have had a typical reaction: there is no evidence in patient records that doctors and nurses ever used twilight sleep again after their brief 1908 experimentation. Not until 1914, when women's magazines presented twilight sleep to the public as a wholly new discovery, rather than a twelve-year-old medical controversy already rejected by most American physicians and hospitals, were American doctors forced to reexamine their dismissal of Dämmerschlaf.[17]

Unsolicited Publicity

The selling of Dämmerschlaf to American women in 1914 proved easy. Some medical techniques are inherently interesting to the public, either because they alleviate a condition that affects many people or because their effect is particularly interesting and easily understood. Twilight sleep was that rare medical treatment that fell into both categories. For women, twilight sleep was especially appealing. It had none of the unpleasantness of ether or chloroform: no odor, no mask, no suffocating feeling, no disquieting recollection of helpless semi-stupor. Instead, the entire birth experience was a blank.[18]

The first *McClure's* article about the treatment intrigued the public. The piece, published in June 1914, quoted a typically enthusiastic American woman who had crossed the Atlantic to give birth. "If I had another baby, I would have it in Freiburg, if I had to walk all the way from California!" Almost immediately, other

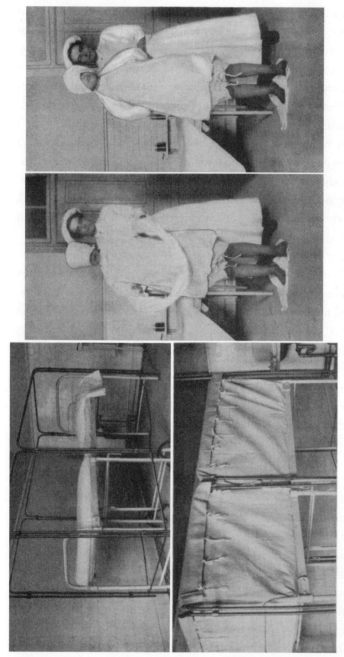

Upper left: screens placed around a labor bed to safely contain a woman under the influence of twilight sleep. *Lower left:* a canvas cover tied to the tops of the screens and surrounding the bed to subdue a woman in the event of delirium due to twilight sleep. *Right:* in addition to the screen and canvas cover, the patient is blindfolded and put into a gown with a continuous sleeve to further prevent her from harming herself in the event she becomes agitated while under the influence of twilight sleep. *Far right:* the continuous sleeve is placed behind the patient's back. *Source:* Bertha Van Hoosen and Elisabeth Ross Shaw, *Scopolamine-Morphine Anaesthesia* (House of Manz, 1915), 40a, 88a.

lay publications similarly characterized twilight sleep as "the new gospel of hope" and criticized American doctors for callously withholding the treatment from mothers.[19]

Enormously offended by the charge, physicians fumed that untutored lay advocates were simplifying the complexities of twilight sleep and overselling it to a gullible public. One doctor tried to explain that no form of obstetric anesthesia— not ether, not chloroform, not nitrous oxide, not twilight sleep—could be safely administered until labor pains were established. Yet women's magazines portrayed the Dämmerschlaf mother as enjoying a long, refreshing slumber throughout labor, eventually waking to find a neatly bundled newborn sleeping peacefully by her side. American physicians criticized the portrayal as unrealistic and dangerous.[20]

The nationalism stirred by World War I heightened doctors' animosity toward the publicity. A Wisconsin doctor complained to the American Medical Association (AMA) that women's magazines had given the public the impression that "it is only these Europian [*sic*] masters of the hypodermic needle that have been capable of such wonderful clinical practises in medication." A Pennsylvania physician wrote a similar letter to the AMA: "Is the McClure *bunch* trying to make the public think such a thing cannot be accomplished in America. Are we to send our Patients to Freiburg or to do the work Ourselves." An Ohio doctor wondered what the American public wanted their physicians to do—establish a chain of twilight sleep hospitals in the United States under German control? He admonished, "We have perhaps more reliable and less dangerous methods *not* 'made in Germany.'"[21]

Doctors' denunciations did not dampen public enthusiasm, however. Social concerns identical to those in the mid-nineteenth century prompted much of the fervor: worry about a low birthrate was as intense in the early twentieth century as it had been fifty years earlier. Anti-immigrant sentiment spurred the latest concern. Josephine Baker, head of New York's Bureau of Child Hygiene and a leading child welfare advocate, warned that if American-born couples continued to have fewer children than their immigrant counterparts, "extermination of the Anglo-Saxon race in this country" was a foregone conclusion.[22] Her sentiment was inspired by the eugenics movement, an influential early-twentieth-century crusade for improvement of the human gene pool through forced sterilization, euthanasia, and segregation of races and ethnic groups. Even the president of the United States weighed in on the looming catastrophe. Theodore Roosevelt charged that the American tendency toward smaller families was a sign of moral disease. He denounced married women who did not have children, or had only a few children, as "criminal against the race." Thus, some in the medical and lay communities alike harbored the same hope for scopolamine-morphine that earlier advocates of anesthesia had harbored for ether and chloroform, anticipating that twilight sleep would encourage culturally desirable women to have more children.[23]

Professionals and laypeople worried, just as they had in the nineteenth century, that women's fear of labor pain was the driving force behind numerous social ills. Van Hoosen explained that experienced doctors "had enough women to make of the doctor's office a confessional" and thus understood precisely how women's terror of labor pain contributed to societal breakdown. Twilight sleep, she contended, had the potential to abolish a host of social problems: "prostitution, abortions, divorces, unwilling motherhood, . . . [and] venereal diseases."[24]

Although this perceived link between labor pain and societal breakdown was reminiscent of why many doctors advocated the use of obstetric anesthesia in the mid-nineteenth century, there was an essential difference between the earlier characterization of the effects of ether and chloroform and the current portrayal of the benefits of Dämmerschlaf. Ether and chloroform gained acceptance in an era glorifying fragile women, but twilight sleep came to public attention when an entirely different view of the ideal woman predominated. The sturdy, bicycle-riding Gibson girl was in vogue, and newspapers and magazines promoted twilight sleep according to this new image. The *New York Times* advised readers that twilight sleep mothers were "sprightly, alert, and in good spirits" immediately after giving birth. A promotional leaflet distributed by the Motherhood Educational Society enticed women by informing them that the Dämmerschlaf mother traversed hospital corridors a mere twenty-four hours after giving birth. In sharp contrast, the "Natural Mother" languished ten days in bed before attempting her "first feeble effort to walk."[25]

The public learned to associate twilight sleep not only with strong, active women but also with healthier babies. As the United States began to define high infant mortality as a preventable social problem for the first time, promoters of twilight sleep touted the treatment as one solution to the country's high infant mortality rate. Women's magazines thus carried suggestive photographs of the robust babies born under twilight sleep. These images of sturdy "Dämmerschlaf children" implied that twilight sleep not only benefited women but also produced better babies.[26]

The public could not escape the deluge of favorable publicity for Dämmerschlaf. *Ladies' World* regaled American women with tales of Gauss's persistent glee in the face of mothers who awoke from twilight sleep unaware their babies had been born; even after being presented with their newborns, they denied giving birth. An amused Gauss claimed, "Some of them declare the child to be ugly and therefore probably the property of the occupant of the next bed." Francis Carmody, the husband of the first American woman to enjoy twilight sleep in Freiburg in the wake of the *McClure's* article, described the details of his wife's "absolutely painless" birth in a letter to a Brooklyn newspaper: "There are no lacerations to heal, no stitches to be removed, no contusions to nurse, and no deranged nervous systems to recuperate." Even the *International Socialist Review* took up the topic, berating "our corrupt capitalistic régime" for forcing women to wait like "beggar[s] upon the good will of Commercialism" rather than "put[ting twilight sleep] at the service of a needy people. The Profit-making germ eats into the very vitals of social progress." News of twilight sleep was so ubiquitous that the *Journal of the Kansas Medical Society* complained that no other topic, save World War I, was receiving as much national attention.[27]

These lay authors, in magazine articles and books alike, urged women to rise up and demand twilight sleep from their obstinate doctors. Hanna Rion, the lay author of a 1915 book about twilight sleep, was typical. She implored her readers "to take up the battle for painless childbirth where I have left off. . . . Fight not only for yourselves, but fight for your sister-mothers, your sex, the cradle of the human race."[28]

The calls to action reflected the enormous influence of women's activism in this period, for causes as varied as suffrage, lowered infant and maternal mortality, abolition of child labor, prohibition, and access to contraception. The assorted movements were part of the flurry of reform now known as the Progressive Era, from roughly the 1890s through World War I, when reformers worked to mitigate the social problems generated by rapid industrialization and urbanization. Given the perceived link between the debilitating effects of "civilization" and middle- and upper-class women's increased difficulties giving birth, many women viewed the twilight sleep movement as a logical addition to the many other efforts aimed at alleviating the problems inherent in urban living. Van Hoosen observed that women's demand for twilight sleep had become so closely allied with other Progressive causes that the arguments against twilight sleep had become incongruously similar to arguments against women's suffrage. Opponents of twilight sleep contended that labor pain was a positive force that made women more courageous and self-reliant. Opponents of women's suffrage contended that allowing women to vote would masculinize them.[29]

The nation's network of women's clubs formed the Twilight Sleep Association soon after the *McClure's* article appeared. Mrs. Francis Carmody, an officer of a woman's club in New York, drew the women in her club into the twilight sleep movement immediately after her son's birth in Freiburg when she sent a letter home detailing her wonderful experience. Word spread and club women nation-wide quickly instituted several activities to encourage medical acceptance of twilight sleep. Most notably, they organized to interview physicians about their willingness to administer twilight sleep and hinted darkly that women's clubs would publish the results of all interviews in order to persuade mothers to patronize only doctors amenable to the treatment.[30]

Audiences soon gathered in public spots to learn more about Dämmerschlaf. Gimbel Brothers department store sponsored a conference featuring Marguerite Tracy (author of the article in *McClure's*) and several Freiburg mothers. In her speech, Tracy listed the New York hospitals offering the Freiburg method: Gouverneur, Jewish Maternity, Lying-In, Lebanon, and Long Island College. Carmody roused the crowd by charging that most doctors were opposed to twilight sleep and so women would have to fight for it. A display of the vigorous babies born in Freiburg was a highlight of the conference.[31]

Enthusiastic patrons lined up at theaters to view movies about Dämmerschlaf. In Plymouth, Massachusetts, an ad in the *Old Colony Memorial* newspaper announced the Moral Uplift Society of America's separate showings for men and women of *Science's Greatest Triumph.* TWILIGHT SLEEP ... *A Boon to Motherhood.* Across the country, Motherhood Educational societies distributed leaflets advertising another movie, this one produced by Hoffman-La Roche Chemical Company, the manufacturer of scopolamine. The photograph of a woman, "tranquility . . . on [her] face" as she labored under the influence of scopolamine, decorated the leaflets. Marguerite Tracy described the Hoffman-La Roche film as "a realization of Edison's dream for the cinema."[32]

In October, four months after the appearance of its original article, *McClure's* ran a second story featuring additional interviews with the wealthy American "Dämmerschlaf mothers" who now formed an ever-present community in Freiburg. These pregnant women traveled to Germany with their older children, placed the children in private day schools, and spent their days socializing with each other and anticipating the painless births of their babies. The article showcased a compelling photograph of an American mother and her two children. The picture's caption explained that the woman's sad-looking six-year-old son was born in the United States, "the old school way." Her four-year-old daughter, already slightly taller than her hapless older brother, was born in Germany under twilight sleep. Physicians gathered at an American Association of Obstetricians and Gynecologists meeting later that year enjoyed ridiculing the photograph and its preposterous message.[33]

Mocking that photo provided doctors with little comfort, however; the criticism implicit in all the publicity stung. The *New York Times* accused physicians of caring more for their own convenience than sparing women pain. The *Times*'s editors likened doctors who eschewed twilight sleep to the now reviled physicians who had ridiculed Viennese physician Ignác Semmelweis in the mid-nineteenth century. Semmelweis had tried in vain to warn his colleagues that their refusal to wash their hands was the source of the childbed fever that killed tens of thousands of women annually. The arrogant doctors who ignored this admonition caused untold suffering; now the *Times* intimated that the reluctance of contemporary doctors to use twilight sleep perpetuated similar agony among women.[34]

Although discussion of medical matters in the lay press was not new, in the decades before the twilight sleep movement, the myriad articles designed to teach Americans about healthy behaviors had been authored mainly by physicians. Now, in sharp contrast, inexpert laywomen and newspaper editors wrote tributes to twilight sleep that audaciously chastised physicians for withholding the miracle from women. For the first time, the medical community faced a consumer movement disparaging medical practice. Doctors were indignant.[35]

Physicians, medical journals, and medical organizations decried the consequences of allowing the laity to dictate medical treatment. *American Medicine* warned that widespread use of twilight sleep would increase maternal mortality. The AMA feared that untrained physicians might succumb to patients' naive demands for scopolamine-morphine and administer twilight sleep with no understanding of its complexity and limitations. One doctor pardoned his young, inexperienced colleagues ("too immature to have searched the literature of ten years ago") for acquiescing to mothers' demands. He accused older physicians who experimented with twilight sleep, however, of inexcusable ignorance "or a willingness to lower professional dignity to secure a fleeting and transient prominence." Even Dr. William Knipe, who spent three months in Freiburg and found some promise in twilight sleep, condemned the "lay gossip" and reported that the unsolicited publicity dismayed Krönig and Gauss.[36]

Discussion of twilight sleep polarized both lay and professional publications, as editorials were "flanked on the one side by enthusiasm and on the other side by skepticism." "It works," the *New York Times* crowed. "With maternity robbed of its horrible tortures and its dreadful perils, this will be a new and happier world. The thought throws a gleam of light through these dark days of war."

Woman's Home Companion scolded both twilight sleep's detractors (for their "pernicious spirit of skepticism") and its proponents (for their "perhaps more pernicious spirit of maudlin enthusiasm"). Opponents of twilight sleep denounced enthusiasts as nervous women who had the money and time to fulfill their every whim. Advocates characterized opponents as dogmatists who dismissed obstetric anesthesia as against the will of God. Discussion tended so much toward exaggeration that one exasperated Denver physician observed that "the honest practitioner . . . hardly knows whether in his efforts he may be considered as a 'benefactor of humanity' or as a 'base impostor.'" Another observer, infuriated, predicted that after hospitals dedicated to twilight sleep appeared around the country, "the latest appeal to nervous and idle women will run its course until the inevitable percentages of mortality and morbidity bring it to a close."[37]

American Physicians Temporarily Change Their Minds

Yet the publicity put immense pressure on doctors to at least reexamine twilight sleep. To wholly ignore women's desires was to put one's medical practice in jeopardy. Disgruntled patients were abandoning cautious doctors and hiring more malleable physicians in their place. As one doctor willing to administer twilight sleep reasoned, "After all, most of the doses of narcotics we give are given, not because we think the patient needs the narcotic, but because he will promptly go to another doctor if we refuse."[38] Physicians began to revisit the treatment. The Central Free Dispensary in Chicago offered clinics, run by a half dozen experienced doctors, including Bertha Van Hoosen, to teach local physicians how to properly administer scopolamine-morphine in obstetrics.[39] Some doctors who had traveled to Germany almost a decade prior only to leave unimpressed with twilight sleep returned to Freiburg. That second visit convinced many that faulty technique prompted their original condemnation.

The new converts cited four common errors committed by doctors who denounced twilight sleep: (1) They combined morphine with every injection of scopolamine instead of only the first. (2) They administered too much scopolamine with each injection. (3) They employed "unstable and deteriorated" scopolamine. (4) They mistakenly believed that twilight sleep abolished suffering when it merely erased the memory of suffering. Alfred Hellman, a gynecologist at Lebanon Hospital and German Hospital Dispensary in New York City, listed other likely reasons for colleagues' dissatisfaction with twilight sleep: physicians did not follow the Freiburg method to the letter; European hospitals had more midwives and physicians available than American hospitals to calm the women

affected badly by twilight sleep; streets around American hospitals were far nois-
ier than in Freiburg, a situation disturbing to twilighted mothers; and "probably,
most important of all, we are not able to have our Kroenigs ten minutes away
from the institutions and our Gausses living in them."[40]

William Knipe was a typical new convert. After his first trials with twilight
sleep ended in disaster, he condemned it. Then he traveled to Freiburg to find out
what generated all the praise. Under the tutelage of Krönig and Gauss, he learned
their technique and reversed his opinion. After he described his epiphany in *The
Modern Hospital*, the *New York Times* noted sarcastically that Knipe's reappraisal
"coincided in practically every detail . . . to those recently set forth in a since
much-scolded lay magazine by two women, also much scolded, who lack the degree of M.D."[41]

After the new medical enthusiasm emerged, some physicians now argued (in
much the same way the medical community had promoted ether and chloroform
decades earlier) that twilight sleep was not only palliative but also therapeutic.
Doctors at Jewish Hospital in Brooklyn contended that the treatment softened
the cervix, hastened labor, and lowered the number of forceps deliveries. Other
physicians reported that twilighted women took "purposeful positions [during
labor] . . . in order to make the best possible use of their muscles." One doctor remarked, "It was as if for the first time I had seen the natural action of a woman
in labor."[42]

These doctors pronounced twilight sleep equally therapeutic for infants. They
cited Ludwig Aschoff, a German anatomist, who credited the morphine in twilight sleep for the lower death rate among Freiburg babies: 1.3 percent versus 3.4
percent in conventional births. Aschoff contended that the opiate temporarily repressed infants' respiration, preventing them from breathing prematurely in
the birth canal. (Subsequent reports confirming that the narcotizing effect of
morphine killed some infants soon negated Aschoff's positive spin on babies' repressed breathing.) At Jewish Hospital in Brooklyn, doctors reported that newborns benefited from their mothers' lessened "nerve exhaustion" and concomi-
tant copious milk secretion. A San Francisco doctor similarly attested to women
emerging from labor refreshed and renewed and ready to focus energetic attention on their newborns. In sum, many doctors now advised, twilight sleep produced "*more* and *better* babies."[43]

Personal experience prompted some physicians to be among the most amenable to twilight sleep. Like Walter Channing sixty years before, these doctors
could be influenced by their wives' births more than by a lifetime of medical
practice. In recalling the birth of his first child, for example, one doctor recalled,

"Everything that a woman could suffer my wife suffered." Of Dämmerschlaf he wrote: "'Twilight sleep' absolutely."[44]

Female physicians could be even more profoundly affected by personal experience. Eliza Taylor Ransom's two harrowing births persuaded her to devote her career to twilight sleep. Ransom remembered that after her first child was born, she preferred death to ever giving birth again. Her belief that every child should have at least one sibling, however, proved stronger than her horror of birth, and her second experience was as intolerable as the first. She recalled, "I had never thought of becoming an obstetrician until I experienced the agonies of childbirth—too terrible to describe. Then I wondered if humanity was worth a woman's anguish. If there was anything in twilight sleep, I proposed to find out all there was to know."[45]

Ransom secured her opportunity shortly before World War I after meeting a rich, elderly man married to a much younger woman. The couple was expecting their first child. "She is such a precious creature and has never known pain nor fear in her life," the man told Ransom. "I'd give all my fortune if I could spare her the inevitable horror." Ransom told him about twilight sleep, and he immediately proposed sending Ransom to Germany. She accepted his offer.[46]

Upon her return from Freiburg, Ransom opened a hospital in Boston devoted to twilight sleep. A year later, at a heavily publicized event at Boston's Cort Theatre, she displayed some of the children born at her hospital. Several of the mothers present had apparently expressed their gratitude to Ransom by making her their child's namesake: more than a few of the babies bore the first name Eliza or Taylor or Ransom. The *Boston Herald*, alluding to the din at the occasion, reported, "The twilight babies . . . proved that the Freiburg method does not injure the lungs."[47]

Ransom long promoted Dämmerschlaf. In 1930 she held a party in the ballroom of the Miles Standish Hotel in Boston. Surrounded by hundreds of adoring ex-patients and their children, she exulted, "Wonderful babies! And they did not cost their mothers a single pain." Her longtime adherence to feminism was evident in her address to the reporters covering the celebration: "Childbirth is excruciating but because no man has ever experienced its pains, many physicians declare that women's anguish is a matter ordained by the Creator. Unless women *demand* relief, they will never get it." A broadside advertising Ransom's practice described the children and mothers who attended the celebration: "There was not one child that was unhealthy. Nor dwarfed. Nor ill developed. Nor of low mentality. There was not one mother who had suffered a single ill effect from childbirth."[48]

Throughout her career, Ransom contrasted her own two miserable postpartum experiences ("lying in absolute quietness, being turned in bed only by the nurse, receiving food from the hands of others . . . enduring unbearable gas pains from constipation due to immobility, and fainting from high enemas") with the freedom and energy afforded her twilight sleep mothers. She encouraged her patients to move about freely immediately after birth, a custom so foreign to American medicine that Ransom's colleagues were horrified. After glimpsing new mothers exercising in Ransom's hospital in a demonstration of what Ransom had dubbed "The Freiburg Gymnastics Postpartum," one doctor shouted, "My Gawd, have you all gone crazy?" Another admonished that allowing women to make social calls within a week of giving birth might be touted by some as evidence of the value of twilight sleep, but in reality the practice indicated only that the much praised Freiburg Frauenklinik persuaded German women to behave like animals. Yet the revulsion of many of Ransom's colleagues soon vanished; after seeing how postpartum exercise benefited women, one initially incredulous physician wondered, "Why wouldn't this be even more beneficial in 'normal obstetrics'?" Mothers of means had long languished for weeks in bed after giving birth—a throwback to the age of fashionably sick women—but twilight sleep now provided grounds for what seemed to be a startling new practice: the resumption of normal activity soon after giving birth.[49]

The Question of Professional Respect

Of all the considerations nudging physicians to think more favorably of twilight sleep in the wake of the twilight sleep movement, the most influential factor was the ongoing dismissive attitude of the lay and medical communities toward obstetrics as a specialty. Most physicians continued to ridicule obstetrics as requiring paltry skill. Charles Ziegler, professor of obstetrics at the University of Pittsburgh, noted with dismay that the word *obstetrics* came from a Latin word meaning "'to stand before' or, as a sneering colleague once observed, 'to stand around.'"[50]

Yet the few women beginning to hire an obstetrician, as opposed to a general practitioner, did not hire a physician with special skills so he could sit by her bed and watch. Frederick Leavitt, assistant professor of obstetrics at the University of Minnesota, told the story of a woman who traveled a great distance so that her first birth would benefit from his expertise. After the birth, however, she refused to pay his fee. He did not deserve payment, she told him: all he had done was "stand around and let nature do the work!" The exasperated Leavitt observed, "Her labor was long and tedious, and I spent hours encouraging her to bear with womanly fortitude a process that was essentially physiological. I admonished, I cheered, I held her hands, I did everything I could, except to put her to sleep and take the baby away." He mused, given patients' attitudes, that no one should be quick to condemn the obstetricians now tempted to "do something" during labor. Patients seemed suddenly unwilling to pay for any services that did not involve instruments or drugs.[51]

Leavitt was hardly alone in his dilemma. Joseph DeLee often faced similar situations. After wealthy Chicagoan Ogden McClurg protested DeLee's fifteen-hundred-dollar fee to attend his wife in childbirth in 1922, DeLee responded, "Any surgeon in my class gets from $1,000 to $5,000 for a simple appendix operation, requiring but a few minutes,—no prolonged care before and afterward." That, he explained, was why the best and brightest doctors eschewed obstetrics. "The work is hard and burdensome, it restricts one's liberty, robs one of rest at night, requires exceptional skill, and withal, it does not pay." The conditions of childbearing women, DeLee chided the irate husband, would never improve until the public willingly paid obstetricians what they deserved.[52]

Obstetricians' despair over the lack of respect afforded their specialty coincided with a crisis in the medical community at large. When the AMA inspected the nation's medical schools in 1906, the organization found half of them inadequate. Alarmed, the AMA prevailed on the Carnegie Foundation for the Advancement of Teaching to conduct an independent investigation of medical education; in response, the Carnegie Foundation hired Abraham Flexner, a Johns Hopkins graduate, to visit and evaluate every American medical school. In 1910 Flexner issued a scathing assessment of American medical education: medical school libraries had no books, advertised laboratories were nonexistent, and schools had no standards for admission. In the immediate aftermath of what became known as the Flexner Report, 36 of the country's 131 medical schools closed.[53]

While his assessment of medical students' general training was blistering, Flexner reserved his harshest critique for obstetric training. "The very worst showing," he wrote, "is made in the matter of obstetrics. Didactic lectures are utterly worthless. . . . The practice is a fine art which cannot be picked up in the exigencies of out-patient work, poorly supervised at that."[54]

Flexner's assessment was corroborated by a 1912 survey conducted by J. Whitridge Williams, professor of obstetrics and dean of the Medical School at Johns Hopkins University, to ascertain the level of training of obstetrics professors in the United States. Williams found that of the 43 respondents to his query, only 9 had seen 1,000 or more cases of labor before becoming professors of obstetrics,

13 had attended fewer than 500 cases, 5 had seen fewer than 100 cases, and 1 admitted he had never attended a single birth before becoming a professor of obstetrics. "Think of becoming a professor of obstetrics," Williams wrote, "with an experience of less than 100 cases!" A quarter of respondents answered the question "Do you consider that the ordinary graduate from your school is competent to practice obstetrics?" with an unequivocal "no." Others responded with revealing provisos: "Well, yes, in a way; that is, some of them." Speaking at a meeting attended by Brooklyn physicians, Williams warned that the average doctor did more harm to women than did midwives, "who are notoriously ignorant." In a pointed reference to general practitioners who delivered babies, Williams said two types of doctors practiced obstetrics, obstetricians who could cope with any obstetric emergency and "men midwives," who could not.[55]

This was the professional atmosphere in 1914 when the entire nation learned about twilight sleep. Despite physicians' outrage at women's demands, and in the face of many physicians' antipathy toward twilight sleep, Dämmerschlaf ultimately proved to be obstetricians' avenue for attention and respect. As William Knipe pointed out in 1915, widespread public interest in twilight sleep at long last signaled "proper appreciation of scientific obstetrics."[56]

Few medical treatments did more to garner lay and professional respect for obstetrics. Gauss and Krönig had long touted their technique as one requiring virtuoso talent to master and valuable time to administer. Dosages of scopolamine-morphine, which demanded administration at difficult-to-ascertain times, had to be so precise that Dämmerschlaf appeared to require techniques only a highly practiced obstetrician could perfect.

At the Frauenklinik, the administration of twilight sleep entailed such unremitting attention that Krönig and Gauss tripled their obstetric staff. Krönig so assiduously tailored treatments to the unique needs of each wealthy patient that he required American women come to Freiburg a month before their due date so his staff could acquaint themselves with the "individual psychology" of each mother in order to determine the precise amount of scopolamine that would best suit her.[57]

The Krönig-Gauss protocol was complex. After a woman went into labor, a nurse or a doctor injected her with a predetermined dose of scopolamine-morphine. Medical personnel then conducted "memory tests" every half hour: they asked the woman how many hypodermics she had received or showed her an unfamiliar object and then showed it to her again a moment later, asking if she had ever seen it before. Impaired memory indicated that the mother had received sufficient scopolamine. Freiburg doctors explained that frequent memory tests were vital to successful outcome; the retention of even minute "isles of memory" allowed mothers to piece together their labors afterward.[58]

Some American hospitals soon mimicked the Freiburg protocol and then some. At the Jewish Maternity and Lebanon hospitals in New York, a doctor or nurse trained in Dämmerschlaf remained constantly at the side of each laboring woman. The staff person's duties included injecting the patient with scopolamine according to the results of repeated memory tests; protecting her from all harsh light and noise; monitoring fetal heart sounds; and checking maternal pulse rates, respiration, papillary reaction, and the intensity and frequency of uterine contractions. To minimize the extreme agitation of mothers so often prompted by scopolamine, hospital personnel wore noiseless felt slippers, employed shaded lighting, decorated labor rooms with "luxurious and harmonious esthetic equipment," and stuffed mothers' ears with cotton soaked in albolene. At the moment of birth, doctors and nurses placed smoked glasses over women's eyes, covered women's faces with a towel, and masked the cries of the newborn with the sound of running water.[59]

Critics enjoyed ridiculing these scenes. One physician wrote, "The chief value of the colored glasses, stuffed ears, and fantastic tests of memory, lies in the fact that no man possessed of common sense is apt to long continue them, and hence, any findings in cases where this foolishness is not practiced can be waved aside as no test of the Freiburg method."[60] But the mockery failed to have the desired effect. Instead, it drew attention to the intricate protocol necessitated by twilight sleep. As women learned that twilight sleep demanded expert attendance and carefully honed proficiency, its complexity elevated the stature of obstetrics, convincing many mothers that obstetrics was indeed beyond the ken of mere general practitioners.

The requirement that virtually every mother desiring a Dämmerschlaf birth be hospitalized enhanced the scientific aura now surrounding the obstetrician. Hospital births were exceedingly rare in the nineteenth century, limited to only a handful of desperate women who had no one to turn to for help except a medical charity. As late as the first two decades of the twentieth century, most physicians still hesitated to encourage healthy women of means to give birth in a hospital. Beatrice Tucker, the first woman resident to serve under DeLee, argued that people were immune to the bacteria in their homes. In the hospital, however, bacteria such as staphylococcus and strep were incessant threats. Despite this ongoing distrust of hospital birth, as early as 1910 the *American Journal of Obstetrics and Diseases of Women and Children* warned that to administer twilight sleep in the home was to court almost certain failure.[61]

Women's desire for twilight sleep thus introduced hospital birth to women of all classes. Now even married, middle- and upper-class women had reason to consider hospital birth. At Wesley Memorial Hospital in Chicago during the heyday of twilight sleep, physicians noted "the delighted eagerness of the mothers who say they 'are coming again.'"[62]

This observation is one of the first indications that births would eventually become a mainstay of hospitals, along with appendectomies, tonsillectomies, and adenoidectomies. Some hospitals even began to advertise in select trade journals, attempting to lure women using Dämmerschlaf as bait. Doctors at Boido Maternity Hospital in Phoenix, Arizona, for example, ran an advertisement in the *Southwestern Stockman-Farmer* in 1914 to inform the wives of local farmers that Boido now provided twilight sleep, "this wonderful medicine," to the mothers of Arizona.[63]

A few doctors did administer scopolamine-morphine in homes. Although most of the beneficiaries of this treatment were wealthy women, one New York City physician claimed he had administered twilight sleep successfully in tenements under the poorest and noisiest conditions imaginable. A Denver doctor who practiced in a rural district similarly described using twilight sleep without a trained assistant for more than one hundred home births. Elizabeth Miner, a Macon, Illinois, doctor, saw no advantage to using twilight sleep in the hospital other than the number of nurses available to help. Miner described her experience to Bertha Van Hoosen, who exulted, "One Roosevelt makes a political party, and this report of Dr. Miner's is a Rooseveltian report in its clean-cut and sweeping success." These doctors insisted that twilight sleep was actually more effective in homes. Hospitals, they argued, were too noisy for scopolamine to work properly and far too busy to justify tethering a nurse to one mother's bedside to supervise twilight sleep treatments.[64]

Perhaps a few physicians administered twilight sleep in the home because hospital birth, despite the appeal of twilight sleep, was by no means a surefire draw in the decade after 1910. Many women continued to find hospitals exceedingly unpleasant places. Lillian Moller Gilbreth, who had already given birth to six children at home, entered the hospital in 1914 to give birth to her seventh child, but she left six hours later because she was lonely and her nurse was "a fiend." That experience was so unpleasant that Gilbreth did not consider hospital birth again until 1922, when her twelfth and last child was born in the Nantucket Cottage

Hospital in Massachusetts. In stark contrast to her first attempt at hospital birth, she deemed that experience splendid: "I would have to wait until my dozenth baby was born to find out how much better it is to have them in a hospital. The nurses here wait on me hand and foot."[65]

As Gilbreth's change of heart suggests, the 1920s was a turning point for hospital birth. During that decade for the first time, many women began to think of hospital birth as an ordinary occurrence even if they did not choose the hospital for themselves. In 1914, for example, when she was pregnant with her first baby, Katharine Kerr Moore wrote to her mother, "I haven't decided yet whether to have my confinement at home or at a hospital. I asked Doc's opinion on the subject and he said that either place would do well enough." One month later she still agonized over the decision: "I am still considering which is best to do—to go to a hospital and be confined, or go through the motions at home." Eventually she had all three of her children at home (her other two sons were born in 1917 and 1921), but shortly before her third son's birth in June 1921 she wrote matter-of-factly to her mother: "Margaret called to me yesterday morning as I was going by, saying that she was having pains and expected to go to the hospital on the 10 o'clock train."[66]

The promise of twilight sleep obviously enticed some women to enter the hospital before the 1920s. The treatment effectively signaled the beginning of the normalization of hospital birth for women of all classes and became the first medical practice to demonstrate that if a woman wanted to enjoy all that modern obstetric care had to offer, hospital birth was a prerequisite. *Scientific American* told readers that twilight sleep worked well, "*but only with every institutional precaution.*" The *Journal of the Kansas Medical Society* noted that a darkened, properly equipped, absolutely quiet delivery room made twilight sleep "a hospital procedure rather than one of universal application." If women had the means to do so, they now increasingly sought out obstetricians, medical professionals who were able to offer the most up-to-date techniques and medications, in stark contrast to the general practitioner or midwife. Within decades, obstetrician-attended, hospital birth became the cornerstone of American obstetric practice.[67]

Side Effects of Twilight Sleep

Yet medical and lay support for twilight sleep turned out to be fleeting, and the very nature of hospitals ironically hastened its demise. The most routine procedures—moving a patient from the labor room to the delivery room, for example—intensified the agitation so often prompted by scopolamine. Physicians complained that twilight sleep was not worth the trouble it caused hospital personnel and, worse, was a potential threat to mothers and babies.[68]

This second round of rejections of twilight sleep, after the first flurry of positive publicity in the lay press in 1914, was soon evident in the medical literature. Franklin Newell, the Harvard physician who wrote some of the most favorable initial reports about twilight sleep in American medical journals in 1907, eventually abandoned the treatment because so many babies in his practice were born asphyxiated, their respiration depressed by the morphine in twilight sleep. Tennessee doctor John S. Beasley observed, "I believe instead of saying it is inhuman for a woman to suffer it is still more inhuman to let infants die." Still other doctors rejected twilight sleep because morphine slowed or halted uterine contractions.[69]

Doctors decried these side effects and more. A Chicago physician reported that in a series of sixty cases at Michael Reese Hospital, more than half the women complained of unquenchable thirst. Dozens of others suffered "intense" headaches for days. He noted, "Women who were rendered so wretched, in many instances for hours and days after delivery, would have gone through a normal confinement of from eight to eleven hours' average duration, and would have been comfortable and happy thereafter, if they had not had the so-called blessing of 'twilight sleep.'"[70]

The side effect reported by doctors most often was uncontrollable delirium. One physician described a woman who became so agitated that she jumped out of bed, climbed out a window, and attempted to leap from the windowsill. Three nurses were needed to subdue her. She remained in shackles for four days. After similar experiences, another doctor began to secure all his twilighted patients at the knee, wrist, and elbow. A Chicago doctor, noting that many physicians who employed twilight sleep put their patients in straitjackets, demanded to know why such a treatment deserved medical acknowledgment, let alone medical sanction.[71]

Hospitals began to abandon the technique along with individual doctors. There was precedence for this rejection: although the Philadelphia Lying-In Charity Hospital used twilight sleep on dozens of patients shortly after its initial introduction in the United States in 1908, nurses and doctors there discarded the treatment within months. Even after the favorable nationwide publicity in 1914, there is no evidence that Philadelphia Lying-In ever employed twilight sleep again. Other hospitals followed the same pattern after the *McClure's* article appeared. After only forty cases, Michael Reese Hospital in Chicago ceased providing scopolamine-morphine to women unless an unusually insistent patient agreed in advance to absolve the hospital of all responsibility. St. Louis Hospital discontinued twilight sleep after only eighteen cases when personnel complained of babies turning blue shortly after birth. After a brief series of cases, Johns Hopkins Hospital termed twilight sleep a "menace to the life of the child."[72]

Reacting to the negative assessments, the Twilight Sleep Association held a meeting in the ballroom of the Hotel McAlpin in New York City to map a strategy to ensure the continued use of the procedure. Eliza Taylor Ransom was one of several speakers who blamed unskilled doctors for any problems. She told her audience that she favored passage of a federal statute outlawing the administration of scopolamine by untrained and unlicensed persons.[73]

Like Ransom, other persistent champions of twilight sleep dismissed every side effect as misunderstanding or incompetence. Asphyxiated baby? Infants were born with breathing difficulties all the time; scopolamine was simply a convenient scapegoat. Extreme thirst? Labor causes thirst. Violence and delirium? Inexperienced doctors administered faulty dosages, precipitating women's hysteria. Prolonged labors? Twilight sleep actually shortened labor, so much so that there was often no time for scopolamine to take full effect. More forceps births? First-time mothers often required forceps. Hemorrhage? How convenient to have a treatment to blame for a postpartum hemorrhage.[74]

Supporters of twilight sleep consistently accused detractors of scapegoating scopolamine. A. J. Rongy pointed out that when three women in a single week developed postpartum psychosis at Lebanon Hospital in New York City, the hospital's neurologist immediately blamed twilight sleep. Yet all three women had received only ether. Other physicians insisted that women who suffered from psychotic episodes would have been difficult to manage under any circumstances. One Freiburg physician noted that, given "stupid" or nervous patients, the most exacting application of twilight sleep often failed.[75]

The End of the Twilight Sleep Movement

Despite a few remaining stalwarts, the twilight sleep movement lasted little more than a year, ending in the same swirl of controversy in which it began. After the outspoken Mrs. Francis Carmody died in childbirth at the Long Island College Hospital in New York in August 1915—only fifteen months after the first *McClure's* article announcing the miracle of twilight sleep—intense lay interest in the treatment effectively vanished. Since Carmody had been a national leader of the twilight sleep movement, her death was widely reported. Although all reports indicated that her death from hemorrhage had nothing to do with twilight sleep, the tragedy nevertheless focused public attention on the dangers of twilight sleep rather than its benefits.[76]

Alice J. Olson, a friend and neighbor of Carmody's, spearheaded a movement to abolish twilight sleep. The mother of eight children, Olson had been deeply shaken by her own daughter's disquieting experience with the treatment. She told the *New York Times* that she had thought of phoning Carmody a number of times to discuss her concerns but hesitated on each occasion. After Carmody's death she deeply regretted remaining silent.[77]

Even Rongy now dismissed twilight sleep. He noted that in the four months before Carmody's death, only one of his patients had requested the treatment. He blamed the Twilight Sleep Association for the technique's quick demise, charging that their excessive enthusiasm had pushed untrained physicians to embrace the treatment. Ignoring his own previous advocacy of twilight sleep, he concluded, "I never advise the twilight sleep treatment and would never give it unless the patient insisted on it. The risks are too great."[78]

Although the twilight sleep movement vanished from the public scene within two years of its appearance, doctors' use of scopolamine in obstetrics, and even the occasional use of the term *twilight sleep,* lasted well into the 1960s. Despite the quick end of both the movement and the elaborate protocol associated with twilight sleep, many doctors continued to use scopolamine in combination with other drugs, most notably Demerol after its introduction in 1939, to erase women's memory of labor.[79]

Indeed, the less attention it received, the more favorably the medical community seemed to assess scopolamine. In 1927 colleagues praised James Tayloe Gwathmey's invention of rectal anesthesia precisely because it created amnesia "as definite as that of scopolamine." In 1932, in reviewing decades of obstetric experiments with assorted anesthetics and analgesics, anesthesiologist Clifford Lull noted that the medications used most often were morphine and scopolamine in assorted doses. The Woman's Hospital in Detroit continued to employ scopolamine in the 1940s, and one doctor there called it the best drug for use during labor. If scopolamine induced hysteria, he administered ether to quell the delirium. By the early 1940s, the Cleveland Maternity Hospital had used morphine in combination with scopolamine in twenty-five thousand births. One Chicago-area obstetrician, who delivered babies from 1946 through 1988, built a large practice in the 1950s and 1960s by promising that no woman in his care would ever remember a moment of childbirth. He used scopolamine to keep that promise.[80]

Despite its short life and quick death as a movement, twilight sleep's legacy remains. The treatment hastened the demise of the generalist who merely dabbled in obstetrics (but who represented the vast majority of doctors who attended births in the early twentieth century) and initiated the rise of the obstetrician, who eventually became a nearly requisite presence at American births.

In this sense, the twilight sleep movement ultimately proved to be not a passing annoyance to obstetricians but a lasting benefit. DeLee's and Williams's efforts beginning in the 1890s to elevate the status of obstetrics had been in vain, and when the first demands for twilight sleep appeared in women's magazines twenty years later, the prestige of obstetrics and obstetricians had not improved substantially. Unlike DeLee's and Williams's futile pleas for more comprehensive medical education, however, women's demands for twilight sleep gave slipshod obstetric practice the public scrutiny it deserved, transforming the image of obstetrics in the process. Instead of the mundane activity of country doctors and lay midwives, obstetrics became, in medical and lay eyes alike, a finely honed skill practiced only by rigorously trained specialists. Twilight sleep was instrumental in quashing the view, as one Huntington, West Virginia, doctor put it, that "any physician and many of the neighbor-women" were competent to render any service needed at a birth. In introducing the concept of standard obstetric protocol to mothers, twilight sleep enhanced the status of obstetrics immeasurably.[81]

The twilight sleep movement also revealed the power of consumers to shape medical practice. Publicity about the technique spread so quickly that a Macon, Georgia, physician complained that before he learned about twilight sleep in medical journals, his patients were demanding he administer it at their next birth.[82] In the medical marketplace, doctors could not afford dissatisfied patients. Thwarted in their desire for a particular treatment, consumers threatened to take their business to doctors and hospitals more amenable to their desires.

Twilight sleep altered numerous habits and perceptions surrounding childbirth, for better and for worse. Because twilight sleep advocates boasted about how well women felt after a Dämmerschlaf birth, the medical community learned that it was safe as well as medically useful for women to get out of bed shortly after giving birth. Women seemed especially gratified that doctors permitted them to eat soon after birth. With the advent of ether and chloroform, many physicians had learned to forbid food to women while they labored and in the aftermath of a birth, fearing that the inevitable anesthesia-induced nausea would result in aspiration of vomit.

Less fortunately, twilight sleep assured that subsequent generations of women would labor in restraints. Although physicians rationalized in later years that this practice prevented women from breaking the sterile field established around the birth canal, twilight sleep was the original (and soon forgotten) source of the restraints, which became ubiquitous.

Despite the quick disappearance of the most elaborate twilight sleep protocols, a woman's distress during labor could now be ignored with impunity. One Chicago physician trained in Freiburg observed during the heyday of twilight sleep that, as long as memory tests regulated the dosage, complaints from women during labor could be dismissed. Most women would be unable to remember significant segments of their labors anyway, and so taking time to comfort and reassure a mother exhibiting distress was now deemed time wasted. A. J. Rongy admitted that under the influence of twilight sleep women certainly suffered—some of his patients could be heard screaming four floors below. The fact that women would be unable to recall their misery, however, made their suffering easier to ignore.[83]

Even twilight sleep's harshest critics, however, failed to specifically criticize the inability of scopolamine to relieve pain. Instead, as William Holt noted, "with the *Daemmerschlaf* [the doctor] does not mind the patient's cries nor the family's remonstrances, being sure that after delivery she will have forgotten all." Nor were women disturbed when they learned that their pain had not been assuaged. Marguerite Tracy quoted one mother who seemed to speak for all Dämmerschlaf mothers: "It makes no difference to me what the doctors say about 'forgetfulness.' For me, it was painless."[84]

One of the few condemnations of this aspect of scopolamine appeared in Sylvia Plath's novel *The Bell Jar*. After seeing a woman give birth under scopolamine in the 1950s, Esther Greenwood, the book's young protagonist, remarked: "Here was a woman in terrible pain, obviously feeling every bit of it or she wouldn't groan like that, and she would go straight home and start another baby, because the drug would make her forget how bad the pain had been, when all the time, in some secret part of her, that long, blind, doorless and windowless corridor of pain was waiting to open up and shut her in again." Plath thus unwittingly made Greenwood reiterate doctors' original rationale for twilight sleep (as well as for ether and chloroform): physicians hoped obstetric anesthesia would ensure that women continued to have babies despite the experience of labor pain.[85]

Ultimately and paradoxically, the solicitous attention that so pleased Stewart at the Frauenklinik eventually prompted the antithesis of thoughtful care. Rather than eliciting more attention and consideration, hospital birth and the increasing use of anesthesia meant women received considerably less. Twilight sleep even stifled simple acknowledgments like Gauss's that Stewart was in severe pain; doctors soon declared labor pain irrelevant because under scopolamine women would be unable to recall their suffering anyway. Since silence increased the odds of keeping women calm while under the influence of scopolamine, doctors also came to believe that women actually benefited from a labor devoid of meaningful companionship. Analgesics and anesthetics and the myriad medical practices and technologies these drugs engendered became substitutes for the comfort and reassurance originally sought by the women active in the twilight sleep movement.

CHAPTER THREE

Developing the
Obstetric Anesthesia Arsenal

The Question of Safety, 1900 through 1960s

*D*orothy Reed Mendenhall, a pediatrician trained at Johns Hopkins University, gave birth to her first child in a Madison, Wisconsin, hospital in 1907. She did not anticipate a difficult delivery. One of her teachers at Johns Hopkins was famed obstetrician J. Whitridge Williams, and he had taught Mendenhall that few births were problematic, particularly if a doctor allowed nature to take its course. She became uneasy only after entering the hospital and meeting the doctor who was about to deliver her baby. His clothes, Mendenhall noted, were "dirty and spotted," and he did not wash his hands before checking Mendenhall's cervix, even after Mendenhall's private nurse followed him around the room with a bowl of disinfectant repeatedly asking, "Wouldn't you like to wash, Doctor?"

After three days of fruitless labor, the physician ordered the exhausted Mendenhall to the operating room, where he intended to turn her breech baby. Just before anesthesia rendered her unconscious, Mendenhall felt boundless despair, turned her head into the pillow, and thought, "This will be the end. I shall die, he doesn't know what to do."

When she awoke, she was back in her room. Her husband told her she had given birth to a "lovely little daughter." Despite this assurance, when Mendenhall finally held her baby, she knew immediately that something was wrong.

Mendenhall's medical and maternal instincts were correct: later that day the baby, Margaret Mendenhall, died of a cerebral hemorrhage caused by what her mother eventually termed "bad obstetrics," probably a reference to the doctor's lack of skill with forceps. Dorothy Reed Mendenhall remained in the hospital for weeks with a raging fever due to puerperal sepsis, fading in and out of consciousness. When her fever finally abated, she left the hospital with damage to her perineum and rectum—also likely due to the doctor's inexpert use of forceps—and unable to control her urine and feces. She blamed the difficult birth on the physician.

Unwilling to trust any doctor in Madison again, when her three sons were born, in 1908, 1910, and 1913, Mendenhall traveled to Chicago, where Joseph DeLee attended the births at the Chicago Lying-in Hospital, the facility he had opened years earlier in conjunction with his home birth dispensary. Despite the death of her daughter and her own suffering during and after Margaret's birth, Mendenhall was not apprehensive when her sons were born. She trusted that DeLee, who "weighed every chance, sterilized his own gloves, and brought them to the delivery room dated," would see her, and her babies, through labor unscathed.[1]

Just as Eliza Taylor Ransom's agonizing births prompted her lifelong work with twilight sleep, the birth and death of Margaret Mendenhall transformed Dorothy Reed Mendenhall's professional interests. Beginning in 1912, Mendenhall served for twenty years in various capacities for the U.S. Children's Bureau, a federal agency established to ensure the well-being of children. She also lectured on nutrition and child care at the University of Wisconsin. She focused her research, writing, and lectures on the relationship between maternal and infant health, ascribing her abiding interest in what she called "safe maternity" to Margaret's needless death. Mendenhall considered every speech she delivered and every article she wrote to be ongoing tributes to her only daughter. In an unpublished autobiography, Mendenhall noted, "Most of my work came out of my agony and grief. *A mother never forgets.*"[2]

Increased Maternal Mortality

Mendenhall's work was part of a concerted, well-publicized, nationwide effort to reduce maternal mortality. One of her employers, the U.S. Children's Bureau, was instrumental in this effort. Officials of the bureau long argued that not only children's health but also mothers' health was their purview because infants' health status depended on their mothers' ability to care for them. Thus the sickness and death of mothers lessened babies' chances for survival.[3]

Mendenhall's disastrous first birth, despite her medical education and the resources that enabled her to hire a private nurse, represented the risk all women faced when giving birth in the early twentieth century. By the time Mendenhall's last child was born in 1913, the situation had not improved. Childbirth remained a leading cause of death among women of childbearing age, second only to tuberculosis. Almost half of the estimated fifteen thousand women in the United States who died as a result of giving birth each year died of postpartum infection, known then as childbed fever, the same disease that struck Mendenhall after Margaret's birth. The illness was almost entirely preventable, if only physicians employed aseptic technique.[4]

Some in the medical community nevertheless dismissed the high maternal death rate as insoluble. Bolstered by eugenic theory, the author of one article in the *American Journal of Public Health* argued, "No nation, except ours, is called upon to face such a racial variation in fitness for motherhood." A lay magazine similarly rationalized, "The American problem is complicated by the Negroes, among whom a very high obstetric death rate prevails."[5]

The vast majority of public health officials, however, did not dismiss the high maternal death rate. They were determined to alleviate it. Every other cause of premature death in the United States had declined precipitously since the turn of the century, yet between 1900 and 1920, when infant mortality plunged 42 percent, maternal mortality rose 27 percent.[6]

Obstetric safety remained so persistently poor that in 1926 the United States placed nineteenth in the lineup of twenty countries then tracking maternal mortality, besting only Chile. This shameful ranking became national news, prompting major lay and medical publications to echo DeLee's longtime demand that all medical students receive rigorous training in obstetrics. *Harper's Magazine* condemned medical schools for treating obstetrics as "an ugly duckling" deserving only token attention. The author of an article in the *American Journal of Public Health* complained that medical school professors apparently believed that obstetrics "can be mastered apparently by inspiration or after the observation of a few normal cases." The *American Journal of Obstetrics and Gynecology* condemned American obstetric training and technique for lagging fifty years behind Germany's.[7]

Obstetric Anesthesia and Maternal Mortality

Numerous studies attributed America's stubbornly high maternal mortality rate to obstetric anesthesia. Dorothy Reed Mendenhall observed in 1917 that antiseptics and anesthesia, "the two things that should make childbirth safer," often did the opposite because both promoted the use of forceps. Given antiseptics, forceps now seemed far less likely to cause infection and, given anesthesia, forceps no longer caused women severe pain during application. Thus even doctors untrained in the use of forceps now readily used the device, thereby increasing the incidence of postpartum infection, which was deadly in the pre-antibiotic era. Even DeLee, who was clearly adept at using forceps, admitted in 1916 that his use of anesthesia resulted in more forceps births and thus an increase in maternal lacerations and hemorrhage. He noted that he had observed this surge in maternal morbidity only in his private practice, not at the Lying-in Dispensary, where he and other doctors rarely dispensed anesthesia or used forceps.[8]

Physicians from other countries often remarked on the tendency of American doctors to overuse forceps. When Mendenhall visited Denmark in 1926, she asked a Danish physician why maternal mortality was so much lower in Denmark than in the United States. He replied, "You interfere—operate too much. We give nature a chance." (In those days, physicians referred to a forceps birth as a "surgical" or "operative" birth.)[9]

In 1933 the New York Academy of Medicine echoed the Danish doctor. In a report on maternal mortality in New York City, the academy blamed maternal death there on the increased use of forceps and the tendency of forceps in unskilled hands to cause puerperal fever. In turn, they attributed the growing use of forceps to the popularity of obstetric anesthesia and its tendency to diminish "the expulsive powers of the uterine musculature." In other words, women incapacitated by anesthesia now relied on physicians' use of forceps to remove their babies from their bodies. Investigators for the New York Academy of Medicine concluded that the cost of alleviating labor pain was prohibitive. *Newsweek* passed this assessment on to the public.[10]

Most physicians already had mixed feelings about forceps, observing that though the instrument could clearly be life-saving, in some circumstances it could also be death-dealing. Charles Meigs had noted in the mid-nineteenth century that, thanks to forceps, he no longer had to use hooks to remove a fetus in a difficult case. Yet he also cautioned that forceps in inexperienced hands often caused great harm. One doctor recalled with horror two tragedies in the 1930s: a colleague had pulled the skin off a baby's head with forceps, and during a breech birth another colleague had ripped a baby's jaw loose. Both infants died.[11]

Mothers suffered similar maiming accidents, as evidenced by the higher maternal mortality rates in countries with more forceps use. In the Netherlands in the 1930s, where doctors applied forceps in only 1 percent of births, 23 mothers died per 10,000 births. In Denmark, where doctors used forceps in 4.5 percent of births, 35 mothers died per 10,000 births. And in the United States, where doctors used forceps in 20 percent of births, 65 mothers died per 10,000 births. When British obstetrician James Young addressed the American Association of Obstetricians, Gynecologists, and Abdominal Surgeons in 1935, he attributed the lower maternal mortality rate in the Netherlands and Scandinavia to the concerted effort in those countries to protect birth from "the surgical stream" embraced by U.S. and British obstetricians.[12] An American observer agreed, charging that the high maternal death rate in the United States had little to do with abnormal labor and a great deal to do with the medical community's lack of regard for "normal spontaneous labor." Anesthesia, forceps, "and a long list of ways of helping nature even in births where nature needs no help" had become common in the United States, often to the detriment of mothers.[13]

The increasingly common use of forceps was not uniform across the country, however. The rate varied from hospital to hospital, city to city, and state to state. In some locales physicians consciously avoided forceps if at all possible. One doctor practicing in rural Arizona in 1946 regretted ever having to use forceps, even during particularly difficult births that clearly demanded them. He used them, he noted, only when he could find no other solution and lamented after one such birth, "I had the worst laceration in my experience. . . . It is always depressing to me when things go badly even though I have no feeling of self censure."[14]

The increased application of forceps was not the only contribution of anesthesia to high maternal mortality. After twilight sleep accustomed select upper- and middle-class women to the hospital, the promise of ever more sophisticated anesthetic techniques was one reason that some women of means continued to be willing to give birth in the hospital. Although in 1900 less than 5 percent of births nationwide took place in hospitals, by 1939 half of all births and 75 percent of urban births occurred there. By 1955, 95 percent of births in the United States occurred in hospitals. With the majority of births moving from home to hospital so rapidly, hospitals had no plans in place to isolate the healthy women admitted merely to give birth. DeLee had long warned that this failure to segregate maternity wards from the rest of the hospital courted disaster, since laboring and postpartum women were uniquely susceptible to infection. To prove that point, DeLee and Heinz Siedentopf of Leipzig, Germany, documented 38 epidemics of postpartum infection in 1933 and traced 35 of the epidemics to the maternity wards of general hospitals. Noting that in New York City the maternal death rate was 5.3 per 1,000 births in hospitals and 1.9 per 1,000 births in homes, Siedentopf argued that home birth, even under the most abject conditions, was safer than hospital birth.[15]

By the late 1940s, two medical innovations unrelated to obstetric practice had lowered the maternal death rate appreciably. Thanks to blood banking and an-

tibiotics, death from postpartum hemorrhage and infection became a rare occurrence. Yet as maternal mortality lessened overall, obstetric anesthesia remained a
leading cause, implicated in one of every eight deaths.[16]

Childbirth between and after the World Wars

Despite the link between maternal death and anesthesia, the brief but intense
public focus on twilight sleep had ensured women's continued interest in physicians' ability to ease labor pain, so much so that articles about labor pain and how
to alleviate it continued to be a staple of popular periodicals through the 1940s.
*The Woman Citizen, Ladies' Home Journal, New Republic, Good Housekeeping,
Reader's Digest, Atlantic Monthly,* and *Woman's Home Companion* were only a
few of the magazines running articles under such enticing titles as "Lifting the
Curse of Eve," "Easier Motherhood," and "You, Too, Should Have Your Babies
without Pain."[17]

Rarely did women's magazines lack news on this topic; between 1920 and 1945
doctors developed almost every obstetric anesthetic technique in use today. Aside
from the old standbys that could be inhaled, assorted drugs were now ingested
orally, administered rectally and intravenously, and injected into different spaces
in and along the spine. Even the forerunner of today's epidural appeared in the
1930s. Lay publications tracked each innovation so avidly that women often
learned of a new offering before physicians read about it in medical journals.
These new drugs and techniques to administer them appeared to be so consistently
promising that one Chicago doctor predicted confidently in 1927 that, though
victory over disease remained elusive, "in no other phase of human suffering is
success so nearly assured as in childbirth."[18]

Given the unremitting public interest, many more doctors now readily promised patients that labor pain would be extinguished. In offering this assurance,
physicians consciously differentiated themselves from their forebears. One typical physician noted in 1927, "The ancient world accepted the inevitability of pain
in labor. Modern obstetricians rebel against this inevitable relation, and have acquired a considerable armamentarium with which to combat it." For a time, authors echoed some form of this sentiment at the start of virtually every medical
journal article on obstetric anesthesia.[19]

Physicians' use of obstetric anesthesia and women's desire for it were becoming
so common in middle- and upper-class circles that, despite Dorothy Reed Mendenhall's medical training, she did not learn that unanesthetized women could
weather labor with aplomb until she visited Denmark in 1926. After viewing an

unanesthetized birth there, she was stunned: "The woman made almost no fuss!" The experience profoundly influenced her. She concluded, "We have developed a fear complex in our mothers as well as a hurry complex in the medical profession to match that of the rest of our people." In ensuing years, American women's fear of labor pain remained so great that Robert Hingson, a prominent anesthesiologist with a special interest in obstetrics, claimed in 1948 that over the years he had received more than four thousand letters from women terrified of giving birth.[20]

Between World War I and World War II, this fear ensured women's ongoing enthusiasm for obstetric anesthesia. One woman, who had previously experienced two difficult unanesthetized labors, said of the rectal anesthesia she received during her third birth in 1930: "Words fail me when I attempt to express what it did for me! . . . Never again will I dread [labor]!" Two Atlanta physicians observed in 1938 that the mere promise of anesthesia allowed a woman to approach labor with confidence and that experiencing an anesthetized birth invariably removed any dread of future labor.[21]

The language physicians and women used to characterize labor both reflected and evoked fear, as it had for decades. Doctors still referred to "the tortures of childbirth." Constance L. Todd, the lay author of the 1931 book *Easier Motherhood*, described childbirth as "racking horror of well-nigh unendurable pain." Dorothy Smith Dushkin, who gave birth to her first child under the influence of ether in 1932, later recalled, "I wanted to know what agony was. I found out, & consider myself most blessed not to have had more of it."[22]

This rhetoric reflected the majority view; most prospective mothers so dreaded childbirth that they had come to prefer unconsciousness or numbness to a felt labor, and most physicians gladly accommodated, even encouraged, that desire. While doctors who attended home births in the nineteenth and early twentieth centuries often admired the easy births of "primitive" women and lamented the invariably difficult births of "civilized" mothers, hospital births and the more frequent use of anesthesia reversed that perspective.

In 1937 physician Roy P. Finney was one of many who deprecated the "primitive" mother "squatting on her bed of leaves . . . suffer[ing] in animal-like silence." In contrast, he lionized the contemporary American woman who gave birth "in a dreamy, half-conscious state . . . awak[ing] in smiles, a mother with no recollection of having become one." Women conjured similar images. In a 1940 *Harper's Magazine* article, one mother ridiculed the "uncivilized," "coarse" pioneer who gave birth to a "baby behind a bush on the Oregon Trail, like that squaw they always tell you about." She was grateful that the torment of birth had "eased a lot since grandma's day" thanks to "Nembutal, gas, cyclopropane, and all the rest."[23]

A tiny but vocal minority did continue to report experiencing (in the case of mothers) or witnessing (in the case of doctors) relatively comfortable labors without anesthesia. Neal Heywood, who practiced osteopathic medicine in Snowflake, Arizona, and established a maternity hospital there in the 1930s, often observed women birthing without fuss. In 1946 one of his patients, a thirty-eight-year-old woman pregnant with her eighth child, waited so long to come to the hospital that when she arrived, hospital personnel did not have time to take her to the delivery room. Heywood reported that the woman had been equally relaxed about previous births: "One time she was just getting into bed when the baby came. I managed to catch it before it hit the floor. She is inclined to delay getting in lest she needlessly troubles somebody."[24]

Yet by the 1930s and 1940s, these types of reports were usually not well received. Angry because another mother had extolled the virtues of an unmedicated labor in *Atlantic Monthly* in 1939, a Virginia woman admonished, "I hoped we had left far behind this mediaeval association of spiritual values with physical mortification." A wealthy Chicago-area woman similarly ridiculed what was soon dubbed natural childbirth: "There is no reason why I or anyone else should become an animal for a few hours."[25]

As these comments indicate, debate about the nature of labor did not end in the nineteenth century. A few physicians still depicted birth as a reliable, safe, and easily endured physiological process in need of only rare medical treatment. The classroom notes compiled by one medical student reflected this notion. During a 1931 lecture, the student dutifully recorded that most women "will deliver ok by themselves" and that the primary duty of the obstetrician was simply "watchful expecting." The professor of obstetrics who delivered the lecture had apparently stressed the latter point so emphatically that the student underlined the phrase "watchful expecting" three times.[26]

Yet between World War I and World War II, a predominant goal of mainstream obstetrics came to be the alleviation of labor pain. Increasingly, even in rural areas, doctors administered anesthesia. When Cecilia Hennel Hendricks gave birth to her first baby in Garland, Wyoming, in 1916, she labored without pain relief and reported later, "everything went beautifully. . . . The doctor was simply fine." She received no lacerations during the birth and credited her physician: "He used only his fingers, no instruments." When she gave birth to subsequent children in 1921 and 1923, however, the doctor administered anesthesia, chloroform during the second birth and ether during the third.[27]

Physicians employed anesthesia in the rural south as well. Between 1931 and 1936 in Pike County, Mississippi, where 75 percent of births still occurred at home, most mothers received pain relief at some point during birth. Twenty-six percent of women received a barbiturate or morphine during first-stage labor and 78 percent received inhalation anesthesia during the second stage. They were given chloroform in the home, and on the rare occasion when a mother gave birth in the hospital, nitrous oxide or ether.[28]

In northern cities, anesthesia use was considerably more widespread. Urban doctors now observed that on the first prenatal visit, virtually every patient asked what would be done to relieve labor pain. A Philadelphia physician described the expectation of the typical pregnant woman in the late 1930s: "She wishes to go to sleep with the first pain and wake with the baby in her arms, and she is sure from her reading that this is not only feasible but it is her rightful privilege."[29]

Women's intense interest in anesthesia helped fuel the move of birth from home to hospital, since physicians and nurses found it easier to employ obstetric anesthesia in an institutional setting. In addition, the nature of hospital maternity wards, where women often labored together in one large room, also encouraged women's growing reliance on anesthesia. Unsettling sounds from nearby beds—groans, screams, cries for help and mercy—exacerbated mothers' fear and pain. In other words, the growing use of anesthesia was both a cause and an effect of the increasing number of hospital births.

Physicians readily acknowledged how disturbing labor wards could be to women. In 1925 Dr. Barton Cooke Hirst, a prominent Philadelphia obstetrician and president of the American Gynecological Society in 1924, noted that though rectal anesthesia worked well on his private patients, it was far less effective for the women laboring in wards, who were constantly subjected to the distress of others, the bustle of nurses, and interruptions by student doctors. Robert Hingson likewise observed that the groans and cries of others agitated even well-sedated patients.[30]

Mothers described the difficulties inherent in laboring within earshot of others. One woman who gave birth in a San Diego hospital in the late 1950s remembered, "Women who are unprepared to face the discomforts of labor frighten women who are having their first child and lead them to believe that they, too, will eventually get to the screaming stage." Women who experienced multiple labors often compared the births, noting that laboring alone could be less intimidating than laboring beside distraught ward-mates. After going into labor with her second child, one woman was immensely grateful to find herself in an empty room because she could labor without the disquieting distractions she had encountered in a crowded ward during her first child's birth.[31]

Another woman similarly recalled laboring in a private room when she gave birth to her first child in Chicago in 1951. Before the birth, on the advice of a friend she had known in college, she read *Childbirth without Fear* by Grantly Dick-Read, the British obstetrician who coined the phrase *natural childbirth*. (Dick-Read and his theories are described in Chapter 5.) Finding Dick-Read's techniques for weathering labor helpful, she relaxed during each contraction and, as he predicted, she needed no pain relief. She labored so quietly, in fact, that nurses did not recognize she was fully dilated until she felt the urge to push. The nurses then panicked, ordered her to stop pushing until the doctor arrived, and eventually rendered her unconscious with inhalation anesthesia to prevent her from giving birth before the doctor made his appearance.

The labors that produced her second and third children in 1953 and 1957, however, were very different. Laboring in wards beside "screaming and howling" women, she quickly abandoned Dick-Read's method and began shrieking in concert with her ward-mates. She recalled, "It was terrible. And it hurt. It was horrible." At some point early in those labors, nurses gave her an injection, rendering her unconscious. On each occasion, she awoke only after the birth was over.[32]

Hospital-Based Obstetric Residencies

Although some women and doctors clearly had ongoing doubts about the safety, and especially the comfort, of hospital birth, the institution and continual growth of hospital-based obstetric residencies between the early 1930s and the early 1940s quickly eliminated the lingering reservations. As hospitals became the exclusive training ground for obstetricians, the steadily growing numbers of obstetrician-attended, hospitalized births hastened the view that, if women wanted access to the most up-to-date obstetric treatment, birth had to take place in the hospital.[33]

Full implementation of hospital-based obstetric residencies took place over a ten-year period. In 1921 the American Medical Association (AMA) Council of Medical Education took the first step in this process when they appointed J. Whitridge Williams to head the AMA Committee on Graduate Training in Gynecology and Obstetrics. Williams's committee made two recommendations, both of which ultimately reshaped the nature of obstetric practice and lay and medical views of birth. First, the committee advised fusing obstetrics and gynecology into a single department in the nation's teaching hospitals; second, they recommended establishing three-year, hospital-based residencies in obstetrics and gynecology, to be completed after internships. To implement these goals, the American Gynecological Society, the American Association of Obstetricians and Gynecologists, and the AMA formed the American Board of Obstetrics and Gynecology (ABOG) in 1930.[34]

The ABOG was the third medical-specialty examining board in the United States. A certifying board for ophthalmology had been first in 1916, and otolaryngology followed in 1924. One of the first acts of the newly created ABOG was to announce that only doctors who limited their practice to women could receive ABOG certification. This move guaranteed that general practitioners would pose only a minimal threat to the livelihood of obstetricians and gynecologists in coming years.[35]

After the ABOG's formation, the growth in obstetric residencies was swift. By 1935, 48 hospitals had been approved for residencies in obstetrics; these hospitals offered a total of 104 training slots in the specialty. Ten years later, 255 hospitals offered 773 obstetric residency positions.[36]

An increase in the number of hospital births paralleled the increase in obstetric residents. Statistics gathered by the AMA in 1939 indicated that half of all American babies were born in hospitals that year. Hospitals celebrated the announcement, some noting that not only were pleased mothers returning to give birth multiple times, but also, for the first time in nurses' and doctors' experience, women who had been born in a hospital were giving birth in a hospital. What doctors once suspected would be a temporary phenomenon based on the demand for twilight sleep was now a multigenerational occurrence. Simultaneously, most physicians ceased attending anything but a hospital birth. In 1920 physician-attended home birth was the norm. In 1940 only 35 percent of births were physician-attended home births. Ten years later, physician-attended home births made up only 7 percent of births.[37]

Unlike home birth, hospital birth by its very nature highlighted the potential for problems, and this new emphasis on pathology occurred just as the ability of the general practitioner to influence birth practices waned. With the growth in hospital-based residencies, the concept of leaving low-risk births to the general practitioner (or to midwives, as is still the common practice in western Europe) and turning over only high-risk births to the obstetrician never took hold in the United States. Instead, with the growing number of obstetricians and the emphasis in their training on birth pathologies, all births eventually came to be defined as potentially high-risk.

The weight now given to the pathological possibilities of birth posed a dilemma. Since few births actually prove to be pathological, obstetricians had to decide how to handle, or even acknowledge, what sociologist William Arney terms the "residual normalcy" of birth. In facing this conundrum, most obstetricians chose to ignore the potential for normalcy in the vast majority of births and instead exaggerate the potential for pathology. By the 1940s, this emphasis permeated all aspects of birth in the United States, from medical practice to lay perceptions of the event. The need for a board-certified obstetrician at all births now seemed a given, as opposed to the lesser-trained midwife or general practitioner, neither of whom presumably had the skill set to handle an obstetric emergency.[38]

Conjoining obstetrics and gynecology reinforced the once-controversial assumption that the salient characteristic of birth is its potential for pathology. By 1946 information gathered from 71 of the 75 medical schools offering a four-year course to obtain the MD degree indicated that 73.2 percent of schools had combined departments of obstetrics and gynecology as recommended twenty-five years earlier by Williams's AMA committee. The new, official link between obstetrics and gynecology ensured that obstetrics would become a surgical specialty; gynecological practice had arisen in the mid-nineteenth century to repair the results of pathological births. The first experimental gynecological surgeries were attempts to fix "accidents of childbirth," particularly the vesico-vaginal and recto-vaginal fistulas caused by prolonged labors due to pelvises malformed by rickets.[39]

As early as 1920, in an influential article in the premier issue of the *American Journal of Obstetrics and Gynecology*, DeLee famously doubted the safety and efficacy of labor's "natural process" and characterized birth as "pathogenic . . . disease producing." He explained dramatically, "So frequent are these bad effects, that I have often wondered whether Nature did not deliberately intend women should be used up in the process of reproduction, in a manner analogous to that of the salmon, which dies after spawning?" Although some of his colleagues immediately denounced this assessment, what the medical community had long condemned as "operative obstetrics" became the norm in ensuing decades. Now that obstetricians were also gynecologists, birth by its very nature became a "pathological process." Obstetric interventions became commonplace, and DeLee became known as the father of modern obstetrics. By the 1940s and 1950s, routine treatments, most notably heavy use of analgesics during first-stage labor and either general or regional anesthesia during second-stage labor, accompanied by a routine episiotomy and a forceps birth, replaced doctors' traditional "watchful expectancy" during labor.[40]

The insular world of hospital-based residencies further ensured that obstetricians would embrace these increasingly standard practices and come to view laboring women as potentially difficult cases to be treated rather than mothers to be seen comfortably through a biological process. As one resident explained, the caseload and associated tasks inherent in medical residencies were customarily so overwhelming that "every second you spend being compassionate means that much less time to sleep. So you become very efficient at not really listening to people—just getting the information you need, and shutting them off." This phenomenon could be especially problematic when treating laboring women, for whom comfort and reassurance might be the most vital—and sometimes the only necessary—part of treatment.[41]

Yet there was no time for the obstetric resident to attend to a laboring woman in that fashion, even if the resident were so inclined. One physician, who was a resident in obstetrics and gynecology at Chicago's Cook County Hospital in 1940, attended well over three hundred births each month of her three-year residency. In the face of this overwhelming workload, she could do no more than arrive in time to "deliver" each baby. Despite their increased education, obstetric residents' view and knowledge of labor and birth was now severely constricted, confined largely to the moment of birth.[42]

Development and Experimentation

Increasingly fearful of birth as they labored without meaningful companionship in an unfamiliar, often crowded, anxiety-producing place, an ever growing number of women looked forward to obscuring the experience with assorted medications. Obstetricians, most of whom now viewed labor as a process to be carefully controlled in order to avert any potential pathology, obliged. Yet, ironically, the growing popularity of obstetric anesthesia also exposed more women and their babies to the dangers of anesthetic side effects, guaranteeing that the medical community would continue to add to the obstetric anesthesia arsenal in their perpetual hunt for safer medications, dosages, and application techniques. The experimentation, in turn, stoked widespread publicity, furthering lay interest.

The search for safer obstetric anesthesia created a paradox that even researchers termed "chaos": the more doctors experimented, the less safe obstetric anesthesia became. One woman, in describing her experience in the early 1930s, inadvertently attested to the sheer variety of painkillers and application methods in use: "This marvelous stuff was given to me; by an injection, by an enema and by mouth and in just a few minutes I could not feel the pains."[43]

Doctors toyed with an array of substances. Barton Cooke Hirst gave marijuana to patients during labor. Noting that when used by adult males, marijuana produced a "sudden outbreak of hilarity, an absence of all sense of time, [and] an indifference to or unconsciousness of . . . surroundings," he observed that these effects were the ones doctors wanted to instill in laboring women. Although there is no evidence that other physicians ever used marijuana in this way, Hirst employed it with some success, prompting in a number of women "a feeling of indifference to pain, a tendency to hilarity, an alcoholic 'jag' in a way, and without the least ill effects upon the infant."[44]

Through the first two-thirds of the twentieth century, individual doctors' strong personal preferences contributed to the uncontrolled experimentation. A Chicago physician remembered in 1931 that during medical school his surgery professor enthusiastically endorsed ether and vigorously opposed chloroform: "I was, therefore, brought up in the ether school." Other physicians just as avidly favored chloroform. An Indiana doctor used chloroform because he often worked by the light of an oil lamp and knew of two explosions caused by the proximity of ether to flame. After use of nitrous oxide became fairly widespread in the second decade of the twentieth century, other physicians condemned both ether and chloroform. Anesthesiologist Virginia Apgar preferred cyclopropane but often worked with doctors who preferred ether. To avoid argument, she religiously placed ether droplets on the drapes in the delivery room. Her colleagues would smell the ether and invariably murmur their approval, unaware that Apgar was using cyclopropane. John Adriani, the longtime director of anesthesiology at Charity Hospital in New Orleans, also preferred cyclopropane, observing that he had never known the substance to cause a single case of liver or kidney damage, as other anesthetics sometimes did. Yet he noted that many hospitals did not meet the standard set by the National Fire Protection Association for the use of flammable anesthetics and so shunned cyclopropane. He thought this unfortunate, noting, "There have been more fatalities from hepatitis from halothane than there have deaths from explosions in operating rooms."[45]

The preference for particular anesthetics varied regionally, often for historical reasons. Anesthesiologist James Tayloe Gwathmey pointed out in 1921 that at Massachusetts General Hospital, where William T. G. Morton first demonstrated the effects of ether during surgery, doctors never used chloroform; in Scotland, where James Young Simpson discovered chloroform, doctors used chloroform almost exclusively. Gwathmey observed that if the location of these discoveries had been reversed, chloroform would be popular in Boston and ether would be the anesthetic of choice in Scotland.[46]

This phenomenon was evident even in James Young Simpson's lifetime. He was well aware that Boston physicians almost without exception eschewed chloroform, and in an 1870 letter to Horatio Robinson Storer, one of the few Boston doctors who preferred chloroform, Simpson condemned the prejudice. "Surely, this is a most strange & narrow . . . policy of the profession of a town like Boston, pretending to be enlightened & living up to the Spirit of the age." Simpson asked Storer, "Are the modern inhabitants of Massachussetts [*sic*] . . . to be curbed & restrained as far behind in the march of intellect regarding the influence of chloroform as their forefathers were with regard to the influence of Tobacco?"[47]

For a time, ethylene oxygen proved popular in Chicago for similar reasons: Chicago was where scientists accidentally discovered its anesthetic properties. When florists asked University of Chicago botanists in the early 1920s to determine why carnations and sweet peas quickly wilted in stores, botanists blamed the ethylene in gas lighting. Arno B. Luckhardt, a University of Chicago professor of physiology, then correctly theorized that ethylene must have anesthetic properties. In 1936 Chicago's Presbyterian Hospital continued to hail ethylene as ideal for use in obstetrics, even though the gas had caused two explosions in hospital delivery rooms, because it relieved pain without retarding labor or harming mother or infant.[48]

As experimentation with obstetric anesthesia mushroomed, doctors increasingly administered multiple substances in a single birth. In the 1920s, Gwathmey was among the first to experiment in this manner. He combined several drugs with ether, starting with a small amount of his mixture and gradually increasing the dosage until it achieved the desired effect. In Atlanta in the 1930s, doctors administered paraldehyde routinely after cervical dilation had reached four or five centimeters. If a woman needed relief before that, they injected her with morphine and scopolamine, Nembutal, or sodium amytal. By the 1940s, doctors at Northwestern University, who customarily used only morphine during labor, also began to give women Benzedrine, an amphetamine, hoping that the Benzedrine would stimulate infants' breathing if it became repressed by morphine.[49]

Just as the medical community found that a promising method failed to live up to expectations, another novel practice would surface, sustaining enthusiasm for further experimentation. Among the most celebrated techniques were James Tayloe Gwathmey's oil-ether colonic method unveiled in 1913, his synergistic method introduced in 1921, and Robert Hingson's 1942 continuous administration of anesthesia through the caudal space in the spine.

Gwathmey did for anesthesiology what DeLee did for obstetrics: under his tutelage anesthesiology became a well-respected specialty in professional and lay eyes. After identifying and then contacting every physician-anesthetist in the country, Gwathmey founded the American Association of Anesthetists (AAA), an organization that assured the eventual recognition of anesthesiology as a medical specialty. He became the AAA's first president in 1912 and subsequently developed tactics to heighten the visibility of anesthesiologists. He refused, for example, to follow long-standing custom and bill the surgeon for his services. Instead, he billed surgical patients directly. There would not be many gynecologists, he argued in 1909 in defense of this scheme, if patients made all payments to the general practitioners who referred them to gynecologists.[50]

In an attempt to vanquish the dangers of inhalation anesthesia, Gwathmey began using rectal anesthesia in 1913. Although a few doctors had experimented with the rectal administration of ether before Gwathmey, he was the first to mix ether with olive oil, a combination that permitted the gradual and even absorption of ether by the colon. Although initially hailed by the entire medical community, rectal anesthesia was quickly confined almost exclusively to obstetrics.[51]

In 1921 Gwathmey promoted with equal enthusiasm his synergistic method, magnesium sulfate and morphine administered hypodermically coupled with quinine, alcohol, ether, and olive oil administered rectally. He explained that each substance either subdued or enhanced the effects of another. Quinine sped contractions that had been slowed by ether and morphine. Magnesium sulfate prolonged the effect of morphine while also diminishing ether-induced nausea. Morphine enhanced the painkilling effect of ether while also reducing the ether-instigated desire to struggle.[52]

Women learned of Gwathmey's synergistic method in one of their favorite magazines. Constance L. Todd explained to readers of the *Ladies' Home Journal* that she had stumbled on the theory of synergism while browsing an article titled "Synergistic Analgesia and Anaesthesia with Special Reference to Magnesium Sulphate, Ether, Morphine and Novocaine" in the *Journal of Laboratory and Clinical Medicine*. She joked, "This title might have been Sanscrit [*sic*] for all it conveyed to me. . . . It seemed to be largely concerned with albino rats." Yet despite her initial bewilderment, she conveyed quite clearly to American women the concept of synergy, that drugs could be used in assorted combinations to enhance and mitigate each other. Reminiscent of the twilight sleep movement's clarion call, she urged her readers to demand "this special dispensation" and reject the doctors who "frighten them off with bogies. . . . Whether or not the extreme agony is forever taken out of childbearing rests with women themselves."[53]

Grateful women all over the country wrote to Todd. One woman reported weeping with joy after reading her article. A Philadelphia mother complained that despite her recent "large, fat" payment to a well-regarded obstetrician, Todd's article taught her that the doctor had not provided her with the best available treatment. She planned to return to that doctor just once more, to tell him that after women learned of Gwathmey's innovation, they would brook no other.[54]

Anesthesiologist Robert Hingson elicited similar lay interest in a new anes-thetic technique in the 1940s. Hingson, who received his medical degree from Emory University School of Medicine in 1938, delivered eighty-two babies as a medical student. They were occasions he later described as accompanied by "full sound effects of the 'Help me Jesus' stage of labor." In 1942, inspired both by these disquieting recollections and by the impending birth of his first child, he and col-league Waldo B. Edwards, an obstetrician, developed continuous caudal anesthe-sia, a method permitting constant small doses of anesthesia to flow into the sacral canal of the spine. The innovation was made possible by development of the flex-ible spinal needle in 1940.[55]

In the years preceding the unveiling of Hingson's innovation, American doc-tors had administered caudal anesthesia with a single injection; the effect of the single-shot caudal lasted for only 45 to 150 minutes, depending on the duration of action of the local anesthetic. The effect of continuous caudal anesthesia, how-ever, lasted as long as the anesthetic flowed and for a time thereafter; it was thus ideal for treating the time-indeterminate but nevertheless finite pain of labor. Physicians had used the single-injection method only at the end of second-stage labor, but colleagues hailed Hingson's continuous method as a long-acting, safe antidote to the pains of first-stage labor as well.[56]

The advantages of continuous caudal anesthesia over inhalation anesthesia were numerous: less toxicity and hemorrhaging, no nausea, and absolute muscle relaxation. The fetus seemed to benefit as well. Continuous caudal anesthesia rendered unnecessary what had become the obligatory inhalation anesthesia in the delivery room, and so the incidence of narcotized babies decreased consider-ably. Hingson claimed that his method cut the death rate of premature infants in half; these babies had difficulty breathing under the best of circumstances, let alone when their mothers ingested or inhaled an anesthetic.[57]

Women seemed to especially appreciate Hingson's continuous caudal anes-thesia. Decca Treuhaft, a typical enthusiast, wrote in a letter detailing her son's birth at Stanford University Hospital in San Francisco in 1944, "Bob [her hus-band] & I sat around playing cribbage & chatting till midnight; I felt no pain at all & was completely conscious throughout. . . . I had this marvelous new cau-dal anaesthetic which numbs you from the waist down but you stay awake all through."[58]

Treuhaft and other expectant mothers likely learned about the continuous caudal well in advance of their labors, since *Time, Newsweek,* and *Woman's Home Companion* published enthusiastic pieces heralding the innovation. In describing her own experience with Hingson's invention, the author of the *Woman's Home*

Companion article likened her labor to a delightful social event. "I was leaning back against the pillows, sipping my coffee and discussing the war with my husband and the doctors. And when Marilyn was born . . . I was as comfortable as if I were sitting in my neighborhood movie theater."[59]

In the 1960s the caudal block fell out of favor, in part because lumbar epidurals proved easier to administer and control. There were other reasons as well. One group of investigators, who set out to prove that continuous caudal anesthesia shortened labor, discovered it did the opposite. It lengthened the labors of first-time mothers by one hour on average and increased subsequent labors by an average of two hours. Doctors' assertion that caudal blocks shortened labor had been a misperception; women were now "awake, comfortable, pleasant, and cooperative" during labor and hence required far less attention from nurses and doctors. Thus women's labors seemed shorter to medical personnel despite their increased length. Further study indicated that the disadvantages of the continuous caudal actually outweighed its advantages. The caudal not only lengthened labor but also demanded constant monitoring, precise technical expertise, and a significantly higher incidence of forceps deliveries. Hospitals began to reject the practice. Even fervent proponents advised further testing.[60]

Who Administered Obstetric Anesthesia?

Despite the increased demand, few training programs for residents in anesthesiology offered anything but minimal experience in obstetrics as late as the 1960s. Between 1961 and 1963, 40 percent of anesthesiology residents attended fewer than fifty vaginal deliveries in the course of their two-year residency; 2 percent attended no vaginal births at all. Even if training in obstetrics had been more comprehensive, the availability of anesthesiologists in maternity wards would still have been minimal. A joint statement written by the American Hospital Association and the American Association of Nurse Anesthetists in 1957 cited a survey indicating that the number of anesthesiologists was barely 30 percent of the total needed in the country. The survey's authors observed that the 3,724 physicians who either limited their practice to anesthesiology or had a special interest in anesthesiology could not possibly administer all the anesthesia needed by patients in the country's 6,959 hospitals.[61]

John Bonica, an anesthesiologist at the University of Washington in Seattle, decried the lack of anesthetic expertise in delivery rooms in 1955. Most anesthesiologists wanted nothing to do with obstetrics, Bonica observed, because of its unpredictable nature. The vast majority of surgeries could be conveniently scheduled, but birth occurred with little notice at any hour of the day or night and on weekends. An obstetrician who graduated from medical school in 1939 and received a fellowship at the Mayo Clinic remembered anesthesiologists' disdain for obstetrics. She recalled their preference for surgery and their treatment of obstetrics as "the stepchild."[62]

Because operating rooms were the priority for anesthesiologists and nurse-anesthetists, John Adriani ordered members of the anesthesiology staff at Charity Hospital in New Orleans to teach obstetric residents how to administer spinal anesthesia and manage its complications. After World War II, because of the nationwide dearth of anesthesiologists, it was becoming the norm for interns and obstetricians to administer the anesthesia in labor and delivery rooms.[63]

One obstetrician recalled how this informal system worked at his hospital. During the first month of his rotating internship at Chicago's Michael Reese Hospital in 1951, he was assigned to anesthesia. For one month he trained under an anesthesiologist and a nurse-anesthetist in the operating room. Afterward, because anesthesiologists and nurse-anesthetists were in short supply even in surgery, he continued reporting to the operating room each morning for a year to administer anesthesia to the first surgical cases of the day. Only later did he report to his then-current rotation in a different part of the hospital. This obstetrician thus became adept at administering ether, nitrous oxide, ethylene, cyclopropane, and pudendal blocks. He pointed out, however, that his expertise was indicative of the cost to pregnant patients. If, after one month's training, an unsupervised intern was responsible for administering anesthesia in the surgical suites of a major metropolitan hospital, maternity wards were served even more poorly. Laboring women, he noted, received "the bottom of the barrel in the way of anesthesiologists. . . . And I'm not talking about 1920 or 1850. I'm talking about 1954, 55, 56."

Eventually, this physician went into private practice in Chicago with two other obstetricians. The three partners often worked as a team in delivery, and given his expertise, this doctor served as the anesthetist. His proficiency remained unusual, however; the patients of other doctors were seldom as fortunate. "I can remember like it was yesterday—somebody else's patient was about to deliver and there was no anesthetist around, you call and they didn't come, and one of the other docs walking in and pouring open-drop ether. . . . I couldn't believe it." Familiar with this reality, obstetricians were likely unsurprised in 1961 when a study of maternal mortality from 1936 to 1958 in Baltimore revealed that 15 percent of maternal deaths were caused by violations of basic, long-standing anesthetic principles.[64]

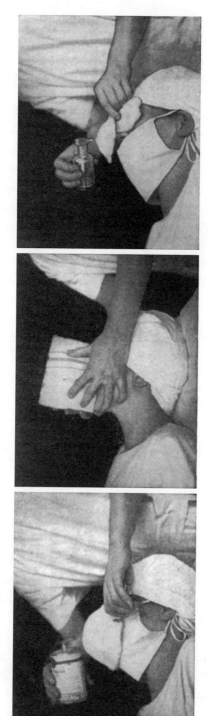

Left: administering ether *via* the open-drop method using a bent safety pin as a dropper. *Center:* administering ether *via* the "closed method," using a paper cone and towel. *Right:* administering chloroform *via* the open-drop method through a moist handkerchief. The patient's face has been covered with "vaselin" to prevent burns. *Source:* Joseph B. DeLee, *Obstetrics for Nurses* (W. B. Saunders, 1927), 186, 188.

Anesthesiologist John Bonica faced one of these life-threatening scenarios when his wife, Emma, gave birth to their first child in 1943. Aware that anesthesiologists avoided obstetrics, Bonica personally trained the chief obstetric resident at St. Vincent's Hospital in New York in anticipation of Emma's labor. When she was ready to deliver, however, the chief resident was performing a cesarean section. Another obstetrician greeted Bonica instead, "just like a typical New Yorker," with a hearty "How ya doing? Emma's doing great. Oh, she's a great patient." To his dismay, Bonica discovered that this obstetrician wanted to avoid anesthesia. He told Bonica, "Look, she has to tough it out. I want an awake baby." But even this wary doctor believed a small amount of ether was necessary at the moment of birth. Thus, when Emma was about to deliver, he hastily summoned an intern and instructed him, "Give her a little drop of ether just to ease her pain." The nervous intern, barely three weeks out of medical school, administered too much ether too quickly. Emma vomited and turned blue. Furious, Bonica pushed the intern aside and stepped in to save the lives of his wife and baby.[65]

From that unsettling moment on, the development of safe obstetric anesthesia became all-important to Bonica. Eventually he became the first anesthesiologist to experiment with the segmental epidural; he pinpointed exactly which portion of the spine needed to be anesthetized during labor and joined the small minority of anesthesiologists interested in obstetrics. He became an outspoken advocate for expertise in obstetric anesthesiology, complaining in the *Journal of the American Medical Association* in 1955 that it was an old custom to assign the least experienced anesthetist and the most antiquated equipment to the maternity ward. Hingson similarly complained that the worn-out anesthetic equipment discarded by surgery was routinely transferred to maternity. He theorized that this was why so many women died of hypoxia while giving birth.[66]

Both Bonica and Hingson long condemned the overall lack of anesthetic skill in obstetrics; Bonica was obviously recalling his wife's near-fatal calamity when he observed that interns, residents, and nurses with no training in anesthesiology were often ordered to administer anesthesia in delivery rooms at the last minute, a situation that would never be tolerated in the operating room. Bonica urged the universal creation of twenty-four-hour anesthesia services dedicated to maternity wards, unheard of then but fairly routine today.[67]

The Question of Safety

The lack of anesthetic expertise in delivery rooms, coupled with the administration of multiple drugs during delivery, resulted in omnipresent danger by the

1930s. One obstetrician recalled that even into the 1970s, when the same doctor who administered the spinal also delivered the baby, nobody monitored maternal blood pressure and breathing. Anesthetized labors and deliveries were even more potentially devastating to infants. Babies were born with blue or purple coloring so often that in a letter to the *Journal of the American Medical Association* in 1941, Yale physiologist Yandell Henderson proposed coining a new word, anarchapnea, to describe a state of uncontrolled respiration in infants after excessive use of barbiturates by their mothers during labor.[68]

Drug-related side effects were so common by the late 1930s that one Philadelphia doctor complained that obstetric treatment had become primarily "treatment of drug confusion." In 1936 Nicholson J. Eastman, a professor of obstetrics at Johns Hopkins University, described an increasingly typical birth. A twenty-one-year-old first-time mother checked into the hospital complaining "bitterly" about pain. During the next five hours she received pentobarbital once, sodium pentobarbital twice, and an ether-paraldehyde-olive oil enema. After her first dose of sodium pentobarbital, she fell asleep, but during contractions she awoke, grimaced, and shrieked. Her discomfort became so pronounced, and the medications administered to alleviate her discomfort rendered her so out of control, that two attendants had to remain by her bedside to keep her from injuring herself, despite restraints. The problem persisted as her labor advanced. During second-stage labor, she remained so unruly that doctors could not persuade her to bear down. They ultimately had to apply forceps. Her baby was born limp and remained so narcotized he could not muster the energy required to breastfeed. Soon he was fed wholly artificially, via a free-flowing bottle. Nicholson condemned the case as exemplifying modern obstetrics.[69]

Yet the multilayered drug regimens were self-perpetuating. Nicholson observed that because virtually every mother and baby eventually went home in good condition and few of the women who had been drugged could recall any aspect of their labor, mothers professed delight with their hospital experience and were soon telling friends about "the 'marvelous green capsules'" they had received. Women's conversation thus ensured the popularity of heavily drugged deliveries.[70]

Through the nineteenth century, doctors worried little about the safety of obstetric anesthesia, believing that the physiology of pregnancy and birth protected women from the anesthetic side effects seen so often in surgery. A Virginia doctor offered a typical observation in 1895: although physicians admittedly gave chloroform to laboring women "often recklessly, carelessly, and copiously," results were nevertheless almost uniformly good. He speculated that the vasomotor and circulatory changes during pregnancy protected laboring women from their doctors' imprudent use of anesthesia. A Minnesota physician theorized similarly that during labor "the heart is hypertrophied and less likely to weaken . . . the uterine contractions aid to some extent the action of the heart and counteract the tendency of chloroform to produce cerebral anaemia." Only a few isolated voices insisted that laboring women did not enjoy immunity from the dangers posed by anesthesia.[71]

Yet even as the majority of doctors in the nineteenth century dismissed the risks of anesthesia to laboring women, these same doctors weighed the relative advantages and drawbacks of individual anesthetics. Initially, they preferred chloroform over ether. Patients needed less of it, it acted more quickly and persistently, and patients were more easily managed under its influence. Physicians noted in particular that, unlike ether, it did not cause a "tendency to exhilaration and talking." Patients, too, usually preferred chloroform; it was cheaper than ether, its smell did not linger, and it irritated the throat and lungs less. Chloroform remained a favorite among physicians into the twentieth century, until abundant evidence indicated that it caused liver damage and sudden death.[72]

Proof that chloroform and ether caused postpartum hemorrhage also accumulated over several decades. In 1850, after one New York doctor administered chloroform for hours to a grateful woman, he reported, "just as I had the child safe, I heard a gush of blood from my patient." He wondered fleetingly if the chloroform had prompted "this flooding" but quickly dismissed the idea. Forty years later, however, evidence pointed to many ill effects of chloroform in addition to postpartum hemorrhage: diminished contractions, an increased need for the use of forceps, and weakening of the heart. In the 1890s a Virginia physician, suspecting that chloroform was the root cause of even the maternal deaths normally ascribed "to heart clot, etc.," urged colleagues to ignore women's complaints during labor and use chloroform only when absolutely necessary, and even then sparingly.[73]

By the early twentieth century, physicians readily acknowledged the dangers of chloroform. J. Whitridge Williams warned in the 1904 edition of his classic obstetrics textbook that chloroform increased the incidence of postpartum hemorrhage and often harmed newborns. DeLee agreed. He had earlier halted all use of chloroform at the Chicago Lying-in Dispensary ("as the women are afraid of the drug"), and he credited that action for the Dispensary's exceedingly low hemorrhage rate.[74]

Indeed, every technique and anesthetic, no matter how enthusiastically celebrated when introduced, eventually evidenced serious drawbacks. Chloroform could prompt postpartum hemorrhage and damage the heart and liver. (When there was a brief move afoot in 1960 to revive the use of chloroform, John Adriani wrote to a New York colleague, "If one survives the chloroform anesthesia, he still has the hepatitis to look forward to.") Ether had its own set of unwelcome side effects: it too could cause hemorrhage, as well as irritate a mother's lungs, damage her kidneys, slow contractions, and asphyxiate the baby. Scopolamine often prompted violent behavior. Doctors came to associate morphine, alone or combined with other drugs, with fetal respiratory distress and death. Cyclopropane decreased oxygen to the fetus. Ethylene was a volatile gas prone to explosion. In Brooklyn, two physicians estimated that one of every three women given sodium amytal exhibited such bizarre behavior that she required restraints— reminiscent of twilight sleep. Unrestrained patients became maniacal, crouched, put their hands in their vaginas, threw aside sterile drapings, fell out of bed, and refused to bear down during delivery. At Michael Reese Hospital in Chicago, 60 percent of women given paraldehyde became so unruly that they too fell out of bed. These falls could be so calamitous that hospital staff worried about broken bones during labor. Barbiturates prompted similar delirium and produced cyanotic babies. Hingson noted that all anesthetics were hazardous to black women because their dark skin camouflaged cyanosis.[75]

Physicians chose a particular anesthetic and application method for many reasons, however. In the first decades of the twentieth century, rural doctors in particular argued that wholly abandoning chloroform was a luxury only urban physicians could afford. Ether, for a long time the only substitute for chloroform, required cumbersome equipment for proper administration; chloroform required little more than a handkerchief. Country doctors thus complained that critics of chloroform were largely physicians attending births in big-city hospitals where they enjoyed the luxury of assistants and readily available equipment. Dr. J. H. Carstens described the plight of the isolated rural doctor: "If you are . . . five miles from nowhere, with nobody in the house but the husband, and he faints and you have to take him by the collar and put him out in the snow and then come back into the house and give that woman an anesthetic all alone, and put on forceps—I would like to see anybody do it and give ether." Carstens acknowledged that chloroform posed risks but pleaded, "Leave chloroform to the general practitioner who has to do the whole work. Do not rob him of that boon. He is very careful and nobody will die from its use in labor."[76]

Ether was not the ideal replacement for chloroform anyway, even given proper equipment. Alice Roosevelt Longworth's reaction to ether in 1924 was a common one. Pregnant at forty-one with her first child, she traveled to Chicago so Joseph

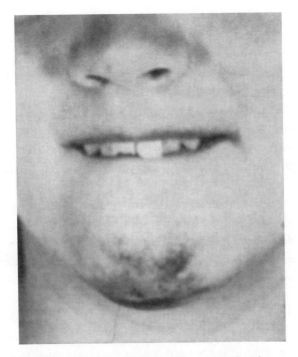

Under the influence of "analgesia [combined] with am-
nesic drugs" (the amnesiac was presumably scopolamine), this woman became agitated, threw herself off
her bed, hit her face on a nearby radiator, chipped her
front tooth, and bruised her chin. "Such patients," doctors advised, "must never be left for a second." *Source:*
Louise Zabriskie and Nicholson J. Eastman, *Nurses
Handbook of Obstetrics* (J. B. Lippincott, 1943), 373.

DeLee could deliver her baby. When she began to hemorrhage, DeLee decided the
baby had to be born immediately. He administered ether and then applied forceps. Longworth reacted very badly to the ether ("choked and turned blue etc."),
greatly alarming DeLee. Neither time nor experience ever alleviated that particular side effect. Another Chicago-area obstetrician, who graduated from medical
school in 1947, remembered walking into the delivery room just in time to see
his wife, who was giving birth to their first child, vomit and turn blue. After that
experience, he forever shunned ether and used only pudendal blocks on his
patients.[77]

The inherent risks of techniques used to administer obstetric anesthesia compounded the hazards of individual drugs. Initially, doctors administered paralde-

hyde rectally; then they found that when they injected it high enough in the rectum to ensure retention and rapid absorption, it irritated the mucosal lining. Giving paraldehyde orally, however, often induced vomiting. And although physicians originally hailed spinal anesthesia after its introduction in the early twentieth century, by the 1940s they associated it with paralysis of motor nerves, decrease in maternal blood pressure, infection, and excruciating postpartum headache. When women described a spinal headache, they often employed the same terminology traditionally used to describe labor pain: "almost beyond endurance." One physician recalled a patient with such a severe headache that she tried to jump out the hospital-room window into the river below.[78]

Doctors also blamed spinal anesthesia for dulling women's ability to push during second-stage labor. In 1925 a woman who had previously undergone two "easy spontaneous deliveries" without anesthesia had a typical experience. When the doctor arrived at her home, he noted "good second stage pains with beads of perspiration standing out on her forehead" and immediately offered spinal anesthesia. She consented to the novel treatment, and he injected a Novocain solution into her sacral canal. Almost immediately, she ceased pushing. The doctor cajoled her, explaining that her baby's head was resting on her perineum and if she just strained a bit the baby would be born quickly. But the seasoned mother was now helpless and responded that she was terribly sorry but her body seemed to have forgotten "how to strain." After a fruitless hour, the perturbed physician lifted the baby's head out of the powerless woman's body with forceps.[79]

This problem proved to be universal. Doctors at Temple University Hospital in Philadelphia reported that 98 percent of patients who received spinals required forceps deliveries. By the 1940s this side effect so troubled Temple physicians that they ordered that spinal anesthesia be given only to first-time mothers and only after the baby's head crowned. In an ironic twist, however, other Philadelphia doctors noted approvingly that while spinals demanded forceps, spinals also alleviated use of the instrument: "Despite the high incidence of forceps delivery, these were greatly facilitated by the complete pelvic relaxation which was obtained."[80]

Increasingly, physicians confused cause and effect: Did the growing use of spinal anesthesia necessitate the frequent use of forceps? Or, as most doctors were coming to believe, did most women, especially first-time mothers, require forceps to give birth safely anyway? Defining medically beneficial treatment became equally problematic: Did the "pelvic relaxation" afforded by spinals prompt easier births, less pelvic floor damage, and hence quicker maternal recovery? Or did pelvic relaxation simply make forceps easier for doctors to use and, given the damage forceps often caused, prolong women's recovery?

As the variety of anesthetics burgeoned, each new substance and method for its administration offered not only a renewed chance for increased safety and comfort but also new threats to health and life. Clifford Lull, coauthor with Hingson of a textbook on obstetric anesthesia, observed that doctors had "enthusiastically endorsed" many procedures for vanquishing labor pain over the years, only to eventually declare each harmful to mother or child in some way. By 1940 University of Wisconsin doctors warned that absolute safety and total pain relief in obstetrics were "reciprocally incompatible": the safer the technique, the less effective the pain relief; the more effective the pain relief, the less safe the technique.[81]

Concerned physicians struggled to identify precisely what made each substance and method of application potentially unsafe. Was it the nature of the medication or the amount used? Was it the way doctors and nurses administered it or when they administered it? Or for how long? Were first-time mothers the most vulnerable to anesthetic side effects? Did anesthesia require specific skills for administration, or could virtually anyone administer it? Could anesthesia be safely administered at home or only in the hospital? Why did mothers seem impervious to some drugs while their babies were born narcotized?

Yet in the mid-twentieth-century United States, a period with clearly delineated gender roles, some physicians dismissed anesthetic side effects and attributed any negative reactions to the annoying proclivities of certain women. Two physicians observed of sodium amytal in 1932, "A patient with an excitable temperament is far more prone to develop restlessness than one in a calm, cheerful frame of mind." Doctors likewise declared the agitation induced by paraldehyde "most pronounced in patients of a highly nervous or excitable temperament."[82]

Physicians also tended to refer obliquely to class and immigration status when assessing patients' reactions to anesthesia. Doctors warned in 1947 that when using obstetric anesthesia and analgesia, "best results are obtained if the mother is of normal intelligence and has no language difficulty." Women occasionally echoed this view. One mother writing in the *Ladies' Home Journal* in 1930 claimed that certain types of anesthesia always worked well, at least among "private patients of sufficient intelligence to cooperate with the doctor."[83]

Most physicians did note that anesthesia worked best on their private patients, women who had seen them for prenatal care. Doctors had the confidence and cooperation of these patients. "Ward cases," in contrast, were doubly handicapped: relegated to disturbingly noisy wards, they were also strangers to the doctors who delivered their babies. If analgesia and anesthesia were more successful for private patients than for the anonymous, working-class women who increasingly labored side-by-side in hospital wards rather than in their own homes, it might have been because the private patients were benefiting from a measure of the so-cial birth that had sustained women in the past. A private patient was not com-pletely alone among strangers; over time she had achieved a rapport with her doctor.[84]

Doctors' consistent observations that certain women did not react well to ob-stetric anesthesia indicate a probable tendency through at least the 1930s and 40s to be more willing to provide obstetric anesthesia to middle- and upper-class, rather than working-class, women. Given their allegedly greater intelligence, not to mention mastery of English, doctors deemed women of means theoretically better able to utilize the full promise of anesthesia. At least some working-class women who wanted anesthesia therefore had to specifically seek out amenable (and affordable) hospitals and doctors well in advance of giving birth. In antici-pation of her second birth, one frightened woman sought the advice of Con-stance Todd, the lay author of *Easier Motherhood*. She told Todd, "I just have a perfect horror of the ordeal ahead of me, still remembering the hours of agony I suffered before and expecting this to be even worse. . . . It has preyed on my mind so much that I really do not think I can survive it." She begged Todd to supply her with a list of hospitals in the Philadelphia area offering "ward cases" the new anesthetic recently described in a magazine.[85]

Physician-attended home birth seldom afforded low-income women the op-portunity for an anesthetized labor either. The medical students apprenticing at the Central Free Dispensary in Chicago, who attended the home births of working-class mothers, were dispatched to these births armed with sacrosanct written instructions. These students were almost always on their own at a birth; only when faced with an emergency did they summon a supervising physician. Thus their directives described even the most mundane procedures to be used, including step-by-step orders for cleansing a parturient's vagina, labia, and cli-toris and arranging medical paraphernalia for ease of use. The only mention of anesthesia on the detailed list was a warning that if ether, the only anesthetic apparently used by the dispensary, was administered during the "perineal stage," that is, as the infant emerged from the mother's body, a physician had to be pres-ent. Yet the directives of home birth dispensaries did vary according to institu-tion and locale. One general practitioner recalled that as a medical student in Indianapolis in the 1920s, he administered ether and chloroform unsupervised, via an imprecise drip method, whenever he attended home births.[86]

There is indeed mixed evidence of working-class women's access to obstetric anesthesia. In the 1940s John Adriani experimented with saddle block anesthesia at Charity Hospital in New Orleans, a hospital that served an almost exclusively

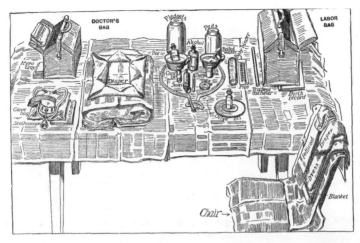

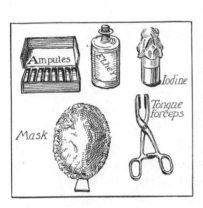
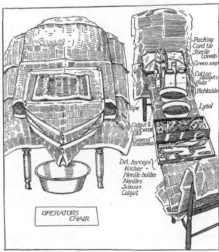

Illustrations of the customary setup for home births attended by doctors from the Chicago Lying-in Dispensary. Note that the primary emphasis at these births was on asepsis, while pain relief was only a tangential consideration. *Source: The Technic of the Chicago Maternity Center Formerly the Chicago Lying-in Hospital Maxwell Street Dispensary*, 1933, pp. 4, 17, 19, American College of Obstetricians and Gynecologists History Library and Archives, Washington, DC.

poor, black population. The records of his experimentation indicate that in addition to a saddle block, the women giving birth at Charity Hospital also received at various times ethylene, Demerol and scopolamine, Seconal and scopolamine, morphine, and phenobarbital. In other words, they received the full array of analgesics and anesthetics made available to paying patients in private hospitals. Even so, Frank Moya, professor and chair of the Department of Anesthesiology at the University of Miami, complained in 1966 that women's economic status, "whether they be white or Negro," dictated their access to obstetric anesthesia.[87]

If some doctors tended to dismiss maternal side effects from anesthesia and attribute them instead to women's class or personality quirks, the medical community neglected the effect of anesthesia on newborns even more. Although physicians complained with the advent of twilight sleep that morphine depressed newborns' breathing, rather than highlighting potential anesthetic dangers to infants, most medical journal articles through the 1930s strove to diminish alarm. A 1936 study conducted at Johns Hopkins Hospital determined that of chloroform, ether, and nitrous oxide, only nitrous oxide depressed newborn respiration to a profound degree. Other physicians dismissed even that danger, noting that nitrous oxide, if properly administered, did not affect the fetus. One Chicago area doctor assured a group of colleagues that he had investigated every case of newborn brain injury in his community, asking "each pediatrist and every psychiatrist" whether the analgesia given to the baby's laboring mother had caused the injury in question. In every case experts absolved the drugs of blame.[88]

The effect on newborns of drugs given to their mothers during labor eventually became impossible to ignore, however. One troubled doctor estimated in 1941 that 30 to 60 percent of babies whose mothers had been given analgesics needed some form of resuscitation at birth. A Philadelphia doctor wondered, "What percentage of 'stillbirths' and deaths in early infancy result from narcotics and anesthetics given to the mother during labor?" Problems were due in part to the high dosages administered to mothers. One physician, a mother of five and the only doctor in a sparsely populated county in Colorado, recalled that when she was a medical student in the late 1950s and early 1960s, "all the obstetricians . . . knocked their patients out with drugs and anesthetics and then they delivered an infant from this inert mother's body which usually had to be resuscitated because the baby was so zonked from too much drugs that it didn't breathe spontaneously." The problem was so prevalent that some doctors began to routinely administer nalorphine toward the end of a labor in order to reverse the inevitable respiratory depression in newborns.[89]

A few obstetricians became so alarmed by anesthetic side effects that they began to experiment with drug-free methods to relieve pain. One Chicago-area obstetrician studied hypnosis in the 1950s. Interested patients came to her office every one or two weeks throughout their pregnancies for labor preparation classes. She developed what she called "a patter" and employed it during these women's labors. Although hypnosis required her presence at births for innumerable hours, this physician did not consider that a disadvantage of the method. She explained, "I never counted the time with the patient." Most of her patients who chose hypnosis were delighted with the experience.[90]

Eventually, anesthesiologist Virginia Apgar, via research too compelling to ignore, permanently alerted the medical community to the effects of obstetric anesthesia on newborns. As the first American physician to prove that anesthetics and analgesics cross the placenta, she was inspired to develop a quick and consistent way to assess infant well-being immediately after birth. The Apgar Score, unveiled in 1952, used five signs—heart rate, respiratory effort, reflex irritability, muscle tone, and color—to judge a newborn's health status. Each sign received a score of zero, one, or two; a total Apgar Score of four or less demanded immediate resuscitation efforts. Doctors were now required to scrutinize every infant at birth to determine the baby's score. Doing so graphically highlighted in delivery rooms across the country the consequences of medications received by mothers during labor. Doctors began to compare the transplacental passage of assorted drugs.[91]

The clarion call represented by the Apgar score did not diminish the use of obstetric analgesia and anesthesia, however. Despite ongoing research demonstrating that analgesics and anesthetics crossed the placenta and entered the fetal blood supply shortly after administration to the mother, doctors continued dispensing multiple pain-relieving medications during labor. In the early 1970s, still attempting to warn the obstetric community that newborns were unable to metabolize the many drugs given to their mothers, two doctors wrote, "Despite these ominous facts, the use of delivery medication in the United States is commonplace, its absence a rarity." The question of safety remained unresolved.[92]

In the 1920s and 1930s, the high-profile public discussion about high maternal mortality and inadequate obstetric training gave women ample reason to continue to anticipate birth with fear. In 1933 Bailey Patterson Sweeny was so anxious about the birth of her first child that she left a letter for her husband, Arthur, to be opened in the event of her death during childbirth.[93]

Women's apprehension increased their desire for anesthesia, which permitted them to be mentally, if not physically, absent from the harrowing event. Even women who approached birth with relative nonchalance welcomed anesthesia. When Dorothy Dushkin gave birth to her fourth and last child in 1940, she exhibited such a "casual attitude & [seeming] lack of pains" that nurses were stunned when they discovered she was fully dilated and ready to give birth. But like her cohorts, Dushkin was "mighty glad to gasp in the gas" in the delivery room.[94]

The twilight sleep movement helped create this eagerness for anesthesia; the interest it aroused guaranteed publicity for every subsequent anesthetic innovation. Women's magazines, which had brought the news of twilight sleep to public attention, continued to describe in detail every development in obstetric anesthesia subsequent to twilight sleep, effectively acting as a conduit for both the fears and the hopes of expectant mothers.

As hospital-based obstetric residencies and women's desire to benefit from the full array of "modern advances" promoted by women's magazines assured the permanence of hospital birth, the tensions inherent in laboring in an institutional setting ensured the increasing use of obstetric anesthesia. Not only were the hospital and its associated medical rituals unfamiliar and intimidating, but when women labored in proximity to one another, their fear was contagious. Even Dushkin, who labored with relative ease even during her first pregnancy in 1932, found the hospital unsettling. After hospital personnel installed her in a private room shortly before her delivery, she was bothered by the moaning and shrieking of other women—"rather a disagreeable introduction." Anesthesia gave women who labored in an unfamiliar setting among strangers a measure of comfort as they anticipated and experienced such a lonely, painful, mysterious ordeal. Hospital birth was thus both an effect of women's and physicians' interest in anesthesia and a cause of their increasing interest in anesthesia.[95]

By the time mothers began to give birth to the baby boomers, birth had become an event to be medically tamed, if not conquered. Physicians arranged births to occur by appointment and mothers completed their labors in a preordained amount of time. Laboring women were, of course, physically present at the births of their children, but in all other respects they were absent. Since women were unconscious during a sizable portion of their labors, doctors now starred in the event. Mothers had become mere supporting players.

CHAPTER FOUR

Giving Birth to the Baby Boomers

The Question of Convenience, 1940s through 1960s

*L*iving in Los Angeles in 1948 and pregnant for the first time after three years of marriage, Alice Munro Isaacs knew almost nothing about childbirth; she was the first in her social circle to become pregnant, and her mother had never discussed birth with her. Yet she was unperturbed by her lack of knowledge and happy to rely on her obstetrician's expertise.

During her pregnancy, Isaacs visited her doctor regularly: once a month in early pregnancy, then twice a month, and eventually once a week as the birth neared. If problems arose between visits, she made additional appointments. When she had morning sickness early in her pregnancy, for example, the doctor advised her to come in weekly for shots to treat the nausea. She never asked what was in the shots.

In February 1949 Isaacs's due date came and went. Because her husband, Jack, worked during the day and attended classes at the University of Southern California at night, the couple moved in temporarily with her parents. Isaacs did not want to risk being alone when she went into labor. Two weeks later, weary of the pregnancy, Isaacs talked to her doctor about labor induction. The obstetrician advised Isaacs that at this point in her pregnancy, consuming castor oil would likely trigger labor. She purchased a small bottle, downed its contents, and waited with trepidation for something to happen. Nothing did.

When Jack came home from work that evening, they ate dinner with her parents as usual. After dinner, Jack left for school. While helping her mother clear the table, Isaacs felt a gush of warm water between her legs. Her parents drove her to the hospital. Hospital personnel wheeled her to the "prepping room," where a nurse shaved Isaacs's pubic hair and prepared to administer an enema. Hoping to avoid the enema, Isaacs explained that she had consumed an entire bottle of castor oil earlier in the day. The nurse told her every woman in labor had to have an enema, regardless.

Following "the prep," someone wheeled Isaacs to a small, dark room and helped her into bed. Almost immediately she felt her first faint contraction. Soon Jack, who had rushed to the hospital after his class, joined her. A nurse came in to give Isaacs a shot and explained to the couple that the injection would either speed up Isaacs's labor or put her to sleep. Although Isaacs did not understand how a medication could prompt one of two diametrically opposed reactions, she explained later, "Jack and I didn't question anything that any medical person said, so he went downstairs and waited and I did go to sleep."

Her next recollection was a voice urging her to push. "Alice," someone said, "you have to push if you want to have a baby. Wake up and push." Isaacs was so annoyed at the disturbance that she pushed just so the faceless intruder would stop bothering her. Apparently satisfied with her response, a medical team wheeled her bed down the hall to the delivery room.

The move from the darkened labor room to the brightly lit delivery room helped awaken Isaacs. A medical team lifted her onto the delivery table and then rolled her onto her side so the doctor could administer saddle block anesthesia. Isaacs explained, "A saddle block was a new kind of thing at the time and they considered this the best thing to do and so that's what I had said I wanted."

She lost all feeling in her lower torso but was aware that the doctor gave her an episiotomy and then used forceps. She remembered, "I really wasn't worried about it. I don't know why." Someone held Isaacs's newborn daughter up for her to see and then whisked the baby away. A nurse kneaded Isaacs's stomach to expel the placenta. She recalled, "No one addressed me and . . . I had the feeling of being so much meat on the table."

A nurse returned Isaacs to her room and instructed her to remain flat on her back and absolutely still to prevent a spinal headache. Jack came to see her and she learned for the first time that she had been unconscious for close to twelve hours before giving birth.

Like the other women in the maternity ward, she remained motionless in bed for three days. At the end of the third day, nurses permitted her to sit up and dangle her feet over the edge of the bed. She did not leave her bed until the fifth day, when she went home.

On the drive home, Isaacs sat on the pillow the doctor advised Jack to bring to ease the pain of her episiotomy. She remembered feeling "awfully uncomfortable and quite disillusioned. Here the birth was all over and I was still having pain from the stitches."[1]

Postwar Attitudes toward Birth

Alice Munro Isaacs was one of the women who gave birth to the cohort known as the baby boomers. Isaacs and her contemporaries reversed a 150-year decline in fertility in the United States. The birthrate had decreased from 7.04 children per white woman of childbearing age in 1800 to 4.24 in 1880, 3.56 in 1900, and 2.4 in 1930; then, in the aftermath of World War II, it rose to 3.2.[2]

This trend does not, however, adequately explain the large bulge in the population that came to be known as the baby boom. The women who reached reproductive age during and immediately after World War II, women born just before and during the Great Depression, were members of the smallest generation born in the twentieth century. How did this relatively tiny group give birth to the largest generation in American history when their average family size was only slightly over three children?

Demographers explain that women born in the 1920s and 1930s gave birth to the boomers by behaving unlike any birth-controlled population before or since. Previous and subsequent generations of American women did not marry and have babies in concert. Some never married. Some married as young adults. Others postponed marriage until well into adulthood. Some married but had no children or only one child. Others had a child every year or two of their reproductive years. Still others had several children but widely spaced their births. The generation that came of reproductive age in the 1940s and 50s, however, behaved with unusual uniformity. Virtually all individuals married. When they married, they customarily married young and then had three or four children during the first few years of their marriages. Most stopped having children by their mid to late twenties. In other words, the women who gave birth to the baby boomers created an unprecedented bulge in the population by all doing the same thing at the same time.[3]

There was strong social imperative for this atypical behavior. In the aftermath of World War II, society characterized childlessness, or having only one child, as both personally tragic and publicly subversive. A "lonely only" child was destined to be a misfit. Large families were characterized as happy families, and happy families created socially responsible, productive citizens.[4]

Uniform matrimonial and reproductive behavior was not the only uncommon trait of the generation that grew up during the Great Depression. This was also the first generation to defer to doctors on most medical matters, and for good reason. Medical miracles now abounded. Antibiotics seemed to have eradicated infectious disease, the ability to store and transfuse blood lessened the dangers of surgery and traumatic injury, and the maternal death rate had plummeted from almost 80 deaths per 10,000 live births in 1920 to 8 deaths per 10,000 live births in 1950.[5]

Of all medical miracles, penicillin was arguably the single most important contributor to the postwar public trust of doctors and hospitals. Penicillin saved the lives of soldiers during World War II; after the war physicians used it to successfully treat civilians suffering from what had been frequent bacterial killers in the past. One physician who attended medical school in the 1920s remembered those days clearly: "That was a very heady experience for a doctor, because while we were busy doing things for people all the time, we weren't really doing any specific curing. . . . Then came the antibiotics, and it got so it seemed we were curing everybody that had a fever and was sick." With the advent of penicillin, medical innovation and its stewards, highly skilled physicians, had become guarantors of health and long life.[6]

Isaacs's attitude toward her obstetric care illustrated the mind-set of her contemporaries: the laity no longer had strong personal opinions about medically related matters. Instead, they customarily embraced doctor-recommended options and considered only doctors' medical knowledge to be truly valid. Professional authority, coupled with what medical sociologist Paul Starr terms "the retreat of private judgment," dictated all forms of patients' medical decision-making and their acceptance of medical treatment.[7]

In this climate of reliance on physicians, women's fear of birth diminished. An Ohio physician was one of many struck by the difference between his current patients' attitudes and women's outlooks a generation before. "As I remember patients years ago, they had a dread of childbirth which at times amounted almost to horror. . . . Contrast this patient with the young woman who has learned from her friends that childbearing is no ordeal, in fact, a practically painless experience and not in the least disagreeable." As this doctor observed, women did learn from friends, and increasingly from their obstetricians, that they would have little to worry about—indeed, they would have little even to do—during birth.[8]

Anesthesia clearly played a salient role in this attitudinal shift. Now that women were psychically absent from birth, ceding authority to obstetricians was only logical. Even mundane conversations between mother and doctor reflected women's relinquishment of power. When Bailey Patterson Sweeny entered the Lenox Hill Hospital for her first birth, she received spinal anesthesia for three hours before being wheeled to the delivery room, where she received "whiffs of gas." Just before she went "out like a light," her doctor assured her, "One more push and I'll have control of it."[9]

Alice Munro Isaacs's unquestioning acceptance of every treatment recommended to her by a doctor or nurse typified this transformation. The host of obstetric treatments now offered by medical personnel seemed to guarantee not only safe birth but also worry- and pain-free birth. Helen Walcott McKenzie, who lived in an affluent suburb north of Chicago along Lake Michigan, recalled the horrifying description of birth she often heard as a child from her mother, who "endured unnecessary agony for twenty-eight hours in a 'normal delivery' without even a whiff of gas." Ominous depictions of birth such as this prompted McKenzie and, undoubtedly, many other daughters to be extremely grateful that they had come of reproductive age in the 1930s and 1940s rather than earlier.[10]

The characterization of birth in the immediate aftermath of World War II intensified the perceived need for anesthesia. As the public became accustomed to applying war metaphors to just about everything, fathers equated birth, as well as their own nervous pacing in hospital waiting rooms, to their recent battle experience. This tendency is graphically reflected in the Stork Club Books maintained by one Chicago hospital in its maternity ward waiting room. The hospital encouraged expectant fathers to record their thoughts in the journals as they awaited the imminent birth of their babies. One young husband wrote in 1949: "I thought Fox holes & army bunks were hard. . . . All I here [sic] from the nurse is your wife is doing good . . . the poor kid I wish she doesn't have any trouble. She's a good soldier & a brave one to [sic] the nurse said." Another expectant father wrote in 1950, "This waiting around is worse then [sic] sitting through the preliminary barrages that preceded the attacks on Cassino. At that time one could expect counter battery fire but now only God knows what will come next."[11]

The anxiety elicited by the Cold War also encouraged acceptance of obstetric anesthesia. At a time when Americans feared domestic as well as foreign threats, some physicians argued that modern obstetric care, including the most up-to-date anesthetic methods, had the power to eventually eradicate all such menaces. In 1950 the president of the American Association of Obstetricians, Gynecologists, and Abdominal Surgeons noted in his presidential address that mothers who were "not mental and physical wrecks as the result of childbearing" had the wherewithal to rear "healthy and happy citizens . . . not . . . Communists, Fascists, or Nazis."[12]

Following the custom initiated by twilight sleep, women's magazines stoked the intense public interest in obstetric anesthesia by religiously informing women about the latest innovations. After an article in the July 1946 issue of *McCall's* heralded John Adriani's work on saddle block anesthesia, interested women inundated the Charity Hospital in New Orleans (where Adriani headed the department of anesthesiology) with inquiries. One woman from Los Angeles sent a Western Union telegram asking Adriani for the names of doctors in southern California who were skilled in saddle block anesthesia administration. Similar pleas came from Gainesville, Florida; Detroit, Michigan; and Stockton, California. A woman from Biloxi, Mississippi, wrote to beg Adriani to accept her as a patient. He responded that the Charity Hospital admitted only Louisiana residents who were unable to pay hospital costs. He did, however, send the expectant mother the names of other physicians in New Orleans who would gladly provide her with saddle block anesthesia if she wanted to travel that far to have her baby. Colleagues from around the country also wrote to Adriani after the article appeared in *McCall's* to complain about "pseudo medical articles" reporting innovations that had not yet received professional scrutiny in the medical literature.[13]

As the letters to Adriani attest, many pregnant women now went to extraordinary lengths to make sure they would have no labor pain. Given the unprecedented guarantees that seemed to come with antibiotics and blood banking, women in the postwar world eagerly sought the most up-to-date obstetric treatments. Accordingly, obstetric protocol became increasingly elaborate, especially in regard to obstetric anesthesia, contrasting sharply with what had been customary practice just a few decades prior.

Birth now took place in the hospital. Upon entering the hospital, women underwent multiple requisite treatments: an enema, shaving of pubic hair, and sometimes labor induction; even when labor was not induced, it was often augmented chemically. Obstetricians were customarily the primary birth attendants but were not normally present while their patients labored. Instead, they arrived shortly before the birth "to deliver" the baby. Virtually all women were heavily drugged throughout labor. The actual birth took place in a surgical suite under full anesthesia. Once a woman was wholly unconscious, her obstetrician performed an episiotomy, applied forceps, removed her baby from her body, and then stitched her up. During five- to ten-day recuperation periods, mothers and babies resided in separate hospital rooms. Nurses brought babies to their mothers every four to five hours for feedings and even then only during daytime hours.

Paternalism and Prenatal Care

Doctors now enjoyed authority in all aspects of health and medicine, but nowhere was physicians' authority more evident than in obstetrics. Frequent prenatal care appointments, as well as women's lengthy postpartum hospital stays, pro-vided an unusual number of opportunities for physicians to both reassure and take charge. Pregnant women customarily saw their doctors a minimum of four-teen times during pregnancy and, as in Alice Isaacs's experience, often signifi-cantly more than that. These visits made women very reliant on their doctors. One mother who gave birth to her first child in 1949 and her second in 1952 recalled of her pregnancies and births: "The doctor was in command. . . . the doctor was God. And when the doctor told you this is how it's going to be, you didn't worry. You let the doctor worry."[14]

Routine prenatal care was a relatively new medical phenomenon. Not until well into the 1920s did women's letters and diaries mention appointments with doctors during pregnancy. Yet by the early 1930s, middle-class women's accep-tance of prenatal care was obvious; their descriptions of new, exacting regimens during pregnancy were manifest. Bailey Patterson Sweeny, pregnant with her first child in 1933, was typical. According to notations in her diary, her doctor carefully structured her diet, forbade her to ride in buses and cars, and ordered her to come to his office three times a week for injections to control nausea. During the first trimester of Sweeny's pregnancy, he also diagnosed a displaced uterus and ordered her to wear a pessary for four weeks.[15]

Two federal programs, the Sheppard-Towner Maternity and Infant Protection Act and the Emergency Maternal and Infant Care Program (EMIC), helped to persuade the nation's mothers of the importance of both prenatal care and hos-pital birth. Sheppard-Towner, enacted by the U.S. Congress in late 1921 and repealed in 1929, provided federal dollars (to be matched by voluntarily partici-pating states) for visiting nurses who dispensed pre- and postnatal advice to women in their homes and for clinics to counsel mothers on infant care. The ser-vices offered by Sheppard-Towner, most notably its popular informational pam-phlets and opportunities for mothers to have direct contact with visiting nurses, primed millions of women to routinely seek prenatal care for themselves and well-child care for their infants and older children.[16]

The EMIC, instituted by Congress in 1943 and terminated in 1949, effectively eliminated any lingering doubts women of all classes might have had about the efficacy of prenatal care. The EMIC provided payment under the Social Security Act for all prenatal and maternity care of the wives of servicemen in the military's four lowest pay grades. During its almost seven-year existence, EMIC paid for one of every seven births in the United States, covering the medical expenses of more than 1.2 million pregnant women. State and local health departments ex-panded the influence of the EMIC by forming EMIC medical advisory committees that recommended standards for prenatal and hospital maternity care and provided lists of competent specialists to mothers. These local committees encouraged mothers to use obstetricians (as opposed to general practitioners or midwives) and to give birth in the hospital. Ninety-two percent of EMIC mothers gave birth in the hospital; in comparison, the overall 1945 rate in the United States was 79 percent.[17]

Even before the EMIC, any middle-class mother who still balked at prenatal care found her uncertainty lessened considerably in 1939 when doctors offered the first laboratory test to confirm a pregnancy. The lure of the "rabbit test," injecting a rabbit with the urine of a woman who suspected pregnancy and then looking for changes in the rabbit's ovaries, virtually guaranteed that mothers of means would now seek out a doctor early in pregnancy and forge a relationship with that doctor. Articles in medical journals began to define obstetrics as "good prenatal care *plus* skilled medical and nursing care during delivery and the puerperium." The frequent prenatal visits that ensued served to transform the relationship between women and physicians.[18]

Women came to rely on their doctors in many ways. Since the vast majority of obstetricians were men and all their patients were women, most obstetricians felt protective of their patients in two culturally significant capacities, as men and as physicians. Given the predominant cultural belief that pregnant women were especially vulnerable to upset, obstetricians came to play a uniquely important role in their patients' lives. One typical obstetrician at the University of Rochester argued that a "dependent type of doctor-patient relationship" benefited pregnant women, and he advised colleagues to use even the most routine aspects of prenatal care to reassure patients. He recommended, for example, that doctors cultivate in mothers a soothing "phantasy of mid-pregnancy" by allowing them to listen to their baby's heartbeat during prenatal exams. Thus, a medical ritual that women today still look forward to, a practice that ostensibly affords women full participation in medical aspects of their pregnancy, had its origins in paternalism.[19]

In instituting this and other procedures, doctors did not intend to infantilize women. Rather, they sought to improve what they feared was pregnant women's precarious mental health, a major medical concern of the time. A typical pharmaceutical company advertisement appearing in *Obstetrics and Gynecology* in 1960—accompanied by a photograph of a slovenly dressed, visibly pregnant woman slumped in a chair with a glum look on her face, cheek resting wearily on open hand—advised obstetricians to prescribe Dexedrine, an amphetamine, to "help encourage normal activity," particularly "when your pregnant patients do little more than sit, eat, and gain weight." Numerous other ads urged obstetricians to prescribe tranquilizers to calm their invariably nervous pregnant patients.[20]

The paternalism exhibited by doctors during prenatal visits persisted through delivery. One man, relegated to the waiting room while his wife was in labor in 1949, learned from his wife's doctor that the baby was breech. Yet the doctor assured the man he would not mention this to his wife, the woman about to have the breech birth, because she "worried too much." Other physicians feared that using the word *spinal* would frighten women already made impossibly nervous by pregnancy. These obstetricians suggested disguising the nature of the treatment by calling it *lumbar anesthesia*, a phrase they assumed was so obscure that no woman would have any idea what they were referring to.[21]

One obstetrician, who graduated from the University of Chicago School of Medicine in 1945, noted that doctors at that time customarily averted women's questions and concerns by responding to every query with a blanket guarantee: "I'll take care of you. Don't worry. I'll do everything." And he observed that obstetricians consciously elicited reverence from nervous expectant fathers as well. He laughed remembering a common scene in his Chicago hospital: "They [obstetricians] had these fathers holed up in this little room and they get through with delivery. . . . and made sure that they had a little blood splatter on their scrubs and they'd say to the father . . . 'That was one of the most difficult deliveries I've ever had but your wife and the baby are just fine.' And it reminds me of an old Mike Nichols/Elaine May kind of a thing, 'Oh God bless you doctor. God bless you.'"[22]

Patients now regarded doctors with such reverence that mothers did not question a medical technique even when it clearly baffled them. One woman who found first-stage labor difficult discovered, like so many women before and after her, that the pain became negligible during second-stage labor. Her baby was about to be born in the presence of nurses in 1953 when the doctor rushed into the delivery room. The woman remember that he immediately "took over . . . told me to take chloroform, and as he was in charge . . . I couldn't very well argue, so I took it." Having felt no pain at the time, she could only guess at why the physician considered anesthesia necessary. She told her mother later, "By the feel of things the head was born by the time I took the chloroform so I suppose the chloroform was to make sure I wouldn't wriggle at the wrong moment." After the birth she greeted her husband by vomiting into a bowl. She blamed "that horrid chloroform" for her postpartum misery.[23]

Cooperative Patients

The numerous appointments required for prenatal care transformed the most basic interactions between obstetricians and their patients. Traditionally, the emphasis in obstetric care had been on labor. Doctors spent many hours by women's bedsides patiently waiting for babies to be born. By the 1940s, however, physicians regarded prenatal exams as a far worthier use of their time and deemed every hour spent comforting and encouraging a laboring woman to be an hour squandered. As the emphasis in obstetrics shifted from attending births to providing prenatal care, physicians no longer had the time to sit by laboring women's beds; thus it became more necessary than ever to give birth in the hospital. Obstetricians now needed the help of an institution to care for laboring women.

This change in priority signaled a fundamental transformation in the medical view of birth. Physicians at the University of Kansas Medical School observed that medical students increasingly judged only the moment of birth worthy of their attention and thus the only portion of labor they had anything to learn from. Women who delivered quickly were consequently prized and praised. In contrast, long labors were considered inherently troublesome labors. This stance encouraged medical routines designed to make labor predictable and to make it progress more quickly. Labor induction, the chemical augmentation of spontaneous labor, the administration of powerful analgesics throughout first-stage labor, spinal or general anesthesia during second-stage labor, episiotomy, and a forceps delivery became the routine.[24]

Sheer demographics helped justify this protocol. The increase in the number of births after World War II sapped hospital services. To compound the problem, most births were to first-time mothers, women who always have the longest labors and require the most attention. Furthermore, many physicians still were on duty in the armed forces, leaving fewer medical professionals to attend these first-time mothers.[25]

Physicians had long alluded approvingly to the tendency of analgesia and anesthesia to make mothers cooperative during labor, but women's cooperation, now defined as requiring negligible attention from nurses and doctors, became especially essential during the baby boom. Physicians confirmed matter-of-factly that analgesia kept laboring women quiet, effectively lessening the demands on busy nurses and doctors. One obstetrician noted during this era, "A good labor floor has been a quiet labor floor." Susan Munro Isaacs's twelve-hour, drug-induced, unconscious state had become typical, exemplifying how overburdened physicians and hospitals handled the overabundance of maternity cases.[26]

Nowhere was this use of drugs illustrated more clearly than in nurses' nickname for Nisentil, an analgesic with a chemical pattern similar to Demerol (but 2.5 to 3 times more potent) and customarily injected subcutaneously in combination with scopolamine. Nisentil's effect on women was so helpful to hospital personnel that they referred to it jokingly as "nice 'n still."[27] Doctors and nurses made similar observations about other drugs. Under Demerol's influence women were "fairly quiet, easily aroused by calling their names, and very cooperative." One physician reported in 1960 to the National Academy Screening Committee on Drug Addiction and Narcotics that phenazocine "produced a generalized quieting effect, almost tranquilizing" on laboring women. Because his nursing staff was so delighted with that result, he worried that objective evaluation of the drug might be impossible.[28]

When doctors discussed new analgesics such as Demerol and Nisentil with their pregnant patients, they were not so crass as to use the word *cooperative*. Rather, they simply and reassuringly associated the drugs with pain relief. Women corroborate this, reporting uniformly that their physicians promised them many times during prenatal visits that their labors and births would be pain-free.

What many women who gave birth in the 1940s and 1950s seem to have been unprepared for, however, was the amount of time during labor that they were unconscious. Given their ignorance of birth and contemporary birth practices, most had not necessarily equated painlessness with oblivion and thus many were surprised to find that they could recall little of their labors, remembering only that at some point, often shortly after hospital admission, they received an injection of some unknown substance and then—nothing. These women tell the same cryptic story about the births of their children: "I was unconscious." "I was out." "I don't know what I had. But whatever it was, it knocked me out." Physicians corroborate mothers' renditions of birth experiences, readily admitting that by the 1950s the largest obstetric practices in the United States were being built "upon the obstetrician's reputation for knocking his patients out cold."[29]

The Question of Convenience

Partly because of their new inability to cope with long labors and fully conscious women, physicians redefined the term *dystocia*, stalled labor. Traditionally, doctors had reserved a diagnosis of dystocia for women with extreme conditions such as large tumors, contracted pelvises caused by rickets, or a fetus weighing more than twelve pounds. By the 1940s, however, obstetricians had expanded the definition of dystocia to include "uterine inertia," an amorphous phrase used to

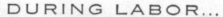

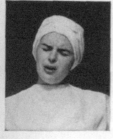 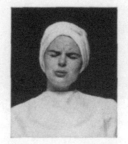 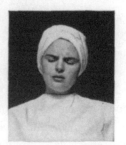

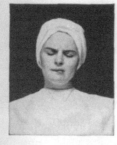 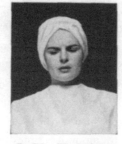 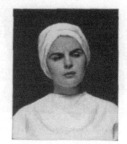

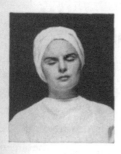 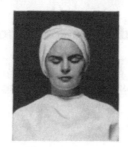 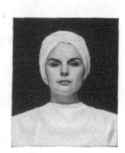

Advertisement for Nisentil marketed directly to obstetricians by Hoffman-La Roche, a pharmaceutical company. *Source: Obstetrics and Gynecology* 3 (January 1954): xxv.

describe lack of appropriate progress during labor. Each stage and substage of labor, this reframing of *dystocia* seemed to imply, should take place in a predetermined amount of time.[30]

The Friedman curve, a graph indicating the average time elapsed during cervical dilation and fetal descent, seemed to justify this redefinition. Emanuel A. Friedman, who eventually became chair of the Department of Obstetrics, Gynecology, and Reproductive Biology at Harvard Medical School, developed the curve in 1953 while a resident at Sloane Hospital. Well accepted for almost fifty years after its introduction, the Friedman curve taught that the cervix normally dilated from four to ten centimeters in about two and a half hours. Although Friedman ultimately complained that his tool was "being abused more than . . . being used appropriately," many physicians nevertheless came to believe the Friedman curve implied that if a woman's cervix took much longer to dilate than the curve indicated, then "prolonged labor" justified medical intervention.[31]

The flood of births that became the baby boom ensured that intolerance for a too-slow labor met not only with medical approval but with social approval as well. When the annual number of births almost doubled between the 1930s and the 1950s, from less than 2.5 million to almost 4.5 million, overworked obstetricians and youthful mothers with multiple children born one or two years apart searched for ways to cope.[32]

Almost overnight, the word *convenient* appeared in the articles published by medical journals and women's magazines that explained and advocated the myriad changes in obstetric procedure. In using this word, doctors were not being cavalier. *Convenient* had become a national buzzword. Preplanned, highly controlled, hospitalized birth was just one of many innovations now embraced by the nation. TV dinners, remote-control television, and pop-top cans were also part of the "convenient" lineup touted by newspapers and magazines. Among a people as hurried and time-conscious as Americans, coveting convenience was probably inevitable; the baby boom only prodded its development. For the millions of Americans now living in suburbs, commuting long distances to and from work and living in households full of babies and small children, the mere notion of convenience became a lifeline.

The first hint that Americans would eventually embrace convenience as a cultural icon appeared in the nineteenth century as the United States underwent rapid industrialization. At that time, Americans welcomed a closely allied concept, efficiency. What became the national obsession with efficiency was an outgrowth of Frederick Taylor's late-nineteenth-century theory of scientific management, a philosophy designed to maximize industrial output and revenue.[33]

Taylor described scientific management as the shortest amount of time needed to complete a job without tiring workers. Frank Bunker Gilbreth, a contemporary of Taylor, speculated similarly that there was one best way to perform every task. Both men's theories were eventually subsumed under the rubric "Taylorism," a philosophy that revolutionized industry. Taylor and Gilbreth linked the benefits of efficiency largely to industry, industrialists, and industrial workers, but Lillian Moller Gilbreth, an industrial psychologist and Frank Gilbreth's business partner and wife, associated the efficient management of industry with the public good, specifically with contented, healthy families. She argued that efficiency promised workers more "happiness minutes," that is, increased occupational safety, lessened fatigue, and more leisure time.[34]

Although obstetricians never expressly acknowledged the philosophies of either Taylor or the Gilbreths as they reformulated obstetric protocol in the 1940s and 1950s, the notions of these industrial psychologists spoke directly to physicians' views of labor and their desire to streamline that bodily process. The unpredictability of labor had posed a difficulty to doctors long before the baby boom. In 1838 one Harvard-trained physician who decried "the haste and impatience of the [birth] attendant" also sympathized with his colleagues: "The hands of the clock move at a sluggish pace, we think of our other patients who have expected our visits for the last twenty four or thirty six hours . . . visions of quiet chambers and downy beds are floating before the mind's eye, and prompting us to interference with the tardy (as they seem to us) operations of nature." This perpetual inability of doctors to formulate even rudimentary schedules whenever they attended a birth prompted a doctor in the 1920s to sympathize with young physicians who hastened labor even in ways that could be life-threatening.[35]

The problem persisted. In 1937 the *Ladies' Home Journal* published an unsolicited letter from a doctor who cautioned his younger colleagues against impatience, admonishing them not to use forceps to shorten labors. "Don't hurry," he warned them. That caveat, however, was far more easily issued than put into practice. To exploit a Cold War term, once efficiency became a core American value, birth became intrinsically un-American. Birth defies the most basic planning: pinpointing precisely when labor will begin is impossible. Even the span of normal gestation varies from 38 to at least 42 weeks. And once in active labor, a woman might deliver within 30 minutes or 30 hours.[36]

The baby boom made coping with these vagaries even more difficult for doctors and families. Preplanned, meticulously managed, "convenient" births seemed the obvious solution. Lay publications soon promoted every change in obstetric protocol as a means of making mothers' and physicians' lives easier and overcrowded hospitals more functional. Magazines even encouraged the practice of getting women out of bed within twenty-four hours after a birth (to prevent blood clots) as convenient for every interest group. Mothers regained their strength more quickly, so they needed less of nurses' attention and could be released from the hospital earlier, making room for other patients. And when these energetic mothers came home, they could immediately resume their household duties, making life easier for the entire family.[37]

Rationales offered to the public for other changes in obstetric protocol—most notably labor induction, heavily drugged labors, and the routine use of episiotomy and forceps—likewise fit the cultural imperative for convenience. The baby boom mandated the perfect application of Taylorism: if women could give birth at a predictable time and in less time and not bother nurses and doctors as they labored, harried young mothers and overworked doctors and nurses could plan ahead, be less fatigued, and enjoy better outcomes. Even hospitals would benefit. By planning when each birth would occur, maternity wards would never be overcrowded.

For individual doctors, this systemization of birth became a virtual necessity. Although a solo obstetric practice is almost unheard of today, it was fairly common before the 1980s and demanded total dedication of the physician. One Chicago obstetrician, who practiced alone for forty years beginning in the late 1940s, learned to mitigate the challenges posed by the baby boom in the same way so many of his colleagues did, by prescheduling patients' births several months in advance. He explained, "Because I had such a large practice I had to get rid of at least 5 or 6 pregnancies a week . . . so that I could live some kind of a life." By inducing all patients on Wednesdays and Saturdays, he was able to limit deliveries to those days, keep reliable office hours the rest of the week, and enjoy Sundays with his family.

He described the protocol he developed in the 1950s. Except for the rare woman who delivered early and missed her long-planned appointment, he induced all his patients with Pitocin on a Wednesday or Saturday morning. After administering "the pit," he injected patients with "rather large doses" of scopolamine and Demerol. He reasoned, not unlike his forebears who practiced in the heyday of twilight sleep, that if his patients were unable to remember anything about their labors, they would be more willing to have additional children. Then, at the end of first-stage labor, he reversed the effects of the scopolamine and Demerol with a dose of nalorphine to prevent respiratory depression in the newborn. During second-stage labor, he aided the mother, who was now unconscious owing to inhalation anesthesia, by greasing her pelvic canal with green soap, performing an

episiotomy, and applying forceps. Even if his patients had not been rendered unconscious as their babies were being born, he still would have aided them in this
fashion, for he feared that pushing during the second stage caused pelvic floor
damage. He explained, "I didn't want my patients to push. I didn't want them
to do anything. . . . pushing was one of the no-nos as far as my practice was
concerned."[38]

Another Chicago obstetrician, who graduated from medical school in 1951,
had a different rationale for a similar protocol: he sought to minimize risk to the
fetus. He administered full anesthesia just before delivery, performed an episiotomy, and then used outlet forceps "to lift the baby's head out of the pelvis and
to protect it from the [mother's] strong perineal muscles." He assured any patients wary of this plan that outlet forceps were decidedly different from the mid-
forceps their mothers had feared and that his way was easier and safer than
nature's way. He told women, "You can imagine the baby's head having to push
through those muscles versus my just making a cut and lifting the baby's head out
through there."[39]

This medical control of every stage of the birthing process became common
countrywide. In 1947, when Decca Treuhaft gave birth to her fourth child in Per-
manente Hospital in Oakland, California, she entered the hospital a week before
the birth. "Most of the time being what they call 'induced,' consisting of a total of
5 big doses of castor oil, 5 Triple-H enemas (so called by the nurse—it stands for
High, Hot & a Hell of a lot) and 45 shots of something or other. Also innumerable pills. The Dr. says it was a very easy birth—which it probably was for him, I
guess it all depends on your point of view."[40]

More than two decades earlier, Joseph DeLee was the first to legitimate these
practices by suggesting in the premier issue of the *American Journal of Obstetrics
and Gynecology* precisely how babies could be born systematically. In what became one of the most influential articles in the history of obstetric practice, he
touted what he dubbed "the prophylactic forceps operation." DeLee's "operation"
consisted of injections of scopolamine during first-stage labor, the administration of ether during second-stage labor, an episiotomy, a forceps delivery, and
manual removal of the placenta with the aid of ergot. He advised that his procedure would both systemize birth and prevent pathological occurrences.[41]

Before publication, DeLee read the article before a group of colleagues. When
he finished, J. Whitridge Williams, long DeLee's philosophical opponent, rose
from the audience to denounce the recommendations. "If his practice were to become general and widely adopted, women would be worse off eventually than
had their labors been conducted by midwives. . . . If I have understood Dr. DeLee

correctly, it seems to me that he interferes 19 times too often out of 20." Another obstetrician concurred, charging that DeLee's procedure was "a hospital 'stunt.'" Yet during the baby boom, busy doctors took DeLee's core philosophy to new heights, making birth systematic and predictable in ways that would have alarmed even DeLee.[42]

During the baby boom, philosophical descendants of J. Whitridge Williams did protest the trend. In 1959 the president of the American Association of Obstetricians and Gynecologists criticized the obstetricians who took on more patients than they could reasonably handle. He admonished, "Instead of sympathizing with the 'dear, overworked doctor,' I am appalled at the harm he does to obstetrics in general." In 1957 *McCall's* similarly condemned the "Tuesday-Thursday-and-Saturday obstetricians" who attended births only at preplanned times. The magazine called Pitocin "potential dynamite." The uterus, *McCall's* warned, sometimes reacted so violently to the drug that it "burst like a balloon, killing mother or child. And yet this drug is being widely used to suit the convenience of a patient or her doctor."[43]

For understaffed hospitals, overworked doctors, and pregnant women with one or more small children at home, however, the proclaimed benefits of induced, anesthetized labors and forceps deliveries seemed to far outweigh any seemingly improbable disadvantages. In lay magazines, doctors offered reassuring descriptions of the new way of giving birth: "Muscles continue[d] to go about their business" while women peacefully slumbered. One new mother was so pleased with her experience that, reminiscent of the women who once vowed to walk from California to Germany to enjoy twilight sleep, she exulted, "I'd much rather have a baby than a bad cold!"[44]

Pitocin and Obstetric Anesthesia

When women's magazines reported on innovations in childbirth during this period, they invariably singled out Pitocin and anesthesia for special publicity and praise. This was no coincidence, since the two treatments were inextricably linked. In spontaneous labor, the intensity and frequency of contractions build slowly. When labor is induced or augmented with substances like Pitocin, however, the onset of pain tends to be sudden and immediately intense. Women complained of such abnormally powerful labor pain after being "pitted" that they needed analgesia or anesthesia to help them withstand the agony. Reports of this phenomenon appeared in the earliest recorded observations of chemically augmented labors.

In 1916, for example, a wealthy woman who had already given birth three times without anesthesia was in labor with her fourth child at Sloane Hospital in New York City. After six hours "with little discomfort, but with increasing impatience on the patient's part to have it over with," her physician decided to augment her labor with an injection of pituitary extract. In minutes, the woman's pain was so great she begged for relief. The doctor immediately administered nitrous oxide. She gave birth one hour later. The woman was so enthralled by the experience—doctors, after all, had quickly and successfully treated her intensified pain—that she donated a gas apparatus to Sloane "so that the poor women in the wards could have the same relief, in their labor, that I did."[45] The common practice during the baby boom of chemically augmenting labor (to speed birth) or chemically inducing labor (so women and doctors could plan well in advance when labor would begin) similarly normalized the use of anesthesia.

In response to reports of greatly intensified pain, some doctors did denounce augmented or induced labors as "violent." DeLee, who obviously did not oppose other medical interventions during birth, likened labor augmentation to setting off a bomb that had the potential to blow up the uterus. Yet doctors who routinely used Pitocin dismissed the intensified pain as better than the alternative. One physician argued that long natural labors destroyed women's morale and stamina far more profoundly than quick, extremely painful labors that could immediately and effectively be treated with anesthesia.[46]

Before the early twentieth century, doctors induced labor only when faced with medical conditions that threatened a mother's life, for example, diabetes or eclampsia. Before pituitary extract and, eventually, oxytocin and Pitocin became available, induction methods included breaking the amniotic sac, placing a bougie between the membranes and the uterine wall, and forcibly dilating the cervix. Given the inevitable side effects of each of these methods, early-twentieth-century doctors associated induction with both infection and premature birth and thus judged the procedures almost as life-threatening as their indications.[47]

The birth of Katherine Shedd Bradley's second child in Chicago in 1920 illustrates prematurity as a dangerous side effect of induction. After Bradley's blood pressure rose, her doctor announced he had no choice but "to take [the] Baby." On April 1 he "inserted a bag to start things." The bougie did little more than prompt a few contractions. Two days later, the doctor anesthetized Bradley so he could insert a second bougie. Bradley's baby, born on April 6 and named David, weighed only three pounds ten ounces.[48]

By 1920, in addition to conditions like eclampsia and diabetes, physicians found an additional reason to induce labor: "postmaturity." Many doctors now labeled large fetuses, weighing more than eight and a half pounds, "postmature," regardless of gestational age. As maternal mortality became a well-defined social problem, doctors worried that large babies made birth more difficult. Thus, some doctors began to plan a woman's date to give birth around the presumed size of an infant, rather than the mother's menstrual history or date of coitus. The smaller the baby, physicians reasoned, the less a mother would "have to huff and pant under an easily avoided avoirdupois."[49]

Before the pressures of the baby boom, physicians specifically resisted elective induction, that is, inducing labor for social rather than medical reasons. DeLee blamed "hysterical magazine and newspaper writers," women, and a good number of his own colleagues for its increasing popularity. He warned, "A streamlined labor can be as safe as a streamlined parachute." In lieu of induction, DeLee ironically recommended his prophylactic forceps operation, the procedure that, in 1920, initiated the very concept of streamlined obstetrics. He advised that his procedure was far safer than "giving a woman a shot in the arm to blast the baby out of her person."[50]

While inducing labor for convenience long remained controversial, augmenting a spontaneous labor with Pitocin to speed it along was well accepted by the 1940s. Obstetricians who worked in large cities recall that by then labor augmentation had become the norm. And although doctors did not recognize that it was happening, this particular use of Pitocin eventually normalized elective induction. If augmenting labor was safe and beneficial, the reasoning went, why not just jump-start labor to begin with?[51]

Even rural physicians began to defend Pitocin. When a doctor had a large territory to cover, they argued, planning when a birth would occur benefited everyone. DeLee, however, continued to oppose the routine induction of labor. He urged his rural colleagues to abandon their sense of urgency. "Let that country doctor go away and come back, even though it is some distance, timing his visits, and if he finds the baby [already born and] in bed it probably won't hurt very much."[52]

Induction intrigued consumers as well as certain physicians, however, ensuring its eventual popularity. As doctors learned during the heyday of twilight sleep, when a medical procedure piques consumers' interest, its normalization is assured even in the face of medical controversy, at least for a time. The enthusiasm of a father who described his wife's experience in a 1938 issue of *Readers' Digest* typified this lay interest. The man explained that his first daughter, born twenty-two years earlier, "came in the old way—the hard way." In contrast, his second daughter, a product of his second marriage, was "born the new way—the easy, painless streamlined way." His wife, who had worried early in her pregnancy that the hour-long ride between home and hospital would be a "mad dash in the dark over a sleety road," was enormously comforted by her doctor's offer of a guaranteed delivery date. "Just like that. It was like ordering something from a store." After checking into the hospital for her long-planned appointment, she received Pitocin along with a simultaneous dose of Nembutal in anticipation of the imminent pain. Later she received scopolamine, then more Nembutal, eventually a third dose of Nembutal, and later a second injection of scopolamine. Awaking after twelve hours, she wondered aloud to the nurse when the baby would finally be born. " 'You've had it,' the nurse told her, 'hours ago. It's a little girl.' " The delighted new mother could not believe it. She mused that a man's suffering during birth was now far greater than a woman's: "I had a rousing good sleep and my husband was up all night pacing the floor and waiting for the phone to ring."[53]

Induction not only provided women and their doctors with the convenience of labors planned well in advance; the treatment also assured mothers that they would not feel a moment's pain because analgesia could be administered simultaneously with Pitocin. Planned due dates also alleviated the potentially deadly effect of anesthesia-induced nausea, for doctors could now instruct women not to eat anything for the twelve hours before their planned labors. Physicians justified elective induction with circular reasoning: induction was of great benefit because women could shun food and avoid one of the biggest dangers of the anesthesia that had become so common due to the painful contractions prompted by labor induction.[54]

Labor Induction and the Baby Boom

Although some obstetricians decried the popularity of Pitocin, most now defended elective induction without shame or defensiveness. This medical approval was not confined to big cities; in 1954 doctors in Galveston, Texas, spoke of the many benefits of birth by appointment. They advised that preplanned birth dates meant that women who lived far from the hospital would never again worry about arriving in time. Hospitals benefited as well, because most women would now be giving birth during the day, when the hospital was better staffed. One doctor argued that a patient's long drive to the hospital or a physician's desire to have patients deliver during "working hours" were both valid reasons to induce labor.[55]

Obstetricians even argued that elective induction was therapeutic, a procedure that allowed a woman to enter the hospital fully prepared mentally and physically. One Los Angeles doctor, who induced all women who were due to give birth while he was on vacation, contended that this too was therapeutic. He explained, "Some patients become so dependent upon us emotionally that our absence creates a situation which is definitely detrimental to their well-being and may exceed the risk of the induction of labor under proper circumstances."[56]

Woman's Home Companion similarly promoted the therapeutic benefits of Pitocin, assuring readers in 1955 that the synthetic hormone often shortened labor by many hours, permitting women (and their babies) to complete birth while still "at their physical best." In contrast, during spontaneous labor, adrenalin coursed through women's veins, "speeding the heartbeat and tensing . . . muscles." Pitocin released the uterus "from the grip of these fear hormones." The *Woman's Home Companion* article also compared the potential dangers of spontaneous labor with the seemingly inherent safety of induced labor. Readers of the magazine learned about Jane, a woman who had relied on her body to initiate labor and whose baby was born on the floor of an all-night drugstore after her desperate husband headed there when he realized they had run out of time to get to the hospital. Pregnant again and now living even farther from the hospital, Jane was in potentially worse straits. She fretted, "What if we get caught in a traffic jam? I just can't have another baby on the road!" Jane's birth-by-appointment not only alleviated her anxiety; it also gave her time to book a babysitter for her older child "and fill a suitcase with nightgowns and lacy bed jackets." When she arrived at the hospital, the "unrushed staff" was able to properly prepare her for delivery at their leisure.[57]

For the many young couples moving from the city to the growing suburbs after World War II, elective induction was a particularly welcome medical innovation. One young husband noted that when their first child was born in 1949, he and his wife lived only seven blocks from the Chicago hospital where his wife gave birth, and so they were able to check into a labor room within twenty minutes of her first labor pain. Two years later, however, they lived in a distant suburb northwest of the city, and traveling to each prenatal exam "seemed like an eternity." They were greatly relieved when their doctor offered to induce labor to alleviate their worries about traffic.[58]

A once-unpredictable event now occurred at everyone's convenience. Nurses took "charge without hurry" and admitted women "in a happy frame of mind without confusion." By eliminating the tension present when women entered the hospital in active labor, nurses could administer the prep in a leisurely fashion. This seemed to transform the nature of the reviled shave and enema. One physician described a prep administered at nurses' convenience as a "careful perineal preparation and a hot soapsuds enema." His terminology was telling; induction was apparently so advantageous that it transformed even the dreaded prep into an experience seemingly akin to deep tissue massage and a warm bubble bath.[59]

Increasingly Elaborate Drug Protocol

As the growing number of inductions prompted increased need for analgesia and anesthesia, the protocol for the relief of labor pain became more elaborate. One common obstetric routine was to administer some combination of Seconal, Demerol, and scopolamine immediately upon hospital admittance and then continue to dispense additional doses of the mixture as needed throughout labor. Despite the short life of the twilight sleep movement and the quick end to the intricate rituals associated with twilight sleep, scopolamine (sometimes still referred to as "twilight sleep" even at this later time) long remained an integral part of obstetric anesthesia regimens. Doctors noted consistently and approvingly that a combination of scopolamine, narcotics, and barbiturates ensured that laboring women would remember nothing of their experience. The mysterious "shot" that rendered Alice Munro Isaacs (the woman whose story begins this chapter) unconscious for twelve hours likely contained scopolamine and several analgesics, and she probably received multiple injections, administered whenever she began to stir, during her twelve-hour unconscious state. According to doctors, the analgesic-amnesiac cocktails given to women during first-stage labor prepared them well for the additional anesthesia they would receive during delivery, either nitrous oxide, a saddle block (what Isaacs received), or a pudendal block.[60]

Ironically, women's heavily medicated states encouraged the use of more drugs. In their attempts to mitigate women's drug-induced confusion and agitation, doctors often administered additional medication. One group of doctors reported, for example, that some patients given sodium amytal and scopolamine became so "maniacal" that medical personnel learned to subdue them with morphine. Similarly, to quiet mothers under the influence of paraldehyde and Nembutal or paraldehyde and sodium amytal, doctors in Atlanta kept ether handy in the delivery room.[61]

Other obstetricians used Thorazine, a tranquilizer synthesized by a French pharmaceutical company, to alleviate women's drug-induced confusion. In Augusta, Georgia, obstetricians regularly administered Thorazine to reduce both women's "maniacal excitement" and their babies' respiratory depression. At Boston Lying-In Hospital, obstetricians administered Thorazine in conjunction with

Advertisement for self-administered Penthrane, which was marketed directly to obstetricians by Abbott, a pharmaceutical company. "As the mother-to-be experiences pain, she lifts the inhaler into place as pictured, and breathes through it.... Using the method described, excessive administration is unlikely.... If she loses consciousness, the inhaler falls away." Note the precaution at the lower right to moderate the customary dosage of additional painkilling medications when also using Penthrane. *Source: Obstetrics and Gynecology* 11 (January 1958): 80–81.

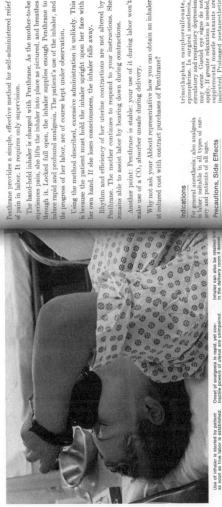
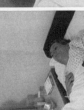

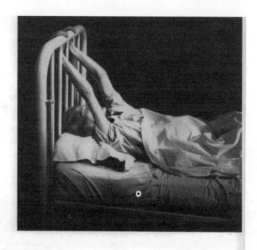

as adjunctive therapy in childbirth, Thorazine®, one of the fundamental
brand of chlorpromazine
drugs in medicine, allays apprehension and agitation; reduces suffering; minimizes the risk of respiratory depression; checks nausea and vomiting.   SMITH
KLINE &
FRENCH

Advertisement for Thorazine, which was marketed directly to obstetricians by the pharmaceutical company Smith, Kline, and French. The photograph implies that women will experience no agonized bed-rail-clutching during labor when under the influence of Thorazine. *Source: Obstetrics and Gynecology* 15 (January 1960): 60.

Seconal and scopolamine (and sometimes Demerol, dilaudid, or large doses of barbiturates) to similarly inhibit mothers' "various states of [drug-induced] mental agitation." Advertisements in obstetric journals for Thorazine called it "one of the fundamental drugs in medicine" and, by implication, in obstetrics.[62]

Physicians who used Thorazine in obstetrics reported uniformly that, of all drugs in use, Thorazine made women the most quiet and cooperative. Injected intramuscularly, it produced such profound "hypnotic sedative action" that doctors observed in laboring women under its influence a "'medical prefrontal lobotomy' effect . . . a torpor, a mask-like facial expression, a quiet phlegmatic acceptance of pain." Mental hospitals soon used it to tranquilize psychotic patients. The drug was so uniquely powerful that it transformed inpatient psychiatric care, converting the nation's locked and barred psychiatric wards into attractive dormitories with drapes and screen doors.[63]

Rather than developing a uniform obstetric drug protocol, hospitals all over the country followed their own unique, intricate regimens. A physician described the protocol at his Chicago hospital in the 1950s: When women "hit the floor," they received Seconal orally, followed thirty minutes later by an intramuscular injection of Demerol and scopolamine. Later, in the delivery room, women received either gas anesthesia, saddle block anesthesia, or a pudendal block. At Sloane Hospital for Women in New York City, the drugs used during first-stage labor included barbiturates ("for apprehension, a symptom common to primiparas, especially those with language difficulty or minimal intelligence"), opiates (for pain), and scopolamine (to erase memory). During delivery, 9 percent of women giving birth at Sloane received a pudendal block, 26 percent received caudal or spinal anesthesia, and 59 percent received inhalation anesthesia. Doctors in other areas of the country used assorted combinations of Demerol, scopolamine, nitrous oxide, ether, Seconal, heroin, and paraldehyde.[64]

Under the influence of so much medication, women were unaware of both their behavior during labor and the behavior of their newborns immediately after birth. Despite their ingestion of several painkilling drugs, women exhibited acute discomfort. They groaned and grimaced throughout the first stage of labor, not unlike the women given twilight sleep injections forty years earlier. The impact on the newborn of so much medication could be even more disturbing. One Chicago obstetrician who began practicing in the early 1950s recalled that some of his colleagues "gave *a lot* of seconal and *a lot* of Demerol [and] those babies would sleep and sleep."[65]

In rural areas, women were given large dosages of drugs less frequently. One physician from Waterloo, Iowa, observed that in his hospital there were rarely depressed babies because of "the parsimony of the doctors with narcotics during labor." Patients in the Waterloo area did receive Demerol intramuscularly once, if they requested it, but one-third of the women received no medication at all, and, the doctor noted, "a patient who is maniacal from excessive scopolamine is never seen." He credited the basic philosophy of Iowa physicians for this: "Iowa women are not stoic peasants by any means . . . however . . . it is far better to undersedate than oversedate and it is a continuing welcome relief to me to note the absence of beds with side rails and restraints in the labor rooms." He said urban hospitals ("where specialists dominate") used too many drugs during labor and did so be-

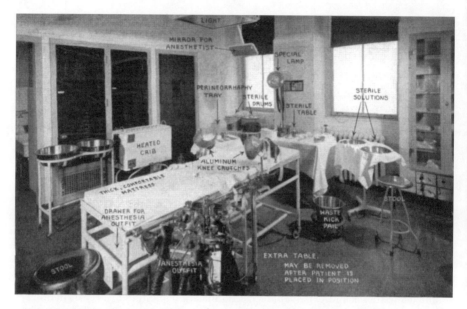

Note the emphasis on anesthesia in this delivery room at Sloane Hospital for Women in New York City in 1943, from the mirror dangling from the ceiling for the convenience of the anesthetist to the anesthesia outfit on the floor. *Source:* Louise Zabriskie and Nicholson J. Eastman, *Nurses Handbook of Obstetrics* (J. B. Lippincott, 1943), 339.

cause of medical competition. He argued that in rural America physicians could afford to be less aggressive.[66]

The Backlash Begins

One indication of the sheer volume of drugs given to women was the amount of medication used even by the doctors who consciously limited drug use. In the late 1950s in Johnson City, Tennessee, for example, obstetricians ended every prenatal exam by warning their patients that when mothers were drugged during labor, their infants were subject to serious risk. "We make every effort," Johnson City obstetricians explained, "to nurture in the patient a will to conscious participation in the birth process." Yet these doctors also left instructions with hospital personnel that if patients exhibited tension or fear, they should receive promethazine intramuscularly, followed by as many injections as necessary of scopolamine and Demerol, followed by trichloroethylene analgesia and a pudendal block during delivery.[67]

Doctors in Johnson City were nonetheless convinced that their educational efforts helped women avoid drugs. At least, they reported with satisfaction, none of their patients required barbiturates or opiates. Women were awake and talking during episiotomy repair, and immediately after delivery they were able to speak with their husbands—exceedingly unusual occurrences in the 1950s and 1960s. More heartening still, their babies were born alert and without breathing difficulties. Johnson City doctors thus urged the country's physicians to spend more time discussing the management of labor pain during prenatal visits in order to persuade women that wholly avoiding pain was a dangerous and unnecessary practice.[68]

This reluctance of some physicians to embrace the popular, widespread drug regimens foreshadowed the resumption of contentious battles such as those between Meigs and Simpson in the mid-nineteenth century and between Williams and DeLee in the early twentieth. Anesthesiologist Robert Hingson intimated the coming battle when he lamented in 1945 that doctors were replacing the comfort inherent in human companionship with drugs: "The psychologic neglect of parturients [is] appalling. In a great many . . . hospitals, less attention [is] paid . . . the labor room than . . . any other. . . . because most of the patients [are] heavily sedated." The president of the American Association of Obstetricians, Gynecologists, and Abdominal Surgeons likewise decried the new emphasis on medical procedures and drugs in lieu of consolation and cheer: "Carefully trained, scientifically stuffed, assembly-line produced physicians" had abandoned the art of medicine. Another critic noted that during the home-birth era, at least doctors had "offered confidence and reassurance along with a whiff of chloroform."[69]

Some physicians began to protest other aspects of the new obstetric protocol. In 1956 Dr. Harry Benaron, who was head of the Chicago Maternity Center, formerly known as the Chicago Lying-in Dispensary, the home birthing service started by DeLee in 1895, told colleagues he had nothing positive to say about labor induction. Like DeLee decades before, he characterized induction as "propelling the infant's brain through the birth passage tumultuously" and cited a study indicating that babies born under artificially stimulated labors had the highest rates of mental retardation. At a meeting of the American College of Obstetricians and Gynecologists in 1958, another doctor presented a University of Iowa study of almost seven thousand labors in which thirty-nine babies died as a direct result of induction. He said the deaths were "a significant price to pay for convenience."[70]

Women's magazines, originally among the most enthusiastic proponents of labor induction for social reasons, began to differentiate between legitimate and frivolous social reasons. *McCall's* listed valid reasons that included having several small children at home, living in a distant suburb, and attempting to avoid "yanking" a weary doctor out of bed in the middle of the night. Unwarranted social reasons included wanting a baby to be born on a specific date such as a wedding anniversary, or before January 1 to ensure a tax deduction, or to accommodate a doctor's upcoming vacation. *Good Housekeeping* provided a similar list, noting that if a woman had small children or lived far from the hospital, inducing labor was often a necessity. This legitimate-frivolous dichotomy proved so compelling that seven months after the *McCall's* article appeared, *Reader's Digest* ran a condensed version of it.[71]

Women's magazines began to print frightening stories of frivolously induced labors gone awry. *Good Housekeeping* described the experience of a woman who had been part of the French underground during World War II. Because her baby was due in July, she asked her doctor ("for sentimental reasons") to induce labor on Bastille Day. The doctor assented. Both the woman and her physician, however, had miscalculated the baby's due date; the infant weighed only four pounds two ounces and soon died of hyaline-membrane disease, the same ailment that had killed President John F. Kennedy's premature son, Patrick, the previous August. The *Good Housekeeping* article also relayed another tragic story, of a woman whose obstetrician, "an inveterate golf player," induced her labor so he would not have to attend her birth on the same weekend he was scheduled to play in a tournament. The woman, however, proved to be unusually sensitive to Pituitrin, and her contractions were so intense and prolonged that they temporarily deprived the fetus of oxygen. The baby was born with brain damage. "Such cases," the magazine admonished, "have become the focal point of the hottest controversy in the field of obstetrics since the thalidomide scandals of a year or so ago." Instead of promoting elective induction, *Good Housekeeping* now dubbed the procedure "possible elective tragedy."[72]

At first, the criticism had only marginal impact. The public, recently introduced to the miracle of antibiotics, tended to equate any new drug or medical procedure with undisputed progress. Pregnant women were especially affected by this idealization of medicine. Two physicians reported in 1963 that doctors prescribed at least one drug to 92 percent of pregnant women and that almost 4 percent of pregnant women ingested ten or more prescribed drugs during the course of their pregnancy. As the *Good Housekeeping* article suggested, however, the revelation that thalidomide had grotesquely malformed thousands of infants in utero eroded the knee-jerk conclusion that medicine and medical innovation were always beneficial.[73]

The growing public skepticism toward medicine soon encompassed the array of medications inhaled and ingested by, transfused and injected into, and administered rectally to women during labor. Virginia Apgar, who discovered—a decade before thalidomide made headlines around the world—that the medications given to laboring women often crossed the placenta, persisted in issuing her warnings that grown women had difficulty enough metabolizing the array of drugs administered to them in the hours before giving birth. A fetus had far worse difficulties.[74]

By the late 1960s, women had ceased accepting the stringent and elaborate medical treatment of birth and were charging that these practices bordered on the inhumane. Magazines began to publish articles describing and lauding "natural childbirth"; the phrase had been coined by British obstetrician Grantly Dick-Read in the 1930s but was little known in the United States until the 1950s and 1960s.[75]

Women's magazines once again exerted their influence, helping to convince mothers that natural childbirth was a viable alternative to heavily medicated labors. *McCall's* told of a physician who had been stationed in Igloo, South Dakota, while in the army. There, he and one other doctor provided all medical care for two thousand civilians. At first this doctor was nervous, since his only experience with pregnancy and childbirth had been in medical school. But his veteran colleague reassured him: "Don't worry about it. . . . there's only one rule to follow: Don't interfere. If you let nature take its course, most of the time your patients will be all right." During the two years he served in Igloo, the anxious doctor followed this advice; he now informed *McCall's* readers that, indeed, women did very nicely with little or no treatment during birth.[76]

Slowly, as a result of such reports, women began to insist on a reversal of the latest obstetric philosophy. Instead of equating elaborate medical treatment with guarantees of safety, women began to vilify heavily drugged hospital deliveries as unwanted and dangerous. The definitions of "necessary," "beneficial," and "risky" obstetric treatments were about to change dramatically once again.

The pressures of the baby boom prompted redefinition of both normal labor and the medical procedures necessary to support normal labor. Strict and elaborate obstetric protocol became standard in order to alleviate the demands made on crowded maternity wards, overworked doctors, and overwhelmed young mothers. Every aspect of the intricate protocol—but most notably induction, episiotomy, and use of forceps—either was spurred by or relied on the heavy use of analgesia and anesthesia throughout labor.

Doctors and mothers alike embraced these highly medicalized births. What had once been condemned as "meddlesome midwifery" now seemed to alleviate risk rather than pose unnecessary dangers. The combination of induction, analgesia, anesthesia, episiotomy, and outlet forceps, doctors argued, spared babies the "prolonged . . . 'pounding' . . . against the perineum [which] may cause brain injury." Mothers were also allegedly well served by the protocol. Stopping the baby's head from acting "as a battering ram against perineal obstruction" was thought to prevent short- and long-term pelvic floor damage and make giving birth a virtually effortless endeavor. The medical sociologist Barbara Katz Rothman has observed of this obstetric philosophy that surgical scissors now prevented babies from ripping their mothers apart while forceps foiled the vaginas and perineums intent on crushing babies' heads.[77]

There were occasional hints of dissatisfaction from women during these years. One mother wrote to DeLee to complain about the beds used in hospital delivery rooms. Calling the beds, with their flat mattresses and stirrups, "medieval," she charged that doctors designed them with one thought in mind, their own comfort. "I had two of my six children on them," she reported, "and—so help me—I'll never go near one again." She chastised DeLee: "It is high time that someone gave a little study to the matter from the mother's viewpoint for after all, tho you would not believe it to read the papers, in the vast majority of cases it is still the mother and not the doctor that has the responsibility and effort of producing the baby." Another disgruntled woman preferred "that final gorgeous burst of speed and effort and agony and knowing everything that is going on . . . [to] any semi-oblivion."[78]

Women began to testify to the discomforts and indignities inherent in the new protocol. Decca Romilly, who gave birth to her second child at Columbia Hospital in Washington, DC, in 1941, was typical. She arrived at the hospital by appointment. At five o'clock the next morning, she consumed "rather a curious breakfast consisting of a whole tumbler full of castor oil," which was followed by an enema. Romilly, who was British and had given birth to her first child in England, then spent the next three hours "scramming to the loo." Nurses came into the room, but instead of acknowledging her discomfort, they "absentmindedly" felt Romilly's abdomen and asked, "Any good contractions yet?" At eleven o'clock a nurse took her to another room, had her don an open-backed gown that barely covered her stomach ("v. indecent"), and then strapped her to "a sort of medieval torture table where they tie your hands & legs down." A doctor came in and punctured her amniotic sac. Then a nurse wheeled her into a ward where she joined six other women. Romilly reported that upon entering the room, "instead of saying 'here comes another patient' or even 'here comes Mrs. Romilly'. . . [the nurse] just shoved me around on the stretcher saying 'here comes another ruptured membrane.'"

According to Romilly, the nurses assigned to the labor ward spent their time chatting with one another and playing cards, "paying absolutely no attention to the groans and writhing going on all around, except occasionally to say sharply to some screaming woman 'Lie down AT ONCE! You're not to sit up.'" Doctors stopped by on occasion to offer Romilly pills to relieve her pain, but each time she declined, "afraid that if I took anything I'd lose control & start screaming like the others were." She eventually took the mysterious pills but remained semiconscious until finally inhaling ether in the delivery room. After World War II, according to most women's and physicians' reports, obstetric practice became even more elaborate and the drug regimen far more severe.[79]

Americans tend to think of the customs of healers in premodern societies as steeped in inconsequential ceremony. Yet anthropologist Robbie Davis-Floyd argues persuasively that the American birth rituals introduced in the 1940s, 1950s, and 1960s, practices that became known in the aggregate as "standard procedures for normal birth," were at least as elaborate as birth traditions practiced in "primitive" cultures and, like many traditional healing ceremonies, served primarily to reassure rather than treat. What came to be the routine medical accoutrements of hospital birth after World War II—the hospital gown, the shave, the enema, the intravenous fluids, the Pitocin drip, the rupture of the amniotic sac, the analgesia, the maternal monitor, the fetal monitor, the anesthesia, the surgical scissors, the episiotomy, and the forceps—were all generally unnecessary to ensure a safe birth. But these elements transformed an inherently uncontrollable biological event into a technological routine, making the vast majority of American women and their physicians more comfortable with birth in the process.[80]

What had been comforting to one generation, however, became galling to the next. By the early 1970s, women were rebelling en masse against what they considered impersonal, unnecessary, even dangerous, medical routines. Whereas mothers of the baby boomers had turned birth over to their doctors, their daughters determinedly reclaimed birth as their own to shape as they saw fit. Whereas mothers of the baby boomers received such elaborate drug combinations that they knew little to nothing about giving birth even after bearing several children, their daughters insisted on knowing and fully experiencing every moment of an event they considered empowering and transformative.

CHAPTER FIVE

Natural Childbirth and Birth Reform

The Question of Authority, 1950s through 1980s

*W*hen Ina May Middleton, a twenty-six-year-old Northern Illinois University graduate student, was pregnant with her first child in 1966, she did not worry about labor pain. Her mother's assurance that labor was not that bad had instilled in Middleton an offhand confidence about birth. She did, however, dread the prospect of unconsciousness. At a routine appointment one week before her due date, she told her obstetrician she did not want any anesthesia during labor. Her doctor was shocked. He told Middleton he could not sanction an "uncontrolled delivery" and explained that when the birth process was left to its own devices the baby's head acted like a "battering ram," often resulting in injury to the mother's perineum and brain damage to her child.

This contention puzzled Middleton. As a child, she had spent summers with her grandmother and her aunts on the family farm in Iowa. There she witnessed many births, and none of the newborn animals seemed brain-damaged. Besides, she wrote later, "My perineum didn't feel like steel to me, and I didn't really believe that brain damage was any more likely to result from perineum pounding than it was from anesthesia or forceps." She left her doctor's office hoping she had persuaded him to let her attempt an unanesthetized birth.

Three days later she went into labor and checked into the hospital. She labored noiselessly, hoping her silence would enhance her chance of avoiding anesthesia. Lying on her side and breathing deeply, she imagined she was a mountain lion. As her contractions intensified, she pictured elaborate patterns on the wall. After a few hours, her obstetrician insisted she have Demerol. She did not argue. A nurse administered the injection.

The Demerol made Middleton nauseous and groggy and did not reduce her pain. Her husband tried to help her relax by rubbing her lower back, but under the influence of the Demerol, she lost her ability to concentrate. By the time her physician and several nurses entered the room with all the paraphernalia needed to administer spinal anesthesia ("they were only with me when they wanted to do something to me"), she had resigned herself to accepting whatever they offered.

After administering the spinal, the doctor and nurses ordered Middleton's husband to the waiting room, lifted Middleton onto a gurney, wheeled her into a delivery room, strapped her down, gave her an episiotomy, and pulled her baby out with forceps, "like a giant wisdom tooth." Sixteen hours later, when she saw her daughter for the first time, Middleton felt "inhibited, ridiculous, and suddenly old." She felt none of the joy and triumph she had imagined. Instead, her most overwhelming emotion was embarrassment.[1]

Four years later, when she gave birth to her second child, much had changed—for the United States socially and politically and for Middleton personally. Martin Luther King and Robert Kennedy had been assassinated, Americans increasingly objected to the Vietnam War, and the activism and social change generated by the civil rights, women's, and antiwar movements were well under way. What many college students dubbed "the cultural revolution" was at its height, and Middleton was in the thick of it. She had divorced and remarried; her second husband was Stephen Gaskin, leader of "the Caravan," three hundred young adults traveling in assorted school buses and vans on a national tour to disseminate Gaskin's spiritual teachings. Ina May Gaskin recalled of the Caravan, "Stephen was always saying in the early days of our church that if we had a platform, it was clean air, sane people, and healthy babies."

Several women on the tour, including Ina May, were pregnant. With extremely limited funds and no health insurance, hospital birth for any of them was out of the question. Besides, the women traveling with the Caravan who had given birth previously in the hospital had been unhappy with their treatment there. Ina May remembered, "We wanted our men to be with us during the whole process of childbirth, and we didn't want to be anesthetized against our will, and we didn't want to be separated from our babies after their births. We were already looking for a better way."

The first Caravan baby was born in a school bus parked in a Northwestern University lot. Ina May and the baby's father rendered aid to the mother. After attending the birth of the second Caravan baby, Ina May began to read everything she could find on delivering babies. The tenth baby born on the trip was Ina May's. Born two months early, he died twelve hours later, probably of hyaline membrane disease. Ina May's interest in midwifery intensified.

In 1971 Stephen Gaskin, his followers, and their children settled on one thousand acres near Summertown, Tennessee, to develop a self-sufficient agricultural collective they dubbed "the Farm," an endeavor that thrives to this day. Quite inadvertently, the Farm became best known not for Stephen Gaskin's teachings but for its Midwifery Center founded and directed by his wife, Ina May. The center soon became a beacon for a nationwide birth reform movement.[2]

Ina May Gaskin and Birth Reform

Ina May Gaskin's first experience giving birth, along with the anger she felt, typified birth for many women in the mid-twentieth century. Obstetricians in the 1940s, 1950s, and 1960s often rebuffed patients' requests, and women's complaints of receiving unwanted treatments had been slowly building in number and intensity since the late 1930s, when the first sporadic critiques of obstetric practice appeared almost unnoticed in magazines amid the far more numerous articles applauding the latest obstetric innovations.[3]

By the early 1970s, around the time Ina May settled on the Farm, these isolated, erratic complaints of forced medical treatment during labor and birth had swelled. In the first issue of *Ms. Magazine,* a woman who had enjoyed her first child's "natural" birth in England described her starkly different experience when her second child was born in a New York hospital. Disregarding her express wishes, the doctor ordered her husband out of the delivery room and tied her legs up in stirrups. When she demanded to be untied, nurses bound her wrists to the table. When she struggled in vain to sit up, the doctor and nurses laughed at her. After the birth, the doctor came to her room to berate her for her "display." Furious, she penned the article for *Ms.* describing her humiliation. She urged American women to pool their energy to "revolutionize the system."[4]

The article was a manifestation of what soon became widespread discontent with American birth techniques. The birth reform movement stemming from this dissatisfaction was an integral part of two broader crusades, the women's movement and the consumers' movement of the 1970s. As women demanded reforms in all aspects of their social, economic, political, and personal lives and consumers demanded better and safer products manufactured by socially responsible industries, a "good" birth came to be defined as a birth controlled by the laboring woman, without unnecessary and potentially dangerous medical treatments. Ina May Gaskin became a well-known advocate for an approach to birth in which trust of women's bodies was paramount.

By then a certified professional midwife, Gaskin wrote and spoke widely about the "spiritual experience" and "sacrament" of childbirth. In her speeches and writings she advocated unanesthetized home birth in the presence of friends and family. At the Farm she encouraged women to remain mobile for as long as possible and to eat and drink as desired throughout labor. By the early 1980s, the Farm's clinic-infirmary boasted nine certified professional midwives, two physicians, a laboratory, a neonatal intensive care unit, two ambulances operated by a state-approved ambulance service that also served neighboring rural communities free of charge, and a stellar record of birth safety.[5]

The path to birth reform symbolized by Ina May Gaskin's work was complex and circuitous. The nationwide, often militant movement for reform was shaped by a confluence of forces that included frustration with the inflexibility of postwar obstetric practice; the willingness to challenge authority that permeated the entire culture in the wake of the civil rights, antiwar, and women's movements; and the profound influence of natural childbirth theoreticians and practitioners in light of the "question authority" tendencies of the 1960s and 1970s.

Mothers Rebel

Long before the women's movement promoted an array of reforms in women's health and medicine in the 1970s, religious groups generated some of women's initial interest in what eventually became known generically as "natural childbirth." The Catholic Maternity Institute in Santa Fe, New Mexico, founded in 1944 by the Medical Mission Sisters, for example, trained nuns and laywomen to be nurse-midwives. These midwives provided full-service medical care to poor Latina women; in doing so, they emphasized emotional support over medical treatment during birth. The Christian Family Movement, an organization championing various family and social-justice issues, likewise spurred interest in changing the relationship between doctors and women. The eight women who in 1957 founded La Leche League (LLL), the international breastfeeding promotion and support organization, were all active in the Christian Family Movement. LLL foreshadowed the gist of the birth reform movement when its leaders urged women to reclaim infant feeding from patronizing physicians, eschew formula, and trust their bodies to produce all the food necessary to sustain their babies.[6]

Religion was initially so important to promoting interest in birth reform that even the pope weighed in on obstetric treatment. In 1949 the Catholic Church designated doctors responsible for mitigating "the sufferings of birth." In a subsequent declaration in 1956, Pope Pius XII also told a group of Catholic obstetricians and gynecologists that the philosophy of Grantly Dick-Read was not immoral. Dick-Read, the British obstetrician who coined the phrase "natural childbirth" in the 1930s, theorized that women who consciously relaxed during labor and avoided feelings of fear could easily forgo anesthesia. The title of one of Dick-Read's books, *Childbirth without Fear*, reflected his basic theory. "Christian obstetrics," the pope assured physicians, did not conflict with Dick-Read's tenets. Three years after the pope's pronouncement on Dick-Read, the Utah Valley Hospital of the Church of Jesus Christ of Latter Day Saints in Provo sponsored one of the first childbirth courses held in a hospital and likely the first such series of classes not on the East Coast. The classes emphasized the centrality of women's efforts in giving birth.[7]

Religion remained an important promoter of natural childbirth. One influential book in this regard was *Natural Childbirth and the Christian Family*, authored by Helen Wessel in 1963. Wessel, who bore six children between the late 1940s and 1961, gave birth to her first three babies under conventional circumstances that included wrist and ankle restraints, both spinal and general anesthesia, episiotomy, forceps, and excruciating postpartum spinal headaches. She did not discover the teachings of Grantly Dick-Read—with whom she later shared a treasured correspondence—until just before the birth of her fourth child in 1954. In her book, Wessel combined Dick-Read's theory of natural birth with basic Christian teachings. She urged readers to have "faith in the rightness and beauty of conception and birth; faith in a loving God who made our bodies as they are. Rest on this faith when labor begins, relax all tensions and cares and wait patiently for love's reward." Wessel eventually became president of the influential International Childbirth Education Association.[8]

Yet religion was by no means the only avenue for spreading Dick-Read's ideas. By the late 1940s, many pregnant American women learned of Dick-Read either through word of mouth or quite by accident when browsing the pregnancy section of bookstores. Dick-Read's theory of natural childbirth elicited such enthusiasm among these women that even their husbands became proselytizers. At Wesley Memorial Hospital in Chicago, where nurses encouraged fathers banished to waiting rooms to record their thoughts in Stork Club Books rather than just nervously pace, one calm entry appeared in 1949 amid dozens of anguished ones. "The birth was quite a natural process," wrote this erudite father. "No anaesthetics because Margaret didn't want any . . . she showed how good it was to have a natural childbirth and explained to the doctors about the 'Read method' while she was in labor. . . . Doctors (generally) know the technicalities of what is happening when a child comes out, but [I] don't think many have much understanding of the psychology. . . . We just have to read 'Childbirth Without Fear' by Read for ourselves and maybe someday bring the hospitals around to the encouragement of natural childbirth instead of dependence on mechanical intervention and not informing the mother or father how the process is going."[9]

Like this new father, critics of American obstetric practice often singled out obstetric anesthesia for special condemnation. One mother explained in *Parents Magazine* in 1948 that after bearing two children, what she had come to dread most when anticipating another birth was "the thought of the anesthetic."[10]

The few organizations in the early 1950s devoted to scrutiny of American birthing practices provided particularly unforgiving analysis. The Maternity Center Association, an organization that helped spark initial interest in natural childbirth in the United States, described American obstetric practice derisively in 1953: "The mother is considered just a pregnant uterus, the baby an impersonal fetus, the father a nuisance—and the miracle of new life just another cold-blooded surgical operation." Yet before the late 1950s, this type of direct, harsh condemnation was rare.[11]

The first wholesale public dissatisfaction with hospital birth did not appear until May 1958, when the *Ladies' Home Journal* published an article titled "*Journal* Mothers Report on Cruelty in Maternity Wards." A letter from a nurse that had been printed the previous November instigated the "report." In her brief but scathing exposé, the nurse described women strapped to delivery room tables with cuffs around their arms and legs and steel clamps over their shoulders and chests. She condemned doctors with "charming examination-table manners [who] show traces of sadism in the delivery room" and implored the *Journal* to investigate "the tortures that go on in modern delivery rooms." An editorial query appeared beneath the letter: Would *Journal* readers care to refute or corroborate the nurse's charges?[12]

Six months later, when the "Cruelty" article appeared, *Journal* editors reported that in the magazine's eighty-year history, only a handful of articles had elicited a comparable "flood" of letters from readers. The article accompanying this observation detailed the pervasive maltreatment of women in maternity wards. Furious mothers complained of "assembly line techniques" and "not [being] treated as . . . a human being." A woman from Kansas wrote that under no circumstance was childbirth pleasant, "but there is no reason to make it a hell on earth." A Detroit mother whose husband was a veterinarian observed, "Even animal maternity cases are treated with a little more grace than is accorded human mothers." A Columbus, Ohio, woman charged that nurses routinely locked women for hours "in lonely labor rooms," only to eventually shuttle them "off to delivery rooms among brusque strangers like sacks of potatoes from the A&P."

Half of the women who shared their stories with the *Journal* accused nurses of preventing them from pushing at the end of second-stage labor—despite an uncontrollable urge to do so—because the doctor had not yet arrived. "I was helpless and at their mercy," recalled a mother from Georgia. A California woman complained that a nurse climbed on the delivery table and sat on her knees to forestall an imminent birth.

Women also condemned mandatory analgesia and anesthesia. "They give you drugs, whether you want them or not," reported one mother. "Modern painkillers and methods are used for the convenience of the doctor, not to spare the mother," complained another. Perhaps most telling was the testimony of a mother who successfully refused a nurse's offer of Demerol and, in doing so, felt "wonderfully *in command*."[13]

Seven months after the article appeared, the *Ladies' Home Journal* ran a second piece expanding on women's grievances. *Journal* editors testified that letters continued to arrive daily, not only from angry mothers but also from husbands, nurses, and even doctors "who had witnessed tortures [in American maternity wards] not very different from those used in Japanese prisoner-of-war camps."

Even more than the first article, this one emphasized the dangers of anesthesia. The piece began with the story of a developmentally disabled nine-year-old named Danny, "the victim of a delayed delivery." When Danny's birth was imminent, the doctor had not yet arrived, so nurses held Danny's mother's legs together and gave her anesthesia for three hours. Danny's mother remained so shaken by the event, and so heartbroken by the result, that she vowed that when her next child was born, she and her husband would travel an extra twenty miles to the only hospital in the vicinity that permitted a husband to be by his wife's side during labor (although not during the delivery). She hoped her husband's presence in the labor room would protect her from reckless nurses and absent doctors. She warned other women, "The responsibility for careful delivery of your unborn child rests on you."[14]

This mother's admonition signified far more than one woman's grief and anger. Fifteen years after her warning, obstetricians found it exceedingly difficult to mandate medical treatment without consulting their patients: women both questioned the wisdom of routine obstetric practices and demanded involvement in medical decision-making. The paternalism of physicians that was rife in the immediate postwar years, when a doctor could unilaterally decide to administer general anesthesia to a laboring woman or deny nutrition to a severely deformed infant and tell the parents the baby had been stillborn, prompted a broad rethinking of American medicine between 1966 and 1976. All physicians were affected by this dramatic change in social thought, but obstetricians experienced the challenge to their authority in a broader, more public forum than did other medical specialists.[15]

The Question of Authority

As critiques of physicians' paternalism became more pervasive, women asked more and bolder questions about standard obstetric practice. Why couldn't relatives and friends stay with them as they labored and gave birth? Why couldn't both labor and birth take place in the same hospital room? Would their doctor be willing to attend a home birth? Why did nurses shave women's pubic hair? Was an enema really necessary during labor? What was the purpose of placing women in restraints? Why did women have to be unconscious during birth? Was labor really that unbearable? What effect did anesthesia have on newborns? Was labor induction safe? Did episiotomies really benefit women? Formulating, asking, and demanding answers to these questions represented a genuine challenge to long-established obstetric procedures.

This challenge did not appear overnight; it developed slowly over about fifteen years. After the two *Journal* articles appeared in 1958, other magazines continued to sow seeds of discontent by publishing positive stories of unconventional births. A thirty-two-year-old Minnesota woman, for example, who reported having a wonderful birth under hypnosis, assured the readers of *Better Homes and Gardens* that she and her husband were not prone to odd behaviors. "We are average people. We go to the House of Prayer Lutheran Church, like to watch television, and when we go out my widowed mother comes over from Saint Paul to baby-sit." Ordinary women like this one, who enthusiastically recommended nontraditional birth practices, lent credibility to the growing disparagement of standard obstetric treatment. Other mothers listened when the average American woman recommended birth "without the fuzziness that comes from getting a drug and gas."[16]

Yet even as women criticized hospital birth in the late 1950s and proposed alternatives, they did not insist on hegemony, as their daughters eventually did in the 1970s and 1980s. Rather than demand an active role in medical decision-making, most women demonstrated their dissatisfaction with obstetrics far more subtly: they began to talk to each other about birth. One woman, who had given birth to seven children in five states, observed excitedly in the second *Ladies' Home Journal* article alleging cruelty in maternity wards that for the first time in her long and varied experience as a mother, "young wives are comparing notes!"[17]

These developments made many doctors exceedingly uncomfortable. In his 1959 annual address, the president of the American Association of Obstetricians and Gynecologists alluded angrily to derogatory articles in lay magazines: "Why do others impugn our knowledge, force advice upon us, and often insist on taking over—except in the delivery room at three o'clock in the morning?" Other physicians dismissed women's charges of maltreatment with sweeping indictments of their own, telling the *Ladies' Home Journal* that most women were "spoiled, hysterical and full of fears" and most husbands were "too emotionally unstable to stay with their wives during labor." These physicians denied there was any validity to women's complaints of maltreatment—accusations that included unwanted anesthesia—with the ironic observation, "The memory of a childbirth experience is unreliable because of anesthetic drugs."[18]

In the early 1970s, the animosity between women and their doctors peaked. An early edition of the feminist health manifesto *Our Bodies, Ourselves* reflected this anger. The book urged women to learn about their bodies in order to wrest medical care from "condescending, paternalistic, judgmental and non-informative" physicians. The counsel went beyond mere words. Beginning in 1969, the Chicago Women's Liberation Union formed a clandestine abortion service. Called Jane because word of mouth informed women who wanted to terminate their pregnancies to call a certain number and "ask for Jane," the group referred women to sympathetic physicians for safe, albeit illegal, abortions. When the women who ran Jane discovered that their most reliable "doctor" had never been to medical school, they decided that they too could learn how to perform safe abortions. Before the U.S. Supreme Court mandated legalization of the medical procedure in 1973, the laywomen who made up the Jane collective performed eleven thousand abortions.[19]

As the story of Jane attests, much of the focus of the women's health reform movement was on self-reliance and self-education, a focus that included childbirth training. The Boston Women's Health Book Collective, the group that authored *Our Bodies, Ourselves*, assured women, "Giving birth does not have to be lonely and frightening. . . . We can prepare ourselves." In citing the significantly lower maternal and infant mortality rates in western European countries where midwife-attended home birth was common, the authors of *Our Bodies, Ourselves* challenged even the bedrock of American obstetric treatment, obstetrician-attended hospitalized birth. As women active in birth reform learned of the outcomes in Ina May Gaskin's home-birth midwifery practice, which were far better than in similar hospital births, this too gave credence to even the most strident critiques of American birth practices.[20]

Yet while natural childbirth and birth reform became well-publicized focuses of the largely white women's health reform movement, similar calls for change did not emanate from the black community. For black women, the changes being forwarded as revolutionary were probably old news: birthing practices among black women had long resembled what natural childbirth advocates now called revolutionary. One study of childbirth folk beliefs in largely black North Philadelphia conducted in the mid-1970s, for example, found that black women preferred to labor at home until the last possible moment. If you go to the hospital too early, one woman contended, "the doctors starts messing you around and it makes the pains worse." Another woman explained that walking around at home, as opposed to lying in a hospital bed, made labor easier. The anthropologist who conducted the North Philadelphia study attributed the tendency of many black women to self-manage their labors to the fact that hospital birth was a more recent innovation in the black community than in the white community. Black women thus were comfortable handling the vagaries of birth in their homes.[21]

"Granny midwives" who attended home births were common in southern black communities through the 1960s. One midwife, who attended three thousand births in Alabama before her retirement in 1981 and never lost a mother, described how she instilled a matter-of-fact attitude toward labor in her clients. "I'd tell them, 'Well, honey child, you're going to have to hurt before your baby's born. . . . If you are going to buck and ram and holler, you ain't going to help you none. You might as well settle yourself down and do the best you can."[22]

The few black women active in birth reform used the movement not only to usher in more humane hospital practices but also to spotlight racist inequities in society. Shafia Monroe, executive director of the Traditional Childbearing Group, an organization of independent midwives who served black neighborhoods in Boston, noted in a 1987 speech that someone once told her it was reasonable for white women to have home births because the homes of white women usually had sufficient heat. Monroe admonished, "What if a [black] woman leaves a cold house to go to the hospital and have a baby? Three days later she'll be coming back to the same cold house with a newborn baby."[23]

While the black community mostly ignored news of birth reform and natural childbirth in the 1970s, the criticism of hospital births emanating from the primarily white, middle-class women's movement became increasingly harsh. As in the 1950s, condemnation focused on the indiscriminate use of anesthesia. The Boston Women's Health Book Collective accused obstetricians of using general anesthesia because they "like their patients to be totally unaware of the obstetrical procedures used," especially episiotomy and forceps. *Our Bodies, Ourselves* then went on to describe the effect of assorted analgesics and anesthetics in detail, so that women could make their own informed decision about the use of pain relief, but the book's position on obstetric anesthesia was clear. The authors warned that "every drug, every method of anesthesia" posed risk to mothers and babies and urged women to remember that although transition (the end of first-stage labor, when women need pain relief most) is "very intense," it is also brief. They advised women to weigh the risks of anesthesia against their ability to withstand "this very last bit" of first-stage labor and not unquestioningly accept doctors' judgment that anesthesia was always necessary.[24]

As the budding women's movement, and soon popular culture, began to celebrate the strength, vitality, and creative ability of women, these words resonated. Natural childbirth became a vehicle to demonstrate women's effectiveness and power. Birth reform organizations sprang up in every area of the country, criticizing standard obstetric methods and educating women about alternatives. Women responded to these organizations in force. They attended childbirth preparation classes, insisted on their husbands' presence in delivery rooms, refused anesthesia, and sought doctors who encouraged and supported physiological labor. Some even gave birth at home.[25]

One woman who had her first child in Detroit in 1968 was cognizant of these developments, and her response to doctors' and nurses' treatment of her when she gave birth proved to be increasingly representative. On learning of her pregnancy, she sought out a childbirth class and prepared for a natural birth. After laboring in the hospital for several days, however, she let a nurse administer Demerol. She remembers: "I'd been in control all that time and breathing. But with the medication on board I could no longer control myself and . . . work with the contractions anymore. And so I found that it was worse than having nothing." Later, as the nurse wheeled her down the hall to delivery, she rallied. Finally, the birth was imminent. But then the nurse, without warning or asking, "just put something in my IV and that was it. I woke up at the end of delivery. . . . strapped to these arm boards that kind of had you spread-eagled so I couldn't lift off the table to even see what they were doing. . . . they completely took over the experience." She responded to this treatment by having her next three babies at home.[26]

Disgruntled mothers like this one embraced birth reform organizations. These groups took many forms. Some were grassroots and stand-alone; others affiliated with national or international organizations such as the International Childbirth Education Association (ICEA), which was first formed from nine local groups in the mid-1950s. The steady increase in affiliates of ICEA heralded the newly massive interest in natural childbirth and birth reform. By 1975 ICEA had 160 local and regional chapters in the United States alone.[27]

Most of the grassroots organizations shared similar analyses of the shortcomings of modern obstetric practice and, given the activism of the 1970s, espoused similar militant tactics for change. Ranging from Birthday, a Boston-area organization, to Birth Community Inc., headquartered in St. Paul–Minneapolis, these groups charged that mothers and their babies were at the mercy of uncompassionate doctors and impersonal institutions and that as a result a frightened, lonely, heavily drugged woman forced to undergo an episiotomy and a forceps delivery and then be separated from her infant for twelve hours or more had become the norm. Leaders of Birthday protested, "The ideal childbirth has become something done to a woman—not something she does." Birth Community Inc. promoted home births avidly; the organization taught women how to apply for birth certificates for babies born at home, fought for the right of lay midwives to practice "whether certified, registered, licensed, or unregulated," and invited Ina May Gaskin to speak at a local church.[28]

Strategies to transform American birthing practices were diverse and imaginative. One tactic was the unauthorized assessment of hospitals by laywomen; the first such "inspection" took place in Tallahassee, Florida, in March 1977. Other, increasingly militant, inspections quickly followed. In July, representatives from two organizations, the Los Angeles Feminist Women's Health Center and Womancare, headquartered in San Diego, toured the maternity ward of the Los Angeles County–University of Southern California Medical Center Women's Hospital. The ensuing exchange between the unsuspecting nurses conducting the tour and the representatives of the two feminist organizations was hostile. In summarizing the visit, members of Womancare and the Feminist Women's Health Center declared labor and delivery at that hospital "probably the least humane any of us had ever seen. . . . The nurses hardly talked to or touched the women. Most of their attention went to the machines." The unauthorized inspectors warned ominously that they planned additional similar visits "to understand the power structure and implementation of procedures at this large institution where 1 out of every 200 babies in this country is born."[29]

Borrowing tactics from the antiwar movement, guerrilla-theater-type confrontations became common. MOTHER (Mothers Of The wHole Earth Revolt) was another California-based organization, whose avowed purpose was "to *demand* changes in the hospital." Part of MOTHER's "nine-month action plan" was to encourage women to share their experiences and confront offending doctors ("let them know we know who they are and what they do to women and babies"). Members of MOTHER declared, "Birth is normal and hospitals are terrible. These facts need no further proof. . . . We are reclaiming motherhood. We will reclaim birth."[30]

The animosity escalated. At the University of Michigan, the books written by J. Robert Willson, chair of the department of obstetrics and gynecology from 1964 to 1978, had to be moved temporarily from the medical library's main stacks to the well-guarded rare-book room after a women's rights group burned one of his coauthored books, *Obstetrics and Gynecology,* on the campus green. The group objected to a chapter in the book titled "Psychology and Life Periods of Women," which was written not by Willson or his coauthors but by two professors at Temple University School of Medicine. The chapter likened women to frightened children and their physicians to protective parents who understood and ably treated women's anxiety. Four years later, in the fifth edition of the same text, the offending chapter had been heavily revised, making it, in Willson's and his coauthors' words, "more appropriate to the rapidly changing attitudes and life patterns of contemporary women."[31]

Displeasure with obstetricians and obstetric practice manifested itself even clandestinely. In the index of the 923-page 1976 edition of *Williams Obstetrics,* placed between "Chancroid" and "Chemotherapy," was the entry: "Chauvinism, male, variable amounts, 1–923." Four years later, when the sixteenth edition of *Williams Obstetrics* appeared, the entry remained, although irritation with obstetric practice had been turned up a notch by the mysterious writer: "Chauvinism, male, voluminous amounts, 1–1102." Jack Pritchard's feminist wife had mischievously slipped the lines into both editions of the standard obstetric text. Pritchard, a professor in the Department of Obstetrics and Gynecology at the University of Texas Southwestern Medical School, was the text's lead author. His wife had compiled the index. By 1985 the tenor of the times had changed enough that in the seventeenth edition of the text, which still bears J. Whitridge Williams's name despite his death in 1931, the line had been vanquished.[32]

When the first "Chauvinism, male" entry appeared in *Williams* in 1976, however, conversations about the nature of childbirth had become a war of words. The individuals and organizations seeking to reshape societal perception of birth deemed a change in vocabulary vital to their mission. The American Society for Psychoprophylaxis in Obstetrics (ASPO), the national organization promoting the Lamaze method, assiduously replaced the word *pain* with *contraction* and the phrase *labor pain* with *work of labor* in all Society literature. Ina May Gaskin rejected both *contraction* and *pain* and substituted the word *rush,* explaining, "I think it describes better how to flow with the birthing energy." A Yale University obstetrician who was a leading proponent of natural childbirth carefully explained the fuss: "The sensation of a 'labor pain' is not comparable to other sensations ordinarily called 'pain,'" and so use of the word "pain" generated unnecessary fear.[33]

As the birth reform movement gained momentum, a few obstetricians did publicly recommend ceding some authority to patients. In a 1974 article in the *American Journal of Obstetrics and Gynecology* (*AJOG*), Irwin H. Kaiser, a New York obstetrician-gynecologist, and his wife, Barbara L. Kaiser, criticized the "masculine stronghold" of obstetrics and gynecology. Noting that the women's movement had recently hailed the legalization of abortion as "finally giving women control over the use of their own bodies as breeding machines," the Kaisers argued that *Roe v. Wade* was one of many signs that physicians sharing authority with patients was inevitable.[34]

Before its publication in *AJOG*, the Kaisers presented their article to colleagues attending the ninety-seventh annual meeting of the American Gynecological Society, where reactions to the Kaisers' recommendation mimicked the contentious public debate. One doctor from Oklahoma City agreed with the Kaisers that the women's health movement had focused appropriately and necessarily on the "demeaning nature of gynecologic care" as one of many examples of the social inequities faced by women. A physician from St. Louis, however, urged colleagues to ignore the exhortations to share authority with patients and not "forsake the women who are the epitome of stability in our society in order to seek the approbation of the militant feminists who seem to be obsessed with a fantasy that somehow all will be Utopian when the top dog is a female."[35]

After the article's publication, some physicians wrote to *AJOG* in support of the Kaisers' suggestion. Whether or not feminists' demands were fair, they noted, women's doctors had to change the way they practiced medicine because discontent with obstetrical and gynecological treatments reflected women's rapidly changing role in society. Women were demanding and receiving the right to participate in the social, economic, and political arenas on a par with men, so doctors could not avoid ceding women greater voice in their own medical care.[36]

As the doctors who supported the Kaisers' recommendations predicted, by the early 1980s birth reformers had achieved tangible success. Hospitals now offered many alternatives to women. St. Joseph's Hospital in St. Paul, Minnesota, was typical. The institution now invited pregnant patients to fill out a form entitled "Your Personalized Birth Plan," allowing them to mark their preferences from a preprinted list of options that included permitting older children to witness the birth of their sibling; playing music during labor; wearing pajamas brought from home instead of a hospital-provided, open-backed gown; photographing or filming the birth; dimming the lights during birth; and using a birthing chair. There was even a space for additional requests.[37]

Hospitals now used the decades-long accusations of inhumane treatment to their advantage. Institutions competed for maternity "center" patients (in the war of words, maternity "ward" sounded impoverished, harsh, and impersonal), each claiming that its smorgasbord of selections was the most comfortable and caring available. The minimal offering was a private, cozy, tastefully decorated room in which to labor, deliver, and recover (that is, a homey "LDR" room). Not all doctors were pleased with this development. One obstetric anesthesiologist ridiculed the new LDR rooms as an "illusion of a home" replete with beautiful damasks and quilts. He found it farcical, not to mention supremely annoying, to have to press buttons to access the cleverly hidden equipment he needed in case of a medical emergency. Hospitals complemented the lovely LDR rooms with "rooming-in," that is, keeping mother and baby together to facilitate bonding and breast-feeding. And, most pleasing to women, hospitals now considered relatives and friends, but especially the male partners of laboring women, vital members of the "birth team."[38]

Women had sought this latter reform for decades. Long before the first stirrings of the women's movement, the request heard most often from laboring women, regardless of their feelings about anesthesia and "the prep," was to have their husbands with them throughout labor and delivery. When one Utah hospital asked women in the late 1950s what would have made childbirth more satisfying for them, more than 40 percent responded, their husband's presence. The forced separation of husbands and wives had been a source of distress for many men as well. One father explained in 1947, "It could be an almost traumatic experience for the husband suddenly to be excluded from the most important happening in their married lives. . . . when I was finally and officially barred from the delivery room, I was quite frankly furious."[39]

Fathers had often been present at home births, but when birth moved to the hospital, physicians steadfastly resisted allowing fathers in delivery rooms, fearing they would disrupt medical routine. One Chicago obstetrician told every patient who asked, "You can have your husband. Or you can have me. . . . I don't like people looking over my shoulder." Other doctors refused to allow fathers in delivery rooms because the notion of a male nonphysician witnessing a birth simply offended them. A Florida woman recalled consulting thirty doctors about permitting her husband to be at their baby's birth and found that most condemned her husband as "a pervert . . . [and] voyeur." A Chicago-area obstetrician similarly noted, "You know what happens when a baby is born? First the head comes through. They [women] pee. And then they crap all over the place. . . . Men don't want to see that in their wives." Yet by the late 1960s doctors could no longer intimidate women. After another woman pressed her doctor to permit her husband to be with her in delivery, the doctor exploded. "You don't really want your husband in there! After all, you don't go into the bathroom when he's using it, do you?" Rather than accept her obstetrician's view, she decided to find a new doctor. "It was his equation of childbirth with defecation that ended our conversation."[40]

When father-attended births did finally become universal in the late 1970s, the transformation seemed instantaneous. Ina May Gaskin recalled watching hospitals change their policies virtually overnight, often after defiant confrontations ended in embarrassing headlines. When doctors ordered one San Francisco man out of the delivery room, he pulled a pair of handcuffs from his pocket and shackled himself to his wife's bed. Gaskin remembered, "Sure enough, he got to be there 'cause he hadn't brought the key, and he didn't faint and that was, of course, the great fear. And after that at that particular hospital and very quickly in San Francisco, dads were welcome in the delivery room."[41]

As mothers became more discerning, hospital administrators learned that attracting and pleasing pregnant women was vital to a hospital's financial success, particularly in an era of savvy consumers and grave discontent with women's medical treatment. A founding member of the American College of Healthcare Architects explained that since women made all decisions about a family's health care, wherever women gave birth became the family's hospital. The opposite was also true: hospitals where pregnant and birthing women had negative experiences were places families learned to avoid.[42]

The Road to Natural Childbirth

The theories of two obstetricians who later became internationally known, Grantly Dick-Read in England and Fernand Lamaze in France, informed the growing militancy of the women demanding reforms. These obstetricians provided the vocabulary and vision American women needed to offer alternatives to contemporary birthing procedures. A fundamental goal of both Dick-Read and Lamaze was to enable women to give birth without the often extreme medical treatments that had become integral to American obstetrics.

Dick-Read's books were the initial tools many women used on both sides of the Atlantic to critique and transform obstetric practice. Beginning as early as the 1930s, but especially in the 1940s and 1950s, many American women, especially those who had been profoundly unhappy with a previous birth, found Dick-Read's books and were inspired by his ideas. He spoke directly to their dissatisfaction by referring sarcastically to the "humanitarian conditions" under which modern women gave birth and urging mothers to demand a return to "the joy that is the reward of natural reproduction." His words gave rise to what became a central tenet of birth reform: women had the right to enjoy conditions that facilitated "natural" birth.[43]

Dick-Read's theory of natural childbirth grew out of a single encounter. Early in his medical practice, he faithfully adhered to prevailing custom and administered chloroform as a baby's head emerged from the mother's body. He ended this practice forever after arriving at one woman's home to find the birthing chamber enveloped in a "quiet kindliness. . . . There was no fuss or noise." During the birth the woman became agitated for only a brief moment—when Dick-Read tried to persuade her to inhale chloroform. After the birth, he asked why she had declined the anesthesia. She appeared puzzled and said simply, "It didn't hurt. It wasn't meant to, was it, doctor?"[44]

After this chance incident, Dick-Read's view of labor changed, becoming strikingly similar to Charles Meigs's stance almost one hundred years before. In his books, Dick-Read postulated that although all women worked equally hard during labor, only frightened women suffered. Much like Meigs's soothing assurance in the mid-nineteenth century that "cheering counsel . . . freed from the distressing element of terror" foretold an easy birth, Dick-Read argued that the nature of labor did not dictate a woman's discomfort; rather, the presence or absence of fear shaped the nature of her labor.[45]

Women acquired from Dick-Read's books a vocabulary, sensibility, and vision that served to level the playing field. One mother recalled that during previous pregnancies doctors had treated her like "a moron," patronizing her with "a distinctly the-less-you-know-the-better-my-dear attitude." But now her newfound knowledge of childbirth, courtesy of Grantly Dick-Read, forced doctors to treat her "like an adult." Another woman, Jan Ruby, from St. Joseph, Missouri, read one of Dick-Read's books and then asked her obstetrician for help in practicing Dick-Read's relaxation techniques. The doctor's response startled her: he did not feel qualified to assist her. This put Ruby in a previously unimagined position. "I realized that except for the regular visits to the doctor for the usual prenatal examinations, I was on my own! The training, the building of confidence, the actual producing of the child, would be my job."[46]

Marjorie Karmel's experience demonstrates how Dick-Read's books transformed even the most skeptical woman's approach to birth. Pregnant with her first child in the 1950s, Karmel returned to the United States briefly with her husband after living for an extended time in Paris. Taking note of her pregnancy, strangers proceeded to annoy her with news of the "beautiful," "thrilling," and "inspiring" notions of Grantly Dick-Read, a person she had never heard of and did not want to know about. Karmel remembered her bewilderment: "Childbirth belonged to the obstetrician, and I didn't see any reason to discuss it at a cocktail party. Obviously American life had changed while I was away." She tried to dissuade the presumptuous conversationalists from further discussion by telling them she didn't like inspirational literature. As she prepared to return to France several weeks later, however, her husband insisted she pack a book by Dick-Read that had been sent to her by one of the audacious strangers. Karmel did so grudgingly, with no inkling of "the emotional dynamite we had so casually flung into our suitcase." In 1959 Karmel's own bestseller appeared, *Thank You, Dr. Lamaze: A Mother's Experience in Painless Childbirth,* about her "joyous and moving" childbirth in France under the guidance of obstetrician Fernand Lamaze. Dick-Read's book, which she read out of boredom on the lengthy cruise between the United States and France, had inspired her to find Lamaze, a doctor amenable to Dick-Read's method.[47]

Newly empowered mothers helped make Dick-Read and Lamaze living legends. These were women who had never anticipated enjoying birth (without anesthesia, no less) and who wanted to share their experience with other women. The *New York Times Magazine* credited Dick-Read with instigating animated discussions among doctors at medical meetings and, even more significantly, among women "over back fences." Before Dick-Read, the magazine noted, many women found that doctors viewed them "paradoxically as a sort of necessary evil in the delivery room." After Dick-Read, women once again recognized that mothers, not doctors, were the central characters at births.[48]

The extreme reactions that Dick-Read still elicits in the medical community—glowing approbation on the one hand, unremitting disapproval on the other—indicate his ongoing influence. Donald Caton, an obstetric anesthesiologist and the author of a 1999 book on the history of the medical and social response to labor pain, suggested in his book that Dick-Read prompted a rift between women and their physicians. A biography of Dick-Read published in 1957 paints a decidedly different portrait, depicting him as a saintly figure who courageously defied conventional wisdom to provide women with information long withheld by an arrogant medical community. The physicians who became Dick-Read's disciples often alluded to his "magnetic and persuasive personality" and the "great personal charm" that encouraged adoring patients to embrace his ideas. His critics, however, believed charisma was all there was to his theories. One obstetrician charged, "Patients wouldn't hurt just to please him."[49]

Indeed, Dick-Read, who essentially built his reputation by unmasking and denouncing the superciliousness of obstetricians, was blind to his own arrogance. He wanted desperately to become a member of the Royal College of Obstetricians and Gynaecologists in the United Kingdom but refused to take the organization's requisite examination because he believed his international prominence was sufficient evidence of qualification for membership. He remained convinced, right up to his death in 1959, that members of the Royal College were simply too jealous to admit him.[50]

Dick-Read often exhibited the very chauvinism and sanctimoniousness that he condemned in colleagues. He contended in his first book, *Natural Childbirth,* for example, that women often felt hostility toward their husbands during labor and thus craved instead the presence of their doctor, "someone upon whose knowledge [they] could lean, and upon whose personality [they] could exercise the woman's prerogative of dependence."[51]

It is particularly ironic that Dick-Read became an icon just as the political scene in the United States focused on civil rights, the empowerment of women, and toleration of difference, for his theory of natural childbirth was based in part on antiquated notions of womanhood, social class, and "primitive races." He theorized, for example, that the "uncomplicated opinion[s]" of "primitive" women allowed them to labor painlessly, while a "tangle of complicated mental influences" burdened their sophisticated European and American counterparts. Dick-Read, who loved anecdotal evidence, offered a story as proof of this theory. He once asked a poverty-stricken mother how many children she had borne and reported that the woman responded unemotionally: "Eighteen, doctor, but I've buried eleven." Dick-Read argued that this woman's "clear" and "uncomplicated" views of birth and death evidenced the "relatively balanced mentality of the uncultured" and the reason they birthed with such ease. Thus in the 1940s and 1950s, when American women first began to take note of Dick-Read, his ideas did not foster feminist aspirations but instead reinforced the postwar stereotype of the ideal middle-class woman: the nurturing, contented, stay-at-home mother. Dick-Read called birth women's highest calling and glorified natural childbirth in particular as "the perfection of womanhood."[52]

Other natural birth theoreticians relied on research rather than anecdote. The relaxation techniques developed by Edmund Jacobson, a University of Chicago physiologist-physician, provided the underpinning of many of the methods eventually honed by the developers of natural childbirth systems, including Dick-Read. In 1929 Jacobson described both the symptoms of what he termed "nervous irritability" ("a general uneasiness . . . tears . . . anguish . . . .rapid pulse and irregular respiration") and its antidote, relaxation. Of particular interest to the few obstetricians searching for alternatives to anesthesia was Jacobson's finding that extreme relaxation mitigated negative reaction to sudden pain. Although he did not specifically study women in labor, the randomly timed electric shocks Jacobson administered to his experimental subjects mimicked the varying intervals between contractions.[53]

Dick-Read was the first person to publicly associate Jacobson's technique of deep relaxation with midwifery, but Dick-Read's lesser-known collaborator Helen Heardman was the first to use Jacobson's technique to alleviate labor pain. Heardman's work was so integral to Dick-Read's ultimate success that one prominent American physician called natural childbirth "The Grantly Dick Read–Helen Heardman Method." Heardman devised exercises to help women prepare for natural childbirth—including breathing, relaxing, squatting, and pelvic rocking—and described those exercises in such clear detail in books and pamphlets that every feature of her techniques, if not her name, became well known to generations of American women. Her study of more than five hundred births demonstrated that "trained" mothers had significantly shorter labors as well as fewer forceps deliveries, perineal tears, episiotomies, hemorrhages, and even stillbirths.[54]

Much of the training developed by Heardman eventually became synonymous with Fernand Lamaze. Indeed, both doctors and women came to use the term *Lamaze class* in a generic sense to refer to all childbirth preparation classes, even though such classes can differ widely in content and underlying philosophy. Although Lamaze's name became far better known than Dick-Read's, he developed his method fifteen years after Dick-Read wrote his first book.

On a trip to the Soviet Union in 1951, Lamaze discovered that Soviet doctors had developed a training program for pregnant women based on Pavlov's theory of conditioned response to stimuli. He had never seen anything like it: women were giving birth in the Soviet Union without drugs and apparently with minimal discomfort. After returning to France, Lamaze modified the Soviet system to his liking, keeping the Soviet physicians' carefully honed method of slow breathing during first-stage labor but adding his own methods of rapid breathing during much of the second stage and panting during birth.[55]

Two laywomen, Elisabeth Bing and Marjorie Karmel (the American living in Paris who wrote about her experience with Fernand Lamaze), were instrumental in popularizing the Lamaze method in America. Initially, Karmel's 1959 book personalized natural childbirth for American women. Eight years later, Bing wrote a book about Lamaze's method, *Six Practical Lessons for an Easier Childbirth*, that sold a million copies. Her bestseller effectively mainstreamed the Lamaze method. In 1960 Bing and Karmel together founded the American Society for Psychoprophylaxis in Obstetrics Inc. (ASPO), now renamed Lamaze International.[56]

By the mid-1970s, the Lamaze method had so permeated American culture that Lamaze classes had become a staple of any television drama or situation comedy showcasing a pregnancy. Thus, most Americans were soon able to describe the fundamentals of Lamaze even if they had never attended a Lamaze class or participated in a Lamaze birth. The TV shows invariably equated Lamaze classes with boot camp and Lamaze "coaches" with drill sergeants.[57]

Pundits soon confirmed this image. Writer Nora Ephron observed in 1978, "The tyranny of the obstetrician is eliminated—and the tyranny of the method is substituted." Lamaze, she charged, could be as rigid and fanatic as the obstetric practices it purported to abolish. Ephron wrote of her own first birth, "It never crossed my mind that I would live through the late 60's and early 70's in America only to discover that in the end what was expected of me was a brave, albeit vigorous squat in the fields like the heroine in 'The Good Earth.'"[58]

Sherwin Nuland, the Yale surgeon and writer, also derisively described the Lamaze classes he attended with his wife in the early 1980s in preparation for the birth of his third (her first) child. During his first marriage, when his older children were born, few Americans had heard of Dick-Read, let alone Lamaze. Now age fifty and about to become a father to an infant once again, Nuland was put off by the class. "Not a very gregarious, chummy kind of fellow," he had no desire to "share" with a group of strangers when asked to do so at the first session by the Lamaze instructor. And when a few of the instructor's former students came one night to discuss their childbirth experiences with class members, Nuland decided that the instructor must have "chosen them using the same criteria developed for selecting TV game-show participants. . . . I thought I would drown in the overflow of verbal corn syrup."

This is not to say that Nuland saw no value in childbirth education or natural childbirth. He recalled both as a physician and as a father that when his first two children were born, "an infant's first view of the world was through the opening in a sterile green surgical drape, as its head slid antiseptically between mother's shaven, germ-free labia and into the highly trained arms of a scrubbed, gowned, and gloved Fellow of the American College of Obstetrics and Gynecology [*sic*]."

He bemoaned that "totally medicalized procedure" and its "moment-to-moment invasiveness" and hailed the women's movement for urging obstetricians to render assistance only to prevent problems "should nature pull one of its infrequent tricks."[59]

Robert A. Bradley, an American obstetrician who practiced in Colorado, devised "husband-coached childbirth," a method that tended to be less rote and autocratic than the Lamaze method that rankled Ephron and Nuland, although enthusiasts of what became known as "the Bradley Method" could be just as dogmatic as Lamaze supporters. Bradley taught men to help their wives relax through first-stage contractions using soothing instructions and comforting mental imagery. One Colorado farm family, the Musgraves, enjoyed "family-centered maternity care" under Bradley's auspices. In 1966 they hailed the Bradley Method as "a far cry from the impersonal obstetrics still favored by some doctors and some hospitals—mother unconscious or numbed from anesthesia, father banished to the waiting room." Frank Musgrave, noting that he never left his farm at calving time, joked, "I figure my wife rates as much attention as the cows do."[60]

Although all purported to help women give birth with little or no medication, there was significant rivalry among the various birth methods. The ASPO implied criticism of Dick-Read in one of its pamphlets: "NATURAL CHILDBIRTH is based on positive thinking, passive relaxation, and a touch of mysticism. The psychoprophylactic method [Lamaze] is based on active participation utilizing scientific principles for dealing with labor." One father, delighted with the birth of his son in 1968, offered a similarly snide critique of Dick-Read: "Lamaze . . . stresses the joy and beauty of childbirth, but avoids the cultish overtones of the Dick-Read method." Dick-Read's and Bradley's proponents, in turn, condemned the ASPO because the organization defended analgesia as one of many tools to be used during labor, if deemed necessary by the physician. "True" natural childbirth advocates condemned this aspect of the Lamaze approach, charging that the Lamaze method deferred far too often to doctors.[61]

Bradley personally joined the fray. He relished the Lamaze epithet "Barnyard Bradley," which alluded to his recommendation (as the son of a veterinarian) that laboring women imitate laboring animals by lying on their sides, closing their eyes, and posing sleep. He readily admitted to "stirring the troubled waters" ("as I am an Irishman") by declaring Lamaze largely ineffective and claiming that more than 90 percent of women who employed the Bradley Method enjoyed "totally unmedicated births." The enmity among natural childbirth proponents persists to this day. Marie F. Mongan, the designer in the early 1990s of Hypno-

Birthing, has criticized Lamaze for so thoroughly abandoning its original precepts that its classes now offer little more than detailed explanations of medical technology and hospital protocol.[62]

Promoting Natural Childbirth

Despite the animosity among proponents of different childbirth education methods, they all, at least initially, aspired to some form of "natural childbirth," even as they disagreed on its precise definition and accompanying protocol. Broadly speaking, a "natural" birth was one with no or minimal medical intervention, in which both the woman and her physician respected and trusted the forces of labor, in which the woman was prepared to work with her body, and in which, accordingly, the doctor did not automatically attempt to manage the woman's body and its powerful functions. As women's right to fully participate in American economic and political life became undisputed, the image of strong, fearless women giving birth without anesthesia or forceps became decidedly appealing. The opposing image—women with wrists bound to operating tables, legs pulled apart and strapped high to stirrups, unconscious or groggy from unwanted anesthetic, their babies yanked from their listless bodies with forceps—became anathema. Thus birth reform and natural childbirth became inextricably linked; birth could not be truly reformed if the medical community (and women themselves) distrusted the ability of women's bodies.[63]

Dick-Read and Lamaze were not the only physician-purveyors of this message. Some American physicians began to spontaneously encourage their patients to become more proactive about birth and medical decision-making. One woman recalled in 1961 that when her first two babies were born, she firmly believed that the less she knew about birth, the less she would worry during her pregnancies, and she reported that her obstetrician encouraged that attitude at every prenatal visit. Five years elapsed between her second and third pregnancies, however, and by then her paternalistic obstetrician had moved, facilitating her introduction to a different sensibility. "When I first stepped into my new obstetrician's waiting room to see a profusion of No Smoking signs and printed commands to Read This, I had the distinct feeling that times had changed."[64]

During her first appointment with the new doctor, he urged her to sign up for his "motherhood course," a series of classes consisting of movies about pregnancy and birth followed by question-and-answer sessions. She was bewildered. "The other doctor had just expected me to produce a baby; he hadn't expected me to ask questions." Initially, she declined the invitation. But her new obstetrician persisted, warning her that he always recognized the patients who skipped his course: "They're twice as scared [during labor] as the others."[65] She eventually agreed to take the class, and much to her surprise she loved it, feeling particularly buoyed after the last session, featuring a movie depicting a natural birth. When the movie ended, the doctor assured his students that they had just witnessed an accurate representation of the vast majority of births and told them, "Things will go pretty much the same way for all of you." By the time she went into labor, this formerly passive mother felt like a "highly trained race horse approaching the starting gate."[66]

Like Eliza Taylor Ransom and Dorothy Reed Mendenhall much earlier in the century, some doctors' own negative birth experiences contributed to their interest in natural childbirth and their desire to empower patients. In 1965, for example, Joni Magee, a twenty-four-year-old medical student, gave birth to her first child. She wanted a natural birth, but her husband was unenthusiastic, so, aware that women needed support if they wanted to forgo medication during labor, Magee dropped the idea. After going into labor and checking into the hospital, however, she found labor endurable until "a little, fat resident huffed into the room" and told her she had only two choices: she could have caudal anesthesia or injections of an unspecified drug that would put her to sleep for ten hours. At her husband's insistence, she opted to sleep. When she awoke, she was in tremendous pain. She begged for a caudal. After receiving it, she ended up with "a forceps delivery, a depressed baby, a sphincter tear, a great deal of blood loss." The experience so unnerved Magee that she decided to pursue the one specialty she had previously rejected, obstetrics. As an obstetrician, she specialized in natural childbirth in nontraditional settings.[67]

Before the advent of the women's movement and nationwide publicity about birth reform, the physicians sympathetic to natural birth were rare exceptions. Particularly in the 1950s, when many doctors viewed any woman expressing even mild interest in natural childbirth as "neurotic," birth reform organizations faced stiff opposition from most physicians. In 1953 *Today's Health* told the story of Susie Andrews, whose older brother had mercilessly taunted her as a child for being "a sissy." To prove her brother wrong, little Susie once leaped impetuously from a top step and broke her collarbone. *Today's Health* attributed the adult Susie's interest in natural birth to this childhood trauma, observing, "Twenty years later Susie Andrews Smith pushed away the hand of a harassed young obstetrician. 'No,' she gasped, 'No, I don't want any anesthetic. I . . . I'm not a sissy, Doctor. I'm not a sissy!'" *Today's Health* explained that "naturally high-strung, anxious or insecure" women (like Susie) could not "safely or wisely" give birth without analgesia and anesthesia. In susceptible Susie's case, neurotic friends had goaded her into being inappropriately courageous.[68]

In an interview with *Newsweek,* Dr. Edward A. Graber of New York's Lenox Hill Hospital also stereotyped some of the women interested in natural birth. He described them as "the compulsives who wear Oxford shoes and walk into the office with a pad and pencil to write down exactly what you tell them—this is the compulsive-neurotic group, the faddists." Another obstetrician offered a similarly derisive description of a patient in a 1956 issue of the *American Journal of Obstetrics and Gynecology.* The forty-two-year-old woman, "interested in 'social problems of the world,'" had "postponed marriage for many years in order to obtain a degree as a Doctor of Philosophy." Her interest in Grantly Dick-Read during her second pregnancy reflected these deviant tendencies, prompting her to become "very demanding and antagonistic" toward her doctor. After giving birth, her hostility increased: while still in the hospital, she accused nurses of preventing her from nursing her infant. The medical staff was indignant, although this was a perfectly reasonable allegation to make in light of the hospital policies in place nationwide in the 1950s that routinely separated breastfeeding mothers from their babies for most of the day and all of the night. Eleven days after her baby's birth, the doctor committed the angry woman to an institution for psychiatric care and blamed natural childbirth for the admission. This doctor also described the case of another woman, whose husband was an infertile alcoholic and who conceived three babies with donor sperm. After the births, her husband refused to help care for their children. Whether his refusal stemmed from his alcoholism, his infertility, both, or neither, the article did not say. But when the exhausted woman "suffered a complete emotional collapse requiring psychiatric care" after the birth of her third child, her obstetrician blamed natural childbirth.[69]

By the 1970s the women's movement was influential enough that this sort of stereotyping and treatment of women had become impermissible. Other social movements similarly contributed to change in perspective about obstetric treatment. The budding environmental movement, for example, aroused concern about water and air pollutants and in doing so drew attention once again to Virginia Apgar's now twenty-year-old finding that pain medication administered during labor and birth crossed the placenta. Suzanne Arms, one of the most articulate and passionate spokeswomen for birth reform, emphasized this fact: "How many times must it be said? *Drugs get to the baby. Drugs adversely affect the baby. Drugs may permanently damage the baby.*" Thus, anesthesia was no longer a magic bullet easing mothers' painful ordeal but a poison administered directly to their babies. Birth without analgesia and anesthesia was now the healthy and so-cially responsible way to labor and give birth.[70]

In this light, natural childbirth became a weighty moral issue, as anesthetics had in the past. Books and articles began to link natural childbirth with every-thing from more stable families to world peace. One natural birth proponent contended that a drug-free prenatal experience inexorably propelled the baby girls produced by such a birth toward "successful motherhood," ensuring cre-ation of the next generation of productive, responsible citizens.[71] A forty-three-year-old man whose first wife had borne three children under anesthesia was now expecting a child with his second wife. He was particularly expansive about the advantages of unmedicated labors. He explained to *Harper's Magazine* that ob-stetric anesthesia ruined not only individual lives but the souls of entire nations:

> The drug . . . gets into the baby, and the infant is born too doped to suckle, even
> if the mother were awake enough to present her breast. During the mother's
> drug hangover, the baby is fed glucose, and loses the will to nurse. . . . So the
> baby stays on the bottle, graduates to pasty canned foods, and grows up with
> its oral needs unsatisfied. And *that* . . . is why so many people smoke too much,
> drink too much alcohol, and need tranquilizers and sleeping pills. This is also
> why we build hydrogen bombs and obsolete aircraft carriers, instead of schools
> and hospitals for the poor. Because we are frustrated from birth, we grow up
> filled with hostility and fear.[72]

Natural childbirth also seemed to ensure preservation of what was deemed appropriate womanly behavior in the post–World War II period. One physician told *McCall's* that because childbirth was the "culmination of a woman's psycho-sexual development," natural childbirth allowed mothers to attain the pinnacle of womanly achievement in a way that medically treated birth did not. Natural childbirth also seemed to guarantee that women would maintain an appropriate appearance and countenance throughout labor, a look and demeanor highly prized and rigidly defined in the 1940s, 1950s, and 1960s. The male author of a *Woman's Home Companion* article typified this view when he met a woman im-mediately after her baby's natural birth and marveled: "Despite all I had been told by some of the country's leading obstetricians about the new technique . . . I still found it hard to believe that the young woman I was looking at had had a child within the hour. Every hair was in place. Powder and lipstick were on just so. Her eyes were shining." Other magazines similarly praised women's ability to main-tain a picture-perfect appearance during and just after birth. A *Look* photo-essay

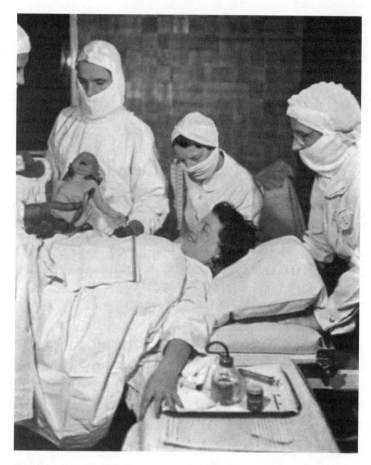

Photograph of a woman immediately after a natural childbirth in
1948, not long after Grantly Dick-Read's book *Childbirth without Fear*
appeared in the United States. In a color version of this photo, the
woman's bright red lipstick and nail polish are readily apparent.
Source: Clifford B. Lull and Robert A. Hingson, *Control of Pain in
Childbirth* (J. B. Lippincott, 1948), 132a.

focusing on the natural childbirth of a serene, fully made-up woman bore the
captions "During labor, an inner calm replaces pain that mothers usually experience" and "The radiant eyes of the mother when the baby finally arrives."[73]

Twenty years later, women's magazines once again described mothers immediately after a natural childbirth in equally approving terms, but this time the
mothers were ideal 1970s women with a decidedly different look: no makeup and

hair unpretentiously askew. And their demeanor was anything but serene: they were panting, and sweating, and orgasmic. The representation of obstetric anesthesia remained allied with both broad social concerns and the ever-changing depiction of the ideal woman.

While mothers once compared their agonizing, unmedicated births with their subsequent heavenly anesthetized births, they now did the opposite, contrasting their dizzy, nauseating, anesthetized births with their thrilling, invigorating, natural births. One woman remembered the "five hideous days of retching aftermath" (likely caused by ether) after her first two births and now hailed the joy of her fully felt, clear-headed third birth. Another mother, "knocked out for hours with anesthetics" during the birth of her first baby, who was "delivered to me next morning like a bottle of milk or the newspaper," had her second baby handed to her "right there in the delivery room and somehow this made him seem completely mine right away."[74]

Even the skeptical physicians who wanted nothing to do with natural childbirth could not help but notice the healthy behaviors exhibited by the infants born to unanesthetized mothers. In Rochester, New York, for example, physicians reported that for the first time in their experience they were examining newborns with excellent color, reactions, and respiration. Until natural childbirth became popular, the medical community had largely ceased recognizing newborn asphyxia as a medically induced problem, "since it was so common."[75]

By the mid-1970s, even some of the physicians who had initially denounced natural childbirth were beginning to accept some of its features, most notably childbirth education classes. An article in *Reader's Digest* titled "Natural Childbirth Comes of Age" quoted Harold Seerveld, an obstetrician at Denver's Lutheran Hospital, who, like most of his cohorts, had once ridiculed natural birth. He recalled his first encounter with the phenomenon, a patient who "entered the labor room followed by an entourage." Her birth attendants "carried how-to manuals, coached her with the ebullience of a cheering squad, and made the doctor feel like an intruder." Seerveld's abhorrence increased after the woman developed complications requiring a general anesthetic. He dismissed the entire event as "a farce." Yet now he steered all his patients to childbirth education classes, advising each that the instruction would cut hours from their labors. *Reader's Digest* informed women that although natural childbirth had once been "a specialized movement, or cult," it was now an activity experienced daily all over the country by ordinary women. Given the favorable assessments, natural childbirth seemed destined to be a permanent fixture on the obstetric landscape.[76]

The Backlash

What seemed to be a nationwide passion for natural birth quickly faded, however, perhaps due to one ironic incentive for the enthusiasm. Early in the debate, Nicholson J. Eastman, professor of obstetrics at Johns Hopkins University and the author of several editions of *Williams Obstetrics,* pointed out that women's willingness to consider natural childbirth was due in part to a generation of women who had been heavily drugged during labor. "They have no gory stories to tell their friends . . . because all they can remember . . . is a pill, a hypodermic injection and oblivion."[77]

That lack of shared knowledge about any aspect of birth likely prompted many women to approach natural childbirth with unrealistic expectations. Even in the 1970s, when enthusiasm for natural childbirth was at its peak, descriptions of mothers' frustration over "failed" births appeared in magazines. One woman wrote in *Mademoiselle,* "Everything had gone beautifully except for one thing— it hurt like hell, worse than anything I had ever experienced." Her anger over the experience increased when her Lamaze teacher explained the alleged reason for her excruciating pain: "You probably had unconscious fears, perhaps some negative feelings about having a baby, so you tensed up." That explanation stoked the woman's fury. "To say that *I* had failed was as if I had taken swimming lessons, learned to swim, and was then told I was a failure because I hadn't been able to continue to swim well when hit by a fifteen foot wave."[78]

The title of Lamaze's book (*Painless Childbirth*) and the subtitle of Marjorie Karmel's book (*A Mother's Experiences in Painless Childbirth*) contributed to women's unrealistic expectations. Both titles conveyed the notion that natural childbirth would render labor a breeze, an impression that ultimately prompted both disappointment and ridicule. Critics pointed out that childbirth was not painless and no natural birth method could make it so. Mothers began to complain that if they did ultimately request analgesia or anesthesia at some point during labor, others later berated them for being weak. One woman lamented in *Glamour,* "It seems as though the first question a new mother gets these days is not, 'Is it a boy or a girl?' but 'Did you take anything?'"[79]

Birth reform advocates were equally dismayed by lay and medical views of natural childbirth for quite different reasons. They feared that mainstream medicine had distorted the meaning of natural childbirth. Rahima Baldwin, a professional midwife and the codirector of the Birth Center in Detroit, complained that women were claiming to have experienced a "natural childbirth" after undergoing every medical procedure short of cesarean section. Baldwin sarcastically quoted an imaginary woman: "I didn't even have anesthesia when they ruptured my membranes and started the Pitocin," or "It was completely natural. All I had was a local for the episiotomy."[80]

Even feminists active in health reform, originally among the biggest champions of natural childbirth, splintered over the issue when some radical feminists denounced birth itself as inherently exploitive of women. An obstetrician explained in 1977 that some of her female colleagues felt that "childbirth is an imposition on the rights of the woman, and they feel that they're being very pro-woman by seeking to remove her from the process as much as possible." This position helped encourage a return to extreme medical treatments.[81]

Among obstetricians, natural childbirth never stopped being a contentious subject, as controversial as anesthesia had been in the mid-nineteenth century. In 1978, in writing a general overview of natural birth methods, two doctors noted that they could not recall such vigorous disagreement among colleagues in decades. This polarization prevented obstetricians from formulating a consensus about the value of and place for natural childbirth. Instead, two irreconcilable views prevailed, a state of affairs reminiscent of doctors' uncompromising views of obstetric anesthesia a century before. According to one group of doctors, natural childbirth was "one of the most significant advances of modern medicine." According to another equally steadfast group, natural childbirth was "a primitive and medically unacceptable practice."[82]

Just as the opposing camps had done in Simpson's and Meigs's day when discussing anesthesia, both sides made extreme claims. Robert Mendelsohn, associate professor of preventive medicine and community health at the University of Illinois, asserted that hospital births had a 99 percent complication rate; when women gave birth at home without medical interventions, the complication rate was 1 percent. At the other extreme, Graham G. Hawks, chief of obstetrics at New York Hospital–Cornell Medical Center, insisted that "babies die from natural childbirth" and argued that its popularity also portended a return to the high maternal death rate of the 1930s. Other doctors did not want to engage in conversation about natural childbirth at all. Joseph Nathanson, clinical professor emeritus of obstetrics at Cornell Medical School, dismissed Lamaze as "utter nonsense." If a woman insisted on using Lamaze, he dismissed her as a patient.[83]

By the 1990s, hostility toward natural childbirth was manifest. Like others before him who had linked the use or nonuse of obstetric anesthesia with societal well-being, Clayton T. Beecham, a Pennsylvania obstetrician with a subspecialty in gynecological oncology, wrote a commentary for *The Female Patient* connecting natural childbirth with rising rates of domestic violence and divorce. Beecham chastised a colleague who scoffed at the claim: "If you think the disfigured vagina [caused by natural childbirth] has no effect on marital contentment, I suggest you take more complete gynecologic histories." The same magazines and newspapers that had touted natural childbirth in the 1970s as beneficial and the wave of the future, denounced it in the 1990s as unreasonably demanding and dangerous.[84]

In retrospect, this turnabout was unsurprising. One of the most celebrated aspects of birth reform was the cozy labor-delivery-recovery room now readily available to most mothers for the asking. These comfortable rooms effectively masked the lack of real change in physicians' approach to birth. Thus, even as hospitals seemed to respond to the demands of birth reformers and obstetricians showed increasing tolerance for the women who refused anesthesia, the cesarean section rate was rising. That two such starkly different phenomena, enthusiasm for natural childbirth and a precipitously rising cesarean section rate, occurred simultaneously was another indication of the vagaries of medical and societal attitudes toward labor and birth. A belief in the need for more sectioned births, rather than the need for more natural births, soon redefined "normal" birth in the United States once again.

Soon after the *Ladies' Home Journal* aired women's complaints about their treatment in American maternity wards in 1958, two physicians writing in the *American Journal of Obstetrics and Gynecology* observed that physicians and women were likely to remain in conflict because each group measured the quality of obstetric care with a different yardstick. Obstetricians gauged success by the maternal and infant death rates. In contrast, women now took obstetric safety for granted and instead judged the quality of care by the compassion and kindness shown them by doctors and nurses in the hospital. "It is an enigma of modern obstetrics," the two doctors noted, "that what passes in the record as a normal labor and delivery may be bitterly remembered by our patient as a terrifying experience." Women's crusade for birth reform in the 1970s, and the contentious discussion the campaign prompted, highlighted like no other episodes in the history of American birth practices the often oppositional forms of knowledge that women and their physicians bring into the birthing room: doctors' medical knowledge of birth and women's anticipation and experience of birth. Each form of knowledge is equally valid, yet each seeks to invalidate, rather than enrich, the other.[85]

Hospitals and obstetricians eventually used women's grievances to their advantage. Given the widespread publicity in the lay press about women's complaints, hospitals began to tout their new offerings: homey birthing rooms; no prep; fathers, friends, and relatives allowed to remain with women throughout labor and birth; and, depending on the predilection of nurses and doctors, facilitation of natural childbirth when a woman requested it.[86]

Labor-delivery-recovery rooms and companionship during labor became permanent fixtures in the nation's hospitals. Natural childbirth did not. As hospitals took over childbirth education in the 1980s, the very classes that had been the foundation of birth reform and natural childbirth (because the classes edified and empowered women) instead became vehicles to acclimate women to hospital protocol and the treatments favored by obstetricians.

Lamaze was an unwitting yet instrumental tool in this development. The hospitals offering in-house childbirth education classes almost always offered Lamaze in lieu of other methods. This proved a clever choice. ASPO guidelines had long recommended that Lamaze instructors stress the potential benefits of medications, medical protocols, and cooperation with doctors. The capstone class in virtually all hospital-based Lamaze classes became a tour of the maternity ward and instruction in maternity ward protocol. "Prepared" childbirth acquired a new meaning. Rather than preparing women to orchestrate their own births, these classes now prepared women to accept doctors' and hospitals' rules, regulations, and treatments.[87]

Despite the movement's waning influence, physicians long remembered feeling unfairly maligned by birth reformers. When Sol Shnider, professor of anesthesia and obstetrics at the University of California in San Francisco, delivered the prestigious Rovenstine Lecture at the annual meeting of the American Society of Anesthesiologists in 1990, he offered an amusing rendition of the history of obstetric anesthesia with special focus on the glorification of natural childbirth in the 1970s. He joked about yearning to form the Society for Prevention of Cruelty to Obstetrical Anesthesiologists when natural childbirth was at its popular zenith and noted that times had changed considerably. In 1990, rather than eschewing anesthesia, most women insisted on an epidural. Shnider was equally amused by this contrasting sensibility, threatening to form yet another fictitious organization, the Society for the Hysterical Use of Epidural and Spinal Opiates in Obstetrics.[88]

By the time Shnider delivered this lecture, natural childbirth had been marginalized. A generation of women who grew up expecting to have full-time jobs in addition to marriage and a family had their own unique image of the ideal birth. Rather than anticipating a sense of strength, empowerment, and transformation from giving birth, young women busy with assorted work and family responsibilities instead sought assurances of comfort, convenience, and a few carefully prescribed and medically orchestrated birth choices.

Epidural Anesthesia and Cesarean Section

The Question of Choice, 1970s to the Present

Anna Dobros, a twenty-six-year-old nurse living in a suburb west of Chicago, was pregnant with her first child in 2003. During her pregnancy she worried about labor pain; listening to friends' stories about birth and watching births on television had frightened her. She talked to her obstetricians about her fear, and they were both very reassuring. They told her, "Oh, you can get through it. You'll be fine." She laughed when she recalled their casual guarantee, noting, "They're both males."

While in nursing school, Anna had witnessed two births. Both women had epidural anesthesia, and she called those experiences "very positive." Yet Anna did not want an epidural for herself. She explained, "When I was in nursing school . . . there was some kind of stigma because there were so many women using epidurals. . . . I wanted things naturally. I'm strong." As a nursing student, she also observed that babies whose mothers opted for an epidural seemed more placid than other babies. "That's why I had it in my mind to gear myself not to have the epidural so I could have this child that doesn't have any drugs in her. And not some sedate look."

During her pregnancy, Anna was too busy to take a childbirth education class. She worked twelve-hour night shifts, and adding a weekly class to that already grueling schedule was unappealing. Besides, she added, "my husband wasn't nuts about it."

At a routine doctor's appointment when she was forty weeks and six days pregnant, one of her obstetricians told her he wanted to wait one more week before considering labor induction. Anna, however, wanted to give birth as soon as possible. Her disability insurance required her to take two weeks off before her due date, and now that she had been off work for almost three weeks, she did not want to fritter away any more precious maternity leave waiting for her baby to be born. Given her predicament, the doctor agreed to induce labor the following morning.

The induction began at 7:00 a.m. Soon Anna had a sensation akin to "bad menstrual cramps." At 2:00 p.m., when her cervix was two and one-half centimeters dilated, a doctor ruptured her amniotic sac. For the next fifteen minutes, Anna did not feel any noticeable increase in discomfort. "And that's when all hell broke loose. . . . I begged and pleaded with my husband to let me have an epidural and get an anesthesiologist in here." Her husband, Mike, repeatedly urged her to hang on for five more minutes. "For 45 minutes he got his way. But I couldn't do it anymore."

When the anesthesiologist arrived, he asked Anna to sit on the edge of the bed. A nurse held her hand. The anesthesiologist instructed her to remain immobile, and Anna remembered trying "to kind of make jokes because here I'm having so much pain but I know I have to stay still." The epidural worked quickly. Anna recalled, "It was just wonderful. I remember going back on the bed and feeling like the biggest load of my life had just been taken off my shoulders." After the anesthesiologist left, Anna simply relaxed. She remembered, "It was nice to kind of like sleep." Nurses came in periodically to turn her and check the fetal monitor.

At 7:00 p.m. Mike went outside to smoke a cigarette. Shortly after he left, nurses and doctors came in to tell Anna that in fifteen minutes she would start pushing. Excited, she called her mother with the news. When Mike returned, Julie, a nurse and friend of Anna's who worked at the hospital, accompanied him. Anna invited Julie to stay for the birth.

Doctors and nurses returned and told Anna to start pushing. As she pushed, Mike held onto one leg and Julie held the other. A nurse held up a mirror so Anna could watch her baby being born. The nurse encouraged Anna: "This is the ring of fire. She's going through the ring of fire. You're doing great." After forty-five minutes of pushing, the nurse told Anna to stop because the doctor had to leave the room for a few minutes. After the doctor returned, Anna's daughter was born.

Anna is pregnant again. She assumes this labor will be induced too, since her disability insurance guidelines for maternity leave have not changed. This time, however, she plans to request an epidural much earlier in the process. "I'm all about the epidural," she says now. "I'm totally for them."[1]

A New Generation Spurns Natural Childbirth

Beginning in the 1970s, as the women's movement prompted unprecedented social, political, and economic gains for women, change was manifest in virtually every area of American life. One sign of the societal transformation was an extraordinary increase in the number of working mothers of infants. Working mothers were by no means a new trend. Even in the 1950s (an era some still mistakenly glorify as the heyday of the devoted, stay-at-home mom) 39 percent of women with school-age children and 18.6 percent of women with children under age six worked outside the home. Yet by the 1990s, these numbers had increased so dramatically that working mothers of children of all ages had become the vast majority. Even more startling to some, most mothers of infants were now workers too. In 1976 only 31 percent of women with children less than one year old worked outside the home; by 1998, 59 percent did.[2]

This development both invigorated and taxed women. In her influential 1963 book *The Feminine Mystique,* Betty Friedan bemoaned society's emphasis on motherhood to the detriment of other avenues for women. Partly in response to this well-publicized criticism and the nationwide activism it spurred, women entered the paid workforce in unprecedented numbers. This dramatic social change did not have the precise impact that Friedan originally anticipated, however. In 1981 she lamented in another book, *The Second Stage,* that in their attempts to juggle motherhood and a full-time job, young women had become more oppressed than their mothers. Friedan urged this overburdened generation to demand governmental and societal support in order "to live the equality we fought for."[3]

Friedan issued this plea because government and society had not responded to the transformation in women's lives with institutionalized support systems. Instead, working mothers of young children in the United States remained on their own. American women were not to enjoy the paid maternity leave, subsidized day care, shorter workweeks, and national health care systems that mothers in other industrialized countries could take for granted.[4]

This lack of societal assistance took its toll. In a *Newsweek* cover story published in 2005 titled "Mommy Madness," Judith Warner described a generation of women "sleep-walking through life in a state of quiet panic." Citing data indicating that 30 percent of mothers of young children suffered from depression, she wondered: "Why do so many of us feel so out of control?" Warner sympathized with her beleaguered cohorts, but she also chastised them: "Good daughters of the Reagan Revolution, we disdained social activism and cultivated our own gardens with a kind of muscle-bound, tightly wound, uber-achieving, all-encompassing, never-failing self-control that passed, in the 1980s, for female empowerment." Women who should have been enjoying the ripened fruits of the women's movement were instead isolated and struggling. Overwhelmed, they accepted without complaint the privatization of their problems, not unlike the women Friedan had profiled decades before in *The Feminine Mystique.* Warner noted, "Instead of blaming society, moms today tend to blame themselves."[5]

Times had changed dramatically since the women's health reform movement enthusiastically promoted natural childbirth. Portrayed in the 1970s as transforming and empowering, labor without analgesia and anesthesia now seemed draining and dispiriting. How could one more punishing activity amid a series of punishing activities be empowering? One mother chided, "In a world where women are constantly proving their worth—in the office, on the playing field, at home—unmedicated childbirth need not be singled out as 'proof' of one's strength."[6] By the 1990s, epidural anesthesia seemed the ideal choice for childbirth, ostensibly offering not only a painless but also a stress-free, even relaxing, way to give birth. Given that alternative, articles in lay publications intimated, why would anyone be foolish enough to choose natural childbirth?[7]

Many obstetric treatments discarded during the birth reform era, including labor induction, met with renewed approval in this environment. An article in the *American Journal of Obstetrics and Gynecology* (*AJOG*) repeated the rationales that made induced labor so popular during the baby boom. Induction enabled busy physicians and mothers to plan ahead. Hospitals benefited as well: if the hospital was unexpectedly crowded on a particular day, personnel could easily reschedule a planned induction. Yet even as they once again advocated medical interventions, doctors continued to pay lip service to the now well-accepted rhetoric of birth reform. Writers of the *AJOG* article, for example, invoked the patient-education, self-help sensibility of birth reformers when they also ironically suggested that another advantage of labor induction was that it allowed a woman to "perform her own labial shave and self-administer an enema at home prior to presenting at the hospital." These authors failed to mention that the women who first advocated this form of self-help had also denounced the ritual shave and enema as unnecessary, demeaning, and exceedingly uncomfortable.[8]

Now that induction was once again couched as convenient, the incidence of the procedure more than doubled nationwide between 1990 and 2003. By 2003, the frequency of elective inductions alone (that is, inductions performed for social rather than medical reasons) ranged from 12 to 55 percent of births among hospitals and from 3 to 76 percent of births among individual physicians. In San Antonio, Texas, induction was so common that the *Express-News* reported that pregnant women now routinely decided when and under what circumstances they would go into labor. Women argued that birth was too significant and time-consuming an event to leave its onset to chance. One mother explained, "You rush through so much of your life, it was nice to be able to schedule something so important as the birth of a child." An article in the *Baltimore Sun* about Maryland's busy Howard County General Hospital echoed the sentiment. Given the increasingly crowded maternity wards at Howard, the hectic lives of pregnant women, and the employers who needed sufficient time to plan for an employee's maternity leave, birth-by-appointment had become a virtual necessity.[9]

Labor induction became the norm in many areas of the country. One obstetrician observed in 2006 that in the large Chicago hospital where she worked, elective induction was so popular that doctors performed them round-the-clock. Women were given appointments not only at the conventional hours of 9:00 a.m. and 1:00 p.m., but also at 1:00 a.m., 2:00 a.m., and 3:00 a.m.—"That's how many we're doing." This physician, who started her obstetric residency in 1973, just as birth reform activists first championed natural childbirth, found the new custom "incredible."[10]

As women came to think of labor as a meticulously planned event (thanks to induction) and easily weathered (thanks to epidural anesthesia), lay publications and television shows increasingly mocked natural childbirth. On the NBC medical drama *ER*, an orderly wheeled a pregnant, recurring character up to delivery while a nurse shouted after her, "Don't be a hero. Get the epidural." A headline in the *New York Times Magazine* similarly characterized women wanting a natural birth as ridiculous: "Advocates of drug-free childbirth tout the experience as if it were an extreme sport—no pain, no gain." Once again, the life circumstances of a new generation moved birth practices in another direction.[11]

Anesthesiologists Embrace Obstetrics

A sharp increase in the number of anesthesiologists helped spur women's interest in and access to the epidural. Before the mid-1980s, an epidural—even if a woman had heard of the treatment and specifically requested it—was not readily available on the labor and delivery floor of most hospitals. Because regional anesthesia needed more training to administer than either systemic drugs or inhalation anesthesia, it usually required the skills of an anesthesiologist, a specialist in short supply. Today, more than thirty-eight thousand physicians in the United States specialize in anesthesiology, nearly four times the number who did so in 1970.[12]

The link between the availability of an anesthesiologist and women's access to epidural anesthesia was evident at Alexandria Hospital in Virginia as early as the 1950s. As one of the first hospitals in the country to routinely offer epidurals in the maternity ward, Alexandria deemed a staff of anesthesiologists on round-the-clock call essential to the service. The obstetricians at the hospital quickly embraced epidural anesthesia, in part because it did mandate the presence of an anesthesiologist. For the first time in their careers, obstetricians at Alexandria could share with another physician the legal and moral responsibility for decisions made in labor and delivery. Alexandria Hospital's obstetricians continued to exhibit enthusiasm for epidurals, eventually noting that in twenty thousand deliveries the method had not caused a single maternal death. In the 1950s, however, the service offered by Alexandria Hospital was rare elsewhere. Most hospitals did not routinely offer epidural blocks in their maternity wards until well into the 1980s or even the 1990s.[13]

Until the 1980s, if a woman did have an epidural, an obstetrician, rather than an anesthesiologist, customarily administered it. A survey conducted in the early 1960s indicated that a board-certified anesthesiologist attended only 14 percent of anesthetized births. One obstetrician recalled that when he was a new obstetric resident at Chicago's Lying-in Hospital in 1972, he and other obstetric residents became adept at administering epidurals because they knew an anesthesiologist was not likely to be available when needed. The department of anesthesiology subsequently asked them to train the anesthesiology residents. Another obstetrician who was also an obstetric resident in the early 1970s, at a different Chicago hospital, described the same scenario: he and his cohorts became more skilled at placing epidurals than the anesthesiology residents. He remembered obstetricians' annoyance at anesthesiologists' unwillingness to work in obstetrics because they disliked being summoned in the middle of the night. "It was a big push on the part of obstetricians to [convey the message to anesthesiologists that] either you're part of the team or you're not part of the team. If you're not part of the team, you know, find another job."[14]

In the absence of an anesthesiologist or an obstetrician adept at anesthetic administration, a nurse-anesthetist would often be summoned to labor and delivery. Nurse-anesthetists were usually so skilled that some doctors preferred them even to anesthesiologists. One obstetrician who began his residency at Chicago's Michael Reese Hospital in 1951 recalled that he could have requested an anesthesiologist for his wife when his first child was born but instead insisted on a nurse-anesthetist, "because she was better."[15]

Through the 1960s, anesthesiologists continued to largely shun obstetrics. The hours were too taxing and the insurance reimbursement too low to attract these scarce specialists in significant numbers. In contrast, surgery offered a relatively predictable schedule and considerably higher pay. On the rare occasion that an anesthesiology resident did express interest in obstetrics, there was seldom opportunity for training. In 1965, when anesthetic mishaps were still one of the four leading causes of maternal death, Sol Shnider, director of obstetrical anesthesia at the University of California in San Francisco, surveyed residency training programs in anesthesiology and found that almost half of the programs completely ignored obstetrics.[16]

Thus, of necessity, obstetricians were often the ones who administered anesthesia at births. A 1969 survey conducted by the American College of Obstetricians and Gynecologists (ACOG) revealed that in 33 percent of cases, when a laboring mother received anesthesia, it was administered by an obstetrician. As available drugs multiplied and the process of administering them in assorted combinations became more complex, obstetricians' multiple responsibilities at births threatened the well-being of mothers and newborns. Authors of an article published in the *Journal of the American Association of Nurse Anesthetists* in 1976 warned that when the obstetrician administered the anesthetic, delivered the infant, and performed neonatal resuscitation, the quality of care suffered. ACOG issued a different admonition. In a 1973 *Technical Bulletin,* ACOG decried the lack of anesthetic expertise in the nation's maternity wards, cautioning that obstetricians and nurse-anesthetists were seldom as adept at administering all forms of anesthesia as anesthesiologists.[17]

ACOG's admonition likely spurred what one obstetrician called "kind of a turf thing" between obstetricians and anesthesiologists. After ACOG issued its criticism, hospitals began to forbid obstetricians to administer anesthesia. In 1981 obstetricians administered 30 percent of regional blocks; in 2001 they administered only 6 percent.[18]

As early as the late 1960s, there were already sporadic signs of anesthesiologists marking their professional territory. This occasional animus was directed in part at nurse-anesthetists. In an exchange between two prominent anesthesiologists who took a special interest in obstetrics (John Adriani, director of anesthesiology at Charity Hospital in New Orleans, and John Bonica, who was then president of the American Society of Anesthesiologists), Adriani suggested that anesthesiologists "take over nurse anesthesia lock, stock and barrel. . . . set up the curriculum, organize the instruction, examine them, certify them, inspect the schools, etc." The desire of the country's anesthesiologists, virtually all of them males, to place a tighter rein on the country's mostly female nurse-anesthetists only intensified with the advent of the women's movement. In an angry four-and-a-half-page, single-spaced, unpublished letter to the editor of *Regional Anesthesia,* Adriani complained in 1983 about the demeanor of the new generation of nurse-anesthetists: "The majority of nurse anesthetists have been aware of their limitations and acted accordingly. However, the contemporary breed of nurse anesthetists that has recently evolved is militant, conceited, and, at times, arrogant. This breed is a menace to the public's welfare. Individuals of this ilk are dangerous because they are oblivious of their limitations."[19]

Anesthesiologists also began to express resentment toward the obstetricians who administered anesthesia. J. P. Greenhill, an obstetrician who assumed authorship of *The Principles and Practice of Obstetrics* after Joseph DeLee died in 1942, also authored *Analgesia and Anesthesia in Obstetrics* in 1952. Yet when he issued a second edition of his book ten years later, anesthesiologists condemned it, arguing that in the decade since release of the first edition, anesthesiology had become such a complex field that obstetricians could not possibly keep abreast of its latest developments.[20]

With the founding in 1968 of the Society for Obstetric Anesthesia and Perinatology (SOAP), obstetric anesthesiology became a visible subspecialty. SOAP members were instrumental in this development, eliciting anesthesiologists' interest in obstetrics by offering numerous presentations as part of the American Society of Anesthesiologists' "Refresher Courses." The SOAP offerings included topics as varied as "Physiology of Pregnancy," "Resuscitation of the Newborn," and "Epidural Anesthesia: Indications, Contraindications, and Complications." The scheduling of five separate professional meetings on obstetric anesthesiology in the United States in 1977 alone evidenced anesthesiologists' growing participation in obstetrics.[21]

With more anesthesiologists dedicated to obstetrics by the 1980s and 1990s and a decidedly different lay attitude toward birth than in the 1970s, women's interest in epidural anesthesia became manifest. Between 1981 and 2001 the incidence of obstetric epidural administration almost tripled at the country's largest hospitals (increasing from 22% to 61% of births) and almost quadrupled at small hospitals (increasing from 9% to 35% of births).[22]

Like other forms of obstetric anesthesia in the past, however, the epidural did not attract uniform favor nationwide. In 1999 Joy Hawkins, then president of SOAP, explained that in New York City women expected to go to the hospital, have an epidural, and enjoy painless childbirth. Her Colorado patients, however, had another vision. "I'm close to Boulder, the 'au naturel' sort of place. The expectations are different." Accordingly, the epidural rate in Boulder was not quite 20 percent; in New York City the rate reached at least 90 percent in most hospitals.[23]

Yet even with this variability in use, by the late 1990s nearly all American women were aware of epidural anesthesia and its effect. One Chicago-area obstetrician recalled in 2005 that more than twenty years earlier, a laboring patient had come to the hospital with a piece of paper pinned to her blouse. She had penned a single word on the paper, "epidural." She feared that without the reminder she would forget to ask for one. Today, he lamented, the epidural was foremost in a laboring woman's consciousness. "I think most [women] are almost calling too early now because they want to make sure they get their epidural."[24]

Women's intensified interest in the epidural solved the perennial problem of low insurance reimbursement for obstetric anesthesiologists. With general anesthesia, an anesthesiologist could care for only one patient at a time, but epidurals allowed anesthesiologists to care for several women simultaneously. The ability of mothers to receive an epidural if they requested one rose accordingly: only 43 percent of the country's busiest hospitals provided the treatment in 1981, compared to 80 percent in 2001. An obstetrician observed in 1999, "Women want it, women demand it, and women receive it!"[25]

As more anesthesiologists specialized in obstetrics and more women requested epidural anesthesia, the epidural received increasingly good press. While their mothers had contrasted their demeaning anesthetized births with their empowering natural births, young women unwittingly mimicked their grandmothers, who glorified anesthesia. A columnist for the *Boston Herald* chided, "More and more women are deciding that there is nothing noble about writhing one's way through labor and delivery. . . . Indeed the most orgiastic moment of the day is more likely simultaneous with that first welcome sensation of anesthetic coursing through one's veins."[26]

In a single generation, the predominant portrayal of the ideal birth had gone from an invigorating, spontaneous, fully felt, athletic event to a nontaxing, carefully scheduled, fully numbed, relaxing event. Busy women reported appreciatively that an epidural block provided them with time to rest in the hours immediately preceding the births of their babies. One typically enthusiastic thirty-two-year-old woman who gave birth to her second child at Boston's Brigham and Women's Hospital alternately read and slept throughout her labor. Before receiving an epidural, she was miserable. Afterward, her sense of humor returned. Another woman told the *Boston Herald* that under the influence of epidural anesthesia, her labor was "wonderful, happy, restful. I was calling my friends, laughing. I was able to enjoy the experience." Another mother agreed: "It didn't enter my mind to go without an epidural. . . . I could watch, not scream."[27]

Epidural Anesthesia and the Question of Choice

Whereas a previous generation extolled natural childbirth because it afforded them control, women now praised epidural anesthesia for the same reason. The meaning of control in the context of birth had changed, however: natural childbirth conferred control by allowing women to take charge of their labors and deliveries and be the central character. Epidural anesthesia, in contrast, conferred control by allowing laboring women to maintain their composure and socialize normally. These different definitions of the same highly valued cultural concept reflected the divergent identities and values of two generations of American women.[28]

Even as epidural enthusiasts abandoned natural childbirth, though, they retained the reproductive-rights rhetoric of the women once active in health reform and portrayed the epidural as a matter of empowerment and choice. In a letter applauding a *New York Times Magazine* article that chastised natural childbirth advocates for discouraging women from having an epidural, one woman observed, "Real 'empowerment' takes place when a woman makes choices that are right for her." An article in *USA Today* echoed that sentiment: "Women's satisfaction with their childbirth experience rests not on how little pain they felt, but on whether their wishes about how to deal with it were respected."[29]

Physicians' professional organizations supported women's-choice epidurals in their official guidelines. When insurance companies began to deny women's claims for epidural anesthesia because there had been no medical need for the treatment, ACOG and the American Society of Anesthesiologists (ASA) issued a joint Committee Opinion in 1993 stating, "Maternal request is a sufficient justification for pain relief during labor." Two years later, ACOG and ASA voiced even broader support for maternal-choice epidurals. Because some studies indicated that administration of epidural anesthesia before five centimeters of cervical dilation increased the likelihood of cesarean delivery, many doctors and hospitals had been refusing to administer an epidural before that benchmark. ACOG and ASA now decried that practice as well, advising that no matter the state of cervical dilation, maternal request was all the indication needed for pain relief during labor.[30]

In the context of reproduction, feminists have advocated what is now termed "women's right to choose" at several junctures in U.S. history. Nineteenth-century feminists were the first to imply reproductive choice in their strong support for ready access to contraceptive devices, a crusade they labeled "voluntary motherhood." Women active in birth reform in the 1970s also invoked the concept of choice. In objecting to the rigid, involuntary nature of postwar obstetric treatments, reformers argued that women deserved not only the right to refuse treatment but also the right to access an array of birthing options. Most famously of late, feminists coined the phrase *pro-choice* to counter the term *pro-life* used by opponents of legal abortion. In invoking this terminology, feminists used *choice* in the same way nineteenth-century feminists used *voluntary*, to assert that life is complicated and everyone needs options, especially in matters relating to reproduction. With the joint ACOG and ASA statements, epidural anesthesia was now ensconced in the historical milieu of reproductive choice as well.[31]

When ACOG and ASA recommended that maternal choice govern all aspects of epidural administration, the organizations effectively paved the way for use of the word *choice* in regard to other medical treatment during birth. Soon after the professional sanction of the maternal-choice epidural, elective cesarean section (what became known in the medical literature as cesarean delivery by maternal request, or CDMR) became another widely touted concept.

The Rise in Cesarean Sections

The contemporary popularity of epidural anesthesia cannot be fully understood without also examining the normalization of cesarean delivery. Public and medical acceptance of the benefit of epidural anesthesia and the need for a high cesarean section (C-section) rate stemmed from the same impulse, the longtime desire of physicians and mothers to maximize comfort and safety during birth. The introduction of the electronic fetal monitor (EFM) in 1965 also linked the increase in the two treatments. The monitor's high false-positive rate for fetal hypoxia raised the cesarean section rate, and, for reasons explained in the following paragraphs, EFM also made physicians less wary of the epidural. The increasing C-section rate also ensured that anesthesiologists would be more readily available in maternity wards to administer epidurals. As one obstetric anesthesiologist noted, when cesarean section rates of 20 percent or more became common, anesthesia coverage became mandatory in labor and delivery. By the late twentieth century, sectioned births and epidurals had come to characterize "normal" birth in the United States, bolstering one another as together they seemed to highlight the risk and excruciating pain inherent in vaginal birth.[32]

The rise in cesarean sections beginning in the 1960s was steep and swift. Between 1965 and 1987, birth by C-section in the United States increased 455 percent, from 4.5 percent to nearly 25 percent of births. In 2006, 31.1 percent of births were abdominal deliveries.[33]

Ironically, the increase was the most precipitous between 1970 and 1981, when natural childbirth was at its zenith in popularity. Thus, for a time, two diametrically opposed attitudes toward birth and the medical treatment of birth prevailed. Compared to the vast publicity surrounding women's appreciation of natural childbirth, however, the rise in sectioned births elicited little initial com-

Cesarean Section Rate, 1910–2006

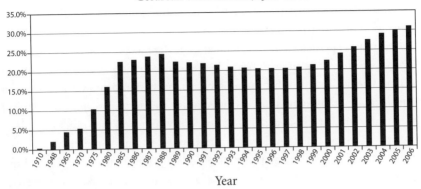

Year

Cesarean section rates began to rise in the United States with the introduction of the electronic fetal monitor, began to taper off when ACOG advised that women with previous cesareans should be urged to attempt a vaginal birth in subsequent labors, and rose steadily again after ACOG recommended that vaginal births after cesareans be attempted only if a physician was "immediately available" to provide emergency care. Since 1998 many American hospitals refuse to allow planned VBACs in their institutions, contributing to the renewed rise.

ment. Not until the late 1970s, as the C-section rate reached 16 percent, did the government, the medical community, and the lay press begin to examine and criticize the trend.

In retrospect, given what turned out to be the fundamental nature of birth reform, it is unsurprising that the ultimate in medicalized birth was being normalized even as natural childbirth enjoyed its heyday. Aside from allowing fathers and friends to remain with women throughout labor and birth, the most ballyhooed response of hospitals to women's demands for a more humane, less medicalized approach to birth was the creation of homey birthing suites—suites designed to hide the medical nature of hospitalized births. The institution of these cosmetic rather than systemic changes in response to mothers' requests for a less technological approach to birth successfully masked the lack of any real change in the American medical community's treatment of birth.

Not everyone was initially complacent about the increase in cesarean sections. The higher rate had long horrified older obstetricians whose careers were ending in the early 1980s, just as the rise was discussed publicly for the first time. These physicians had come of age during the gas-inhalation, pre–blood banking, pre-antibiotic era, when the risks associated with C-section were enormous. When these doctors trained, a low section rate was a sign of skill; a high rate (normally defined as anything even approaching 4%) signaled incompetence. They were thus critical of what they perceived to be the rashness and lack of skill of the new generation of obstetricians.[34]

The most experienced doctors tended to be the most critical of the high rate. One typical obstetrician, who began his residency at Cook County Hospital in 1943 and delivered his last baby in a Chicago suburb in 1987 and whose C-section rate throughout his forty-four-year career was a steady 2.5 percent, characterized young obstetricians this way: "They know everything and they don't know how to apply a forceps. And they do sections, sections, sections on the slightest provocation. If a mother is stuck at 4 centimeters dilation for 3 hours they go ahead and do a cesarean section. If they were to stop and realize what it takes for a cesarean section to occur—the loss of blood . . . the anesthetic risk, the operative risk. It's appalling. It's appalling to me anyway." J. Robert Willson, the recently retired chair of the Department of Obstetrics and Gynecology at the University of Michigan and a former ACOG president, expressed similar dismay in a 1981 address to the Obstetrical Society of Philadelphia. He predicted that because young obstetricians had come to rely so heavily on sections, soon no obstetrician would have the skill to use forceps in an emergency or to provide appropriate aid at breech deliveries. Although Willson lauded the technology now available to obstetricians, he also warned that doctors should never point to technology to justify the unwarranted assumption that it had become unnecessary to hone their hands-on clinical skills.[35]

When obstetricians like Willson learned to perform cesarean sections, the knowledge that once a woman had a C-section, all her subsequent births would be by C-section compounded doctors' wariness about performing the initial section. In 1916 Edwin B. Cragin, professor of obstetrics and gynecology at Columbia University, famously declared, "Once a Caesarean, always a Caesarean," a dictum that served as the medical rule in the United States for the next seventy years.

In Cragin's day, physicians performed sections using the classic cut (vertical and high on the uterus) instead of the low transverse cut (horizontal and low on the uterus) that is almost always used today. Cragin's warning reflected the fact that a sutured uterine wall after a classic cut is weak and prone to rupture during labor. In 1916 the indications for cesarean section were widening to include placenta previa, eclampsia, and hemorrhage, and Cragin was alarmed. He argued that only dystocia, defined as blocked labor caused by large tumors or severe pelvic contraction, warranted a cesarean section. In Cragin's day, almost every doctor saw cases of pelvic contraction caused by rickets developed in childhood.

By the time the C-section rate began its precipitous rise in the 1960s, obstetricians had broadened the definition of dystocia to also include "failure to progress" during labor, a diagnosis that increased in frequency in coming years and that critics of the high section rate termed "vague" and "catch-all."[36]

Despite Cragin's 1916 warning, the indications for cesarean section continued to widen. In the 1928 fifth edition of Joseph DeLee's *Principles and Practice of Obstetrics*, DeLee agreed in essence with Cragin and listed only contracted pelvis as an "absolute" indication for a sectioned delivery. Yet DeLee also listed other potential justifications, including cord prolapse and multiple previous stillbirths. He termed other indications "subjective." The 1951 edition of the same text, however, listed seventeen indications for cesarean section, including "definite disproportion between the baby's head and the pelvic inlet," "extreme narrowing of the pelvic outlet," a previous cesarean, pre-eclampsia, total placenta previa, severe cases of placental abruption, and breech presentations in first-time mothers older than forty. The wording of these broadened indications remained telling, though. Except for a previous cesarean and pre-eclampsia, every indication was qualified: *definite* disproportion between the baby's head and the pelvic inlet; *extreme* narrowing of the pelvic outlet; *total* placenta previa; *severe* placental abruption; breech presentations *in first time mothers older than forty.*[37]

Given obstetricians' reluctance before the 1960s to perform sectioned births, the national cesarean section rate remained well below 4 percent. One obstetrician, who was one of only four obstetric residents at Chicago's Cook County Hospital in 1940, recalled that during her tenure there, although there were fifteen hundred births monthly at the hospital (among a population at high risk for poverty, poor nutrition, and lack of prenatal care), if a resident did more than four cesarean sections a month, case reviews and serious scolding ensued. Supervisors painstakingly reassessed the need for every cesarean section performed by a resident, and, this former resident remembered, "you were told, you didn't do this, you didn't that" to avoid the section. Another physician, who truncated his obstetric residency to go into family practice in the 1940s, recalled that his chief resident in obstetrics was "very interventive": he routinely administered anesthesia, performed episiotomies, and applied forceps. Yet, in keeping with prevailing medical thought of the day, this "interventive" obstetric chief also "felt that a cesarean section rate of about 2 percent was about right."[38]

The increase in this "about right" rate began in the mid-1960s, as the baby boom ended. Observers speculated that the new trend toward smaller families conferred greater value to each newborn and that physicians were performing more sections to enhance fetal outcome. This rationale, used to justify what was then only a slight increase in the number of C-sections, contributed to the medical and lay belief that performing a cesarean section ensured fetal well-being in a way that vaginal birth could not. Five years later, as the section rate increased rapidly, this unproven justification rose to the level of medical and cultural truth and so continued to legitimate the rise. In 1979 an article in the *American Journal of Obstetrics and Gynecology* called for obstetricians to define "the proper level of trade-off" between the lowered infant morbidity and mortality allegedly due to the then 16.5 percent C-section rate and the potentially higher rates of maternal morbidity and mortality prompted by so many sectioned births.[39]

Most obstetricians dismissed this concern, however. There was 1 maternal death in 10,000 births in the United States in the late 1970s, as opposed to almost 70 deaths in 10,000 births in 1930, and so physicians often cited lowered maternal mortality as one of the great success stories of modern medicine. Yet with so few maternal deaths overall, hospitals and physicians saw no difference between sectioned and vaginal births; they would have had to examine hundreds of thousands of births to make that comparison. Interviews conducted with one hundred obstetricians in the mid-1970s about their views of cesarean section reflected how readily physicians dismissed the potential danger of sectioned deliveries to mothers. Only two of the doctors interviewed mentioned maternal risk in relation to cesarean section; all mentioned their concern for the fetus as a reason for performing a section.[40]

However, when a 1977 study published by *Obstetrics and Gynecology* revealed the potential risk to mothers of the rising C-section rate, the public health community took note. That study—of cesarean section and maternal mortality in Rhode Island from 1965 through 1975—reported that maternal death in the state had been twenty-six times greater in sectioned deliveries than in vaginal ones. Researchers wondered, of course, what precisely triggered the higher death rate: cesarean sections or the complications that prompted the sections. They ultimately concluded that 44 percent of the deaths were due to the cesarean section per se.[41]

This conclusion generated enough alarm that two federal agencies issued reports to ward off the feared rise in maternal deaths. In 1979 the Department of Health, Education, and Welfare (HEW) commissioned a report on the causes of the increase in sectioned deliveries and how to reduce the number of C-sections. Two years later, the National Institutes of Health (NIH) issued a similar report. Both agencies released the studies just as birth reform organizations were receiving vast and favorable nationwide publicity for their condemnation of American obstetricians' technological approach to birth. The tone of the reports reflected this unique atmosphere in that both were highly critical of contemporary obstetric practice in general and the high cesarean section rate in particular.[42]

The doctors interviewed for the HEW report cited the threat of a malpractice suit as the primary reason for the rise. After the interviews, however, the author of the HEW report noted that only a slim minority of these physicians had been sued or knew a colleague who had been sued. Rather than having faced a lawsuit personally or even vicariously, these obstetricians practiced "defensive medicine" because of a recent, steep increase in the cost of malpractice insurance.[43]

There have been three medical malpractice "crisis points" in U.S. history; the "crises" refer to rapid increases in malpractice premiums or award size or both. The first crisis occurred in the mid-1970s, the second in the mid-1980s, and the most recent at the start of the twenty-first century. Obstetrician-gynecologists have been affected by these "crises" even more than other physicians; the National Association of Insurance Commissioners estimated in 1975 that compared to other physicians, obstetrician-gynecologists faced ten times the risk of being sued and as a result paid four times the prevailing malpractice insurance rate.[44]

How obstetricians' malpractice liability fears affect cesarean section rates, however, is unclear. Studies have resulted in contradictory conclusions. Some indicate that the higher risk of liability claims decreases the probability of delivery by cesarean. Others conclude the opposite, that there is a correlation between increased insurance rates and more cesarean sections. Still other research finds no association between malpractice experience and cesarean deliveries in low-risk obstetrics.[45]

There are many possible explanations for the different outcomes of these studies. Most notably, each examines a different time period and a different area of the country; obstetric training, obstetric practices, population characteristics, and state laws governing insurance and malpractice premiums have changed over time and differ geographically as well. In any event, the author of the HEW report pointed out that the cesarean section rate began to rise almost ten years before the first medical malpractice crisis point, when lawsuits for failure to perform a cesarean were virtually nonexistent. Thus, she concluded, malpractice threats could not have played a significant role in the initial, precipitous increase.[46]

The HEW report also criticized contemporary medical training. Although few doctors would speak on the record about that factor, obstetricians complained anonymously to the report's author that obstetric residents were no longer trained in methods to encourage and support normal labor, a phenomenon that prompted an increase in the number of C-sections.[47]

An obstetrician who supervised residents at a large Chicago hospital explained how, in her experience, the focus on everything that could go wrong during birth dampened most residents' desire to encourage normal labor. She was acutely sensitive to this phenomenon because when she began her residency in 1992, she and her cohorts acquired a very different view of birth, thanks to the midwives then working at the hospital. Enormously curious about midwives' practices, those residents had followed midwife-attended births daily, "from the sidelines." In doing so, they internalized midwives' sensibilities. She recalled, "We loved our midwives. . . . we would page them when we were in labor and delivery saying, 'This patient's xyz is happening. What is the thing that you guys do to make the baby turn?'" She noted that the hospital's current residents had no midwives to learn from; the hospital had shut down its midwifery service several years prior. Midwives spent more time with their patients than obstetricians did, seeing roughly twelve patients per day as opposed to obstetricians' customary thirty, and the relatively low revenue they generated made paying their malpractice premiums difficult for the hospital.

The obstetrician who learned so much from midwives during her residency now viewed their firing as an incalculable loss: "I'm sad for our [obstetric] residents [today], because they don't get that kind of thing anymore. That there's another way . . . a way to approach labor as a natural life event." She shook her head in disbelief as she described the demeanor of current residents whenever they cared for a patient undergoing a vaginal birth after a previous cesarean (VBAC). Their focus on the possibility of uterine rupture was so unrelenting, she noted, that "[they] act like the patient's about to blow up."[48]

Shortly after release of the HEW report and its critique of medical training and lack of support for normal labor, the NIH convened a conference to develop its own consensus statement on the high cesarean section rate. The NIH panel concluded that because creation of the neonatal intensive care unit (NICU) coincided with the initial rise in C-sections in 1965, the medical community had mistakenly associated infants' improved chances for survival (due to NICUs) with the increase in cesareans. The NIH panelists also contended that NICUs had been so successful in lowering infant mortality that obstetricians and pediatricians alike began to apply the high-risk label to all infants in an effort to improve outcomes even further—an approach that normalized belief in the need for more C-sections. In essence, the NIH panel charged, an emergency mentality had taken over obstetrics.[49]

Epidural Anesthesia, Cesarean Section, and Electronic Fetal Monitoring

Introduction of the electronic fetal monitor (EFM) likewise fostered the emergency mentality that permeated obstetric and neonatal medicine in the mid-1960s. When Dr. Edward Hon of Yale University developed the device to monitor a fetus's heartbeat during labor, he intended for it to be used only when warranted by a woman's health history—if a mother suffered from diabetes or toxemia, for example. In celebrating the advent of the electronic fetal monitor, however, lay publications never mentioned Hon's admonition that the monitor be used only in potentially life-threatening situations. Instead, magazines portrayed all births as inherently risky and fetuses as so incessantly threatened that the very process of birth begged for relentless supervision of the fetus.[50]

A 1969 article in *Life* magazine about Hon's new tool portrayed birth and the safeguard provided by EFM this way: "The woman [pictured] above is in the throes of labor, a period of danger. . . . The fetus must struggle to survive the strains and pressures being put upon it. For years attending doctors have had no reliable way—nothing better than a stethoscope—to tell precisely when the fetus was in trouble." But thanks to EFM, *Life* and other lay publications intimated, a physician was now able to closely supervise every moment of the fetus's perilous descent through the suffocating birth canal, with scalpel poised to save the baby on a moment's notice.[51]

This portrayal proved so compelling that by 1979 American hospitals electronically monitored half of all births, a development that affected obstetricians' traditional behaviors. One obstetrician who had opened her private practice in Chicago in the late 1940s remembered how profoundly EFM altered her demeanor and practice. The monitoring, this seasoned and formerly relaxed physician remembered, "made me crazy with the patients." J. Robert Willson, a former ACOG president, complained in particular about the monitor's effect on young doctors and nurses who would never know what their pre-EFM behavior and knowledge might have been: "One of my concerns is that there is a whole generation of medical students, nurses, and house officers who are learning to rely more and more on fetal monitors as they learn less and less about labor."[52]

The relationship between physicians' EFM-induced vigilance and the increase in cesarean sections did not become the subject of national discussion, however, until 1985, when ACOG warned in its policy and procedure literature that fetal monitors were "highly sensitive but with low specificity." In other words, the meaning of the many changes in fetal heart patterns recorded by monitors was

unclear even as doctors persisted in making medical decisions based on the neb-
ulous messages. Hon, too, criticized what had become the customary use of his
monitor, protesting that "most obstetricians" did not use his invention properly:
"They're dropping the knife with each drop in the fetal heart rate."[53] Yet by the
time ACOG issued its warning, virtually every American hospital had acquired
fetal monitors and employed them in the vast majority of births.

The medical community accepted the need for EFM so quickly that the professional climate would not permit criticism of the device. Despite lack of evidence, most physicians insisted that the benefits of EFM were palpable. One typical doctor observed, "It is unlikely . . . a truly objective double-blind study in
either high or low-risk patients will—or should—ever be completed." When
birth reform efforts prompted some women to reject EFM, because the monitors
tethered them to beds throughout labor in much the same way restraints once
had, another obstetrician denounced what he characterized as the complaints of
selfish women. "Our task is to help these patients . . . recognize that they are introducing their own hedonism into a 12-hour event that may affect the 70–80
years of life of the infants they bear." The image of the steadfast electronic fetal
monitor guarding the perpetually imperiled fetus contributed to the view that
natural childbirth was at best a naive and at worst a reckless approach to birth.[54]

As the electronic fetal monitor became a compulsory diagnostic tool, it ensured the widespread use of the epidural. Because an epidural often lengthened
labor, physicians had customarily augmented these labors with oxytocin. Yet doctors were also well aware that oxytocin prompted its own undesirable side effects,
most notably, intense and irregular contractions that sometimes caused fetal distress. Thus, before the advent of EFM in the mid-1960s, doctors administered
epidurals prudently. The electronic fetal monitor, however, alleviated physicians'
wariness: they were now confident that continual surveillance of the fetal heart
rate would signal any problems prompted by the oxytocin administered to counteract the side effects of an epidural.[55]

Consequently, even as 1970s birth reformers made well-publicized headway in
their demands for a more humane, less technological approach to birth, the
NICU and the EFM were setting the stage for the normalization of epidural anesthesia and a nationwide cesarean section rate of 30 percent. The positive portrayal of natural childbirth turned out to be short-lived. Within a decade, nationwide discussion turned to an opposing presumption, that the birth process by its
very nature endangered babies and harmed mothers. The specter of risk in relation to vaginal birth soon loomed large.

Cesarean Section and the Question of Choice

In 1980 an article in *Glamour* magazine advised that some doctors now felt that unless a woman had a quick and easy vaginal birth, a cesarean section was preferable. The authors of the article portrayed cesarean section as a tender, simple procedure: "Your doctor will carefully cut your uterus. The doctor then reaches in and gently begins to remove your baby." That same year an obstetrician at the University of North Carolina reminded *Newsweek* readers that when he first studied obstetrics in the 1940s, every cesarean section required careful review at monthly staff meetings. Now, he reported, the opposite was true—the vaginal birth had to be justified.[56]

Outspoken critics of the C-section rate nevertheless remained. In 1992, when the C-section rate hit 22.3 percent, the U.S. Public Health Service (USPHS) issued *Healthy People 2000,* a compendium of national health targets for the millennial year. Among the listed goals was a cesarean section rate of 15 percent. For a time, lay and medical publications discussed that target and the reasons for it. The approving tone ended in 1999, however, after the *New England Journal of Medicine* published an opinion piece charging that the 15 percent USPHS goal was "an authoritarian approach to health care delivery" that implied that "women should have no say in their own care."[57]

The dual charges of authoritarianism and misogyny appealed not only to the obstetricians who believed the high percentage of sectioned births was justified, but also to a new generation of feminists, the segment of the population that twenty years earlier had advocated a less technological approach to birth. Given these two powerful lobbies, the charges published by the *New England Journal of Medicine* succeeded in silencing critics and quashing the few remaining attempts to lower the section rate while simultaneously introducing a new concept, maternal-choice cesarean section. Shortly after the article appeared, Benson Harer, the president of ACOG in 2000, used his pulpit to personally sanction elective cesarean sections.

Employing the rhetoric first developed by women's rights activists in the 1970s, Harer equated maternal-choice sections with an array of hard-won women's rights: owning property, suffrage, and access to safe, legal abortion. Many female physicians specializing in women's health quickly joined Harer in endorsing CDMR. Although the feminists who originally advocated birth reform never guessed that their demand for a wider array of birthing options would one day include elective cesarean section, times had changed.[58]

In the 1970s women active in health reform decried the "masculine strong-hold" of obstetrics, implying that more women obstetricians would mean a less medicalized approach to birth. As the number of female obstetricians approached parity with male obstetricians, however, it became clear that gender did not affect a physician's approach to birth. Moreover, when they endorsed the cesarean section as legitimate elective surgery, female physicians proved to be uniquely persuasive, for they spoke with a dual authority—as highly trained medical specialists and as women.[59]

Female physicians soon used a number of venues to make their case for CDMR. Michele Gerber, an obstetrician-gynecologist from suburban San Diego, told a *Washington Post* reporter that in her practice she often saw urinary incontinence, a condition she attributed to vaginal delivery. She thus sanctioned elective cesarean delivery so women could avoid such an undesirable postbirth condition. Other female doctors shared their personal decisions to give birth by cesarean. Kim Warner, a Denver obstetrician-gynecologist, told *USA Today* that she decided well in advance of her first pregnancy to deliver all her babies by cesarean. Like Gerber, she had performed many gynecological surgeries on women "who had delivered the old-fashioned way," and she hoped to escape their medical problems by avoiding vaginal birth. Female physicians discussed their personal choices on television as well. On a 2002 episode of ABC's *Good Morning America,* one of the show's regular medical experts, urologist Jennifer Berman, who was five months pregnant, announced her plans for an elective cesarean. She blamed vaginal birth for the incontinence and prolapsed uteruses she saw daily in her patients and confided "a dirty little secret" to viewers: most female physicians preferred cesarean section to low-risk vaginal birth.[60]

The few existing studies on the attitude of female physicians toward birth support Berman's view. Apparently her "secret" was not merely anecdotal. A greater percentage of female obstetrician-gynecologists, urogynecologists, and maternal-fetal medicine specialists than the population at large do prefer an elective cesarean as opposed to a low-risk vaginal birth for themselves. Another study indicated that this inclination leads to more cesarean sections for their patients as well; the study demonstrated a relationship between a physician's personal preference for birth and the percentage of that physician's patients who deliver abdominally.[61]

There is no evidence that in 1921, when the AMA Committee on Graduate Training in Gynecology and Obstetrics, headed by J. Whitridge Williams, first recommended melding obstetrics and gynecology into a single department in the country's teaching hospitals, Williams or his colleagues considered the effect of such a pairing on obstetric philosophy and practice. Yet though obstetrics and gynecology seem an eminently logical duo today, traditionally the two specialties had contradictory underlying assumptions. Obstetrics presumed physiology. Gynecology presumed pathology. The union thus inadvertently allowed the sensibility of the gynecologist to trump the sensibility of the obstetrician—a genuine loss when the obstetrician and gynecologist are the same person. The promotion and acceptance of elective cesarean section is only the most recent consequence of automatically linking pathology to birth.[62]

Affording Choice or Diminishing Choice?

This presumption of pathology has proved especially easy to accept in a culture that has long equated birth with unfathomable pain. A recent *Boston Globe Magazine* story epitomized the equation. The article's author, Darshak Sanghavi, an assistant professor of pediatrics at the University of Massachusetts Medical School, likened any woman eagerly anticipating natural childbirth to a suicide bomber. He explained, "It's an interesting secular variation on a religious narrative where unbearable pain suddenly transmutes to boundless joy . . . just as men blowing themselves to bits with suicide bombs think they will immediately appear in a paradise of virgins." Why, he wondered, would any sane woman choose excruciating pain in lieu of epidural anesthesia?[63]

In the 1970s birth choices had been many and varied, but Sanghavi's view that there are only two types of births—one dominated by unspeakable agony and the other dominated by a soothing epidural or, increasingly, quick, easy surgery—typified how birth options had been recast. A new generation of women (and their doctors) now characterized a felt labor as an unnecessary distraction: "All things being equal, why not avoid the pain and focus more on the miraculous experience of your baby's birth?" Indeed, in assessing vaginal birth, like Sanghavi, women too now implied that not choosing an epidural was irrational. One new mother noted, "Having the epidural was the best decision I've made in my whole life. The whole time I was in labor, I kept asking the nurse, 'Why doesn't everyone have one of these?'"[64]

Vocal physicians and laywomen promoted cesarean section as another "right" choice. A New York plastic surgeon who scheduled an elective cesarean section for the birth of her second child explained her rationale in the *Pittsburgh Post-Gazette:* "My feeling is, it should be an option. . . . there's this whole crazy movement, and there has been for a while, toward natural childbirth—getting no anesthesia, getting no medicine, because somehow medicine is bad. So women are forced to go through this barbaric ritual, and I think it's insane." In what was becoming the prevailing tone in both lay and medical discussions about choice in relation to birth, this doctor championed choice and then immediately condemned any choice other than her own, sanctioning elective cesarean section in the process.[65]

ACOG joined the fray. In 2003 the premiere professional organization of obstetricians and gynecologists officially defended the right of well-informed patients to choose a cesarean section in the absence of medical indication. Despite later studies indicating that elective cesareans, when compared with low-risk vaginal births, resulted in higher infant morbidity and mortality and more than triple the maternal mortality (as well as a significant increase in life-threatening placental anomalies in subsequent pregnancies), the organization has not revisited its stance. And despite its defense of maternal-choice cesareans, ACOG has never issued a similar statement defending the right of well-informed patients to choose a VBAC or a vaginal breech birth, even though studies show these procedures to be relatively safe. Use of the word *choice* in relation to birth had come to paradoxically mask the circumscription of choice.[66]

Compared to vaginal birth, a cesarean section had come to represent a birth with a seemingly guaranteed good outcome. The chair of the Department of Obstetrics and Gynecology at Sloane Hospital for Women in New York City was one of many experts who now implied that a cesarean section was devoid of risk. He observed in a *New York Magazine* article, "Patients have been very demanding in saying, 'If there's absolutely *any* question of risk, I want you to do a cesarean.'" A mother said of sectioned birth in the same article, "The certainty—knowing how it's going to go—is a good thing. With labor, you have absolutely no control— you don't know when it's going to happen; you don't know how it's going to go."[67]

The notion that cesarean section epitomized safety and predictability was not new. In 1983 Nicholson J. Eastman, chief of obstetrics at Johns Hopkins University, ridiculed this view, which was becoming increasingly common. "I gather the impression that, except in our own clinic, nothing ever goes wrong with a patient who has a cesarean section. Anesthetic mishaps are never mentioned, nor does appreciable blood loss or need for transfusion seem to occur. . . . These sectioned patients in the literature . . . appear to be immune to pulmonary embolism, and the ubiquitous staphylococcus passes them by." More than twenty years later, the concept of "choice" in relation to cesarean section made discussion of the many risks of cesarean section, for both mother and infant, even less frequent than Eastman had implied.[68]

With choice now the watchword in labor induction, epidural anesthesia, and cesarean section—and with each choice increasingly portrayed as "good" or "bad," "risky" or "safe"—the balance of authority between mothers and physicians began to tip once again. In the heady early days of the women's movement, support for patient choice gave patients a meaningful voice in medical decision-making, but promoting choice in relation to birth in the late 1990s had the opposite effect. The simplistic depiction of the seeming dangers of vaginal birth and the safety of cesarean section allowed doctors to steer their patients once again toward doctors' own personal preferences, an interaction that occurred most easily and frequently between female obstetricians and their patients. While male obstetricians, given the lessons of the women's movement, tended to be wary about heavy-handedly recommending particular treatments, female obstetricians, especially if they had given birth themselves, were far less hesitant to promote their vision of the sensible way to give birth.

One Chicago obstetrician (who recalled that during her own first birth, she "could not go without an epidural past one centimeter") "strongly push[ed]" all her patients to have an epidural "because sometimes it just helps them relax and they dilate." She described one recalcitrant patient, pregnant with her first child, who initially rejected this advice. After cervical dilation had not progressed for several hours, however, the doctor "talk[ed] her into the epidural." The epidural did not hasten cervical dilation as predicted, however, and the doctor eventually delivered the baby by cesarean section. After the surgery, in reviewing the course of the birth with the new mother, this female obstetrician intimated that the mother's initial refusal of an epidural inexorably led to the sectioned birth. She chided her patient, "Now, next pregnancy, what are you going to do?" The chastened mother responded: "I'm going to get an epidural right away."[69]

An obstetrician practicing in suburban Chicago explained why she thought so many of her colleagues exhibited frustration when confronted with patients who wanted to forgo assorted obstetric treatments: obstetricians accustomed to medical technologies became dependent on them. Her unique background informed this observation. She had begun her residency in 1982 in Vermont and later moved to Virginia and eventually Chicago. She was grateful that Vermont (she termed the state a "crunchy granola" area) had been her training ground because obstetricians there were less reliant on technologies and medical treatments than obstetricians in either Virginia or Chicago. She found herself constantly telling colleagues in these higher-tech departments: "We don't have to do that, it works okay if you don't do that." Yet she also understood why colleagues dismissed her reassurances. Although she had no trouble accepting obstetric technologies after practicing without them in Vermont, her colleagues, she explained, found it much harder to "go the other way": from a place "where everybody got internal monitors . . . an IV [and] was strapped to the bed" to a place "where people were walking around [and] . . . didn't have IVs."[70]

The dependence on technology that J. Robert Willson decried in the early 1980s when he observed that a generation of physicians and nurses were learning to rely on electronic fetal monitors as "they learn[ed] less and less about labor" soon spread beyond practitioners' reliance on EFM. In 1990, doctors writing in the medical journal *Birth* observed that with the increase in epidural anesthesia administration, nurses working in labor and delivery had lost their clinical ability to support women who preferred to forgo an epidural; nurses asked to do so would become "noticeably uncomfortable." Thus, although physicians and laywomen invoked the concept of choice in the early twenty-first century at least as often as health care activists did in the 1970s, choice in relation to birth had come to mean acceptance or rejection of three routine treatments—labor induction, epidural anesthesia, and cesarean section—and even in the case of these few treatments, a patient's refusal was not always a realistic possibility. This constriction was certainly not the doing of physicians alone. Mothers and their doctors had long done a complex dance, and the new generation of women, with their own unique concerns and burdens, helped shape the latest reality in American birthing practices, aided, ironically, by a new ingredient: a preponderance of females in the latest generation of obstetricians.[71]

Many birthing options had ceased to be options. Between 1997 and 2007 at least nine stand-alone birth centers and midwifery practices closed in the Washington-Baltimore area alone. One mother, who decided to give birth to her second child at home after the birth center where she planned to give birth closed, told the *Washington Post* that her first birth in the hospital had been unpleasant because she was constantly surrounded by medical personnel anticipating problems. She noted that the hospital "changes the experience. It doesn't promote the kind of . . . relaxed, normal experience I think birth should be."[72]

Those who condemned the lack of birth centers and midwifery practices in the DC area blamed rising malpractice rates and poor insurance company reimbursement for the closures. Unlike the obstetricians who also practice gynecology, midwives could not offset low insurance reimbursement for prenatal care with high-priced gynecologic surgeries. In other communities witnessing similar closures, however, midwives' supporters saw more sinister motives. In Salem, Oregon, a women's clinic sued a local hospital for antitrust violations, accusing the hospital of deliberately denying physician backup to midwives in an effort to put them out of business. Others recognized that such closures were a sign of the latest development in the medical marketplace. After St. Luke's Hospital in San Francisco dropped a popular midwifery program, supporters of that program blamed the perceived need for increased medical treatments to assure safe and comfortable birth, particularly the normalization of epidural anesthesia and cesarean section, treatments midwives were not permitted to perform.[73]

Midwives were not the only providers driven out of the birthing business in the 1990s. As doctors specializing in family practice faced ever higher malpractice premiums, birth choices were further constricted because family physicians found themselves increasingly unable to afford to provide obstetric care to women with low-risk pregnancies. In 1986, 43 percent of family physicians attended births; in 2004 only 22 percent did. As the midwives and family physicians specializing in low-risk obstetrics became increasingly scarce, so that in many parts of the country obstetricians were the only remaining medical personnel practicing obstetrics, these obstetricians saw increased opportunities to treat more pregnant women as high-risk, simply because that was their training and focus.[74]

Given the newly limited options in both birth location and birth practitioners, women who wanted to avoid medically unnecessary treatments were finding it increasingly difficult to give birth in the manner they chose. Sandra Steingraber, an ecologist in her late thirties when she was pregnant with her first child in 1998, was typical. Despite going to considerable lengths to avoid Pitocin, anesthesia, and episiotomy, she ultimately managed to avoid only the anesthesia.

Older than most women at their first pregnancy, Steingraber had come of age during the heyday of natural childbirth. Consequently, she anticipated that the childbirth education course she and her husband, Jeff, had signed up for would be a celebration of the power of labor. She teased Jeff as they drove to Boston's Beth Israel Hospital for their first class: "Do you think our instructor will make us roar like lions?"[75]

Steingraber quickly discovered that childbirth education had undergone a fundamental transformation since the 1970s. Hospital-affiliated classes had become the norm, and their primary purpose was to familiarize women with hospital routine. One mother, who in 1991 gave birth at age nineteen to her first child in California, recalled her experience in one of these classes. Rather than teach pregnant students about the nature of birth and ways to weather contractions, her childbirth instructor spent class sessions explaining what nurses and doctors did to and around laboring women: "Now you're in the birthing room, and they're gonna bring in this stuff, and it's gonna be on trays, and it's gonna sit there, and the doctor will come in."[76]

Steingraber's class was similarly constructed; the first class immediately disabused her of any romantic notions she had retained about childbirth education and birthing practices. She was especially stunned by her cohorts' negative attitude toward birth. She recalled of that first meeting, "What unites the class—and separates Jeff and me from the rest—is fear." During routine introductions, one young woman admitted, "I'm just really scared," and then burst into tears. Another woman explained that all she wanted to learn from the class was when she could have anesthesia. By the third week, the once enthusiastic Steingraber was "the sullen one with the attitude problem in the back row, notebook kicked under my chair."[77]

She especially resented the emphasis in the class on medical interventions, noting that the instructor consistently referred to narcotics and epidurals as "the good stuff." Steingraber observed, "Getting chummy with all the latest drugs, technologies, and surgical techniques has the effect of making them seem harmless, normal, and expected." The teacher devoted the majority of class time to describing everything that could go wrong during birth, an approach that reinforced the fear young women brought into the class. Steingraber complained, "Reviewing all injuries that could possibly occur is probably *not* the tack that coaches take with their star athletes right before the big game."[78]

The class did serve to warn Steingraber that if she wanted to evade unnecessary treatments, she would have to take matters into her own hands. After inviting a friend, a retired Canadian nurse-midwife, to come to Boston for the birth "as a kind of . . . courageous presence," Steingraber also hired as her private nurse a labor and delivery nurse who enjoyed working with women who preferred natural childbirth. The nurse promised to "keep the anesthesiologist from sneaking in the door" and eventually fulfilled that vow.[79] At one point in Steingraber's labor, when the anesthesiologist stopped in, "peddling his wares," the nurse listened impatiently until the anesthesiologist apparently crossed a line from describing an epidural to advocating one. "You can't say that," the nurse bellowed as she ushered the doctor from the room. "You are NOT allowed to say that. And we won't be needing your services."

Steingraber did not avoid a Pitocin drip, however. "I don't think we can get away with that," her private nurse told her, and at that point in her labor, Steingraber did not think to question why. "The showdown with the anesthesiologist," she later recalled, "was my last act of resistance." She did not escape an episiotomy either. Despite specifically telling her obstetrician that she preferred a first-degree tear to an episiotomy, at the doctor's prodding Steingraber consented to an episiotomy at the last minute—a distracted decision she regretted for months.[80]

Within twenty years of the instigation of birth reform and the heyday of natural childbirth, medicalized birth was back—and then some. With feminist rhetoric now part of mainstream culture, physicians and mothers alike justified the many treatments and technologies by invoking "women's choice." In stark contrast to the depiction of natural childbirth a generation before, birth had been recast as a dangerous and excruciating venture, much of which women could "choose" to avoid. They could plan when their labor would begin and ensure that they would have no physical sensation of labor; alternatively, they could forgo labor altogether and opt to have the baby surgically removed.

Epidural anesthesia and elective cesarean section (as opposed to the call of 1970s feminists to learn about and trust your body and enjoy a fully felt vaginal birth) had come to represent the essence of female empowerment in relation to birth. In an era of negligible maternal mortality, the once common medical phrase "low-risk vaginal birth" had, ironically, become an oxymoron. To paraphrase Tolstoy: In the early-twenty-first-century United States, all sectioned births are alike; every vaginal birth is risky in its own way.[81]

This latest irony in the history of obstetric practice is a predictable outgrowth of the hyperbole that has long infused medical and lay discussions of childbirth in the United States. The predominant medical and social portrayals of birth have always been extreme and contradictory: menacing torture on the one hand and buoyant uplift on the other. These persistent exaggerations have created what would otherwise be many incomprehensible situations: during much of the history examined in this book, many women went through labor, including the most difficult phase, without medication, only to be rendered unconscious at the moment of birth; mothers lobbied for twilight sleep because it seemed to provide women with solicitous care, only to find that twilight sleep led to rote obstetric treatment and the isolation of laboring women; women who were completely unaware of their agitation and expressions of pain during their heavily drugged births denied that they had experienced any discomfort; after the introduction of spinal anesthesia, physicians were increasingly forced to use forceps because spinal anesthesia made women incapable of giving birth without instrumental aid, yet doctors praised spinal anesthesia because it triggered pelvic relaxation and made the application of forceps easier; as physicians experimented with obstetric anesthesia to make it safer, the experimentation decreased obstetric safety; doctors tended to mitigate mothers' drug-induced agitation with more drugs; and physicians and mothers alike advocated planned inductions because they permitted women to forgo eating and avoid the vomiting caused by the anesthesia, which was increasingly administered because induction prompted such painful contractions. Ultimately, the normalization of obstetric anesthesia has taught women to view themselves as helpless victims of a bodily process rather than as the most important participants in that process. Today the ironies persist. When a sizable segment of the lay and medical communities consider low-risk vaginal birth risky despite historically low maternal and infant mortality, equate major abdominal surgery with a risk-free birth, and condemn vaginal birth without an epidural as fanaticism, a certain consistency can be seen in mothers' and physicians' equating diminished choices with empowered women.

The persistent paradoxes of American obstetric practice can be understood only in light of the cultural tendency to equate birth with unfathomable pain. Physicians unwittingly relay this notion to patients in subtle ways. When academic physicians help medical students master the difficult task of gauging the severity of a patient's pain, for example, they normally suggest that students use a scale from one (easily ignored discomfort) to ten (the worst pain ever experienced by the patient). In many American medical schools, physicians also advise that if the patient is a woman who has given birth, then "ten" should automatically be likened to labor pain, assumed to be the worst pain ever experienced by that particular woman. This indirect message has profound effect. Living in a culture that identifies childbirth as the zenith of human physical suffering primes all mothers in that culture to anticipate birth as an experience best avoided via abundant medical treatment.

The history of the formulation, use, and public and medical perception of obstetric anesthesia is essential, perhaps even the key, to understanding obstetric treatment in the United States. As this book demonstrates, the widespread promotion and acceptance of anesthesia can be linked directly to the normalization of many controversial obstetric practices: forceps use, labor induction, labor augmentation, episiotomy, electronic fetal monitoring, and a high cesarean section rate. Indeed, anesthesia during childbirth is so inextricably connected to these treatments that the more popular obstetric anesthesia has become, the less women and their doctors have been able to tolerate the mere notion of physiological birth. The history of obstetric anesthesia is thus a tale of how some medical treatments have come to be defined as "necessary" and, concomitantly, how both the medical and the lay communities have come to view potentially dangerous treatments as beneficial. Perhaps most of all, the ever-changing representation of obstetric anesthesia reveals how the cultural, social, and political concerns of the moment, all seemingly far removed from the world of medicine, constantly shape the medical treatments offered by physicians and the medical decisions made by the public.

ACOG *see* American College of Obstetricians and Gynecologists.

albolene a moisturizing cleanser.

American College of Obstetricians and Gynecologists the professional organization of obstetricians and gynecologists. Only physicians who restrict their practice to women can be members.

American Society for Psychoprophylactics in Obstetrics the national organization (eventually renamed Lamaze International) that promoted the techniques of French obstetrician Fernand Lamaze. *See also* Lamaze.

amphetamine a prescription stimulant first introduced as the pharmaceutical Benzedrine and originally used to fight fatigue and increase alertness.

analgesia a drug that diminishes pain without total loss of sensation or loss of consciousness.

anesthesia a medically induced state in which the patient experiences no pain. Anesthesia may be brought about through either loss of consciousness or loss of sensation. The term *anesthesia* is most commonly used to describe the drugs that induce the state. *See also* anesthetic.

anesthesiologist a physician specializing in the administration of anesthetics and other pain-relieving medications.

anesthetic a drug or drugs capable of inducing anesthesia. *See also* anesthesia.

ASA American Society of Anesthesiologists.

ASPO *see* American Society for Psychoprophylactics in Obstetrics.

barbiturates a group of sedative-hypnotic drugs that depress the central nervous system. A barbiturate lessens anxiety, decreases inhibitions, and induces sleep. Correct dosage is difficult to predict. Barbiturates can be highly addictive and can cause coma and death.

Benzedrine *see* amphetamine.

bougie an object used to dilate a bodily passage or bypass an obstruction in the body. In obstetrics, physicians sometimes placed a bougie in or near the uterus to induce labor.

Bradley Method also known as husband-coached childbirth. Colorado obstetrician Robert A. Bradley developed this method in the late 1940s to help couples prepare for childbirth without drugs. The Bradley Method teaches women to follow the model of other mammals and relax and pose sleep during labor with the help of a partner-coach.

caudal anesthesia injection of a local anesthetic into the caudal canal of the vertebral column. Also known as caudal block.

caudal block *see* caudal anesthesia.

CDMR cesarean delivery by maternal request. *See also* cesarean delivery by maternal request, primary elective cesarean section.

cephalic pertaining to the head; the normal position for a human birth is the cephalic position (head down).

cervical dilation the opening of the cervix, usually during childbirth. *See also* cervix.

cervical effacement the thinning of the cervix, usually during childbirth. *See also* cervix.

cervix the bottom portion of the uterus where the uterus meets the vagina; the cervix shortens and opens during labor to permit vaginal delivery. *See also* cervical dilation, cervical effacement.

cesarean delivery by maternal request cesarean section in the absence of medical indication, also known as elective cesarean section. *See also* cesarean section, primary elective cesarean section.

cesarean section delivery of a baby through an incision in a mother's abdomen and uterus. *See also* cesarean delivery by maternal request, primary elective cesarean section.

childbed fever *see* puerperal sepsis.

chloral a combination of chlorine and alcohol that reacts in water to form chloral hydrate, a hypnotic sedative. In its pure form, chloral is soluble in ether.

chloroform an inhalation anesthetic first discovered by American physician Samuel Guthrie in 1831, when he combined whiskey and chlorinated lime and determined chlorine's affinity for alcohol. James Young Simpson discovered the anesthetic properties of chloroform and popularized its use. Chloroform can cause heart, kidney, and liver damage. *See also* inhalation anesthesia.

cholera infantum infant diarrhea, usually a deadly ailment before antibiotics and intravenous rehydration therapy.

cord prolapse an obstetric emergency occurring when the umbilical cord drops through the cervical opening before the fetus begins descending into the vagina. If the fetus subsequently presses against the cord during descent, the fetal oxygen supply will be cut off.

cyanosis blue coloration of the skin due to decreased oxygen in the blood.

cyclopropane a colorless, highly flammable gas (chemical formula C_3H_6); once used as an inhalation anesthetic. *See also* inhalation anesthesia.

Demerol *see* meperidine.

dilation *see* cervical dilation.

dilaudid a highly addictive narcotic analgesic, customarily administered in tablet, liquid, or suppository form.

doula from the Greek, literally a woman who acts as a servant to another woman. In obstetrics, a doula provides emotional support and comfort to women during labor and birth.

dystocia traditionally, blocked labor caused by a tumor or a deformed pelvis. Today dystocia is more generically defined as abnormal, difficult, or prolonged labor.

eclampsia *see* pre-eclampsia.

effacement *see* cervical effacement.

EFM *see* electronic fetal monitor.

elective cesarean section *see* cesarean delivery by maternal request.

electronic fetal monitor an electronic device invented by Dr. Edward Hon in the mid-1960s, used to record the fetal heart rate during labor in order to assess fetal well-being. False positives for fetal hypoxia are common and can result in unnecessary surgical intervention, i.e., cesarean delivery.

epidural anesthesia injection of a local anesthetic into the epidural space of the vertebral column. Also known as epidural block and lumbar epidural.

epidural block *see* epidural anesthesia.

episiotomy an incision in the perineum to widen the vagina before giving birth.

ergot a fungus that grows on rye and other grain; given by mouth, intravenously, or intramuscularly as a fast-acting uterine stimulant.

ether an inhalation anesthetic, synthesized when Valerius Cordus mixed sulfuric acid with alcohol to form a colorless, explosive liquid. It was first demonstrated publicly by William T. G. Morton at the Massachusetts General Hospital in Boston in 1846. *See also* inhalation anesthesia.

ethylene a chemical compound with the formula C_2H_4, once used as a general anesthetic.

first-stage labor the initial portion of labor when the cervix effaces and dilates to allow passage of the fetus into the vagina. The first stage of labor ends with complete cervical dilation. *See also* transition.

fistula *see* vesico-vaginal fistula, recto-vaginal fistula.

forceps instrument designed to manually extract the fetus from the birth canal.

Friedman curve a graphic standard, developed by Emanuel A. Friedman in 1953 while a resident at Sloane Hospital, for the average time needed for "normal" cervical dilation and fetal descent.

general anesthesia the state of complete unconsciousness due to administration of drugs. General anesthetic is rarely administered today for vaginal delivery because of the risk of pulmonary aspiration of stomach contents; still used for emergency cesarean section.

halothane a nonflammable, general, inhalation anesthetic designed to be a replacement for volatile anesthetics like ether and cyclopropane. *See also* inhalation anesthesia.

husband-coached childbirth *see* Bradley Method.

hyaline membrane disease known today as respiratory distress syndrome. This disease, commonly suffered by premature babies, is caused by lack of surfactant in the lungs. The fetus does not begin to produce surfactant until sometime between 24 and 28 weeks gestation; surfactant remains insufficient until about 35 weeks gestation, and thus the lungs in premature babies do not inflate properly. Artificial surfactant became available in the 1980s and is now routinely used to treat premature babies suffering from respiratory distress syndrome.

HypnoBirthing a method of childbirth education developed by Marie Mongan in the late 1980s. HypnoBirthing is a form of self-hypnosis achieved with the aid of a partner; it helps women give birth without arbitrary or unnecessary medical intervention.

hypoxia shortage of oxygen in the blood.

iatrogenic resulting from medical treatment.

indication a sign or circumstance pointing to the need for medical treatment.

inhalation anesthesia anesthesia achieved by inhaling an anesthetic. *See also* general anesthesia.

Lamaze a childbirth preparation method developed by French obstetrician Fernand Lamaze in the early 1950s. The Lamaze method is based on Pavlov's theory of conditioned response to stimuli. *See also* American Society for Psychoprophylactics in Obstetrics.

LDR room Labor, delivery, and recovery room; the maintenance of LDR rooms has been one of the few enduring responses to the birth reform movement of the 1970s. LDR rooms allow women to stay in one room throughout labor and birth and the aftermath.

lumbar epidural *see* epidural anesthesia.

magnesium sulfate a chemical compound with the formula $MgSO_4$; when used medically, magnesium sulfate can reduce smooth muscle tone or contractions; used in the treatment of pre-eclampsia and preterm labor.

MANA *see* Midwives Alliance of North America.

menarche the first menstrual period in a girl's life.

meperidine an opioid analgesic used to treat moderate-to-severe pain and delivered via tablet, syrup, intramuscular injection, or intravenous injection. Demerol is the brand name.

Midwives Alliance of North America an organization founded in 1982 to promote midwifery as an integral part of the maternal-child health system in the United States. MANA has become an umbrella organization for midwives, instrumental in setting educational and professional standards for the profession.

morphine the principal active ingredient in opium, a potent analgesic.

multipara a woman who is pregnant and has had previous children; a woman who has given birth two or more times.

nalorphine a derivative of morphine that reverses the effect of morphine and other narcotics; used during labor to mitigate the effects on the fetus of narcotics ingested by the mother.

naloxone a medication used to treat neonatal respiratory depression caused by narcotics ingested by the mother during labor.

narcotic opium or any derivative of opium.

natural childbirth the phrase coined by British obstetrician Grantly Dick-Read to describe childbirth without medicine or medical intervention.

Nembutal   *see* pentobarbital.

NICU   neonatal intensive care unit.

Nisentil   an opioid analgesic chemically related to meperidine but more potent, faster acting, and of shorter duration. *See also* meperidine.

nitrous oxide   a colorless, nonflammable gas; also known as laughing gas. It is used both as an analgesic and as an anesthetic.

nullipara   a woman who has never given birth.

oil-ether colonic method   *see* rectal anesthesia.

opiate   a drug derived from opium.   •

opioid   any synthetic narcotic that has opium-like qualities but is not derived from opium.

opium   a narcotic extracted from opium poppies; a powerful painkiller.

oxytocin   a hormone released naturally by the pituitary gland after distension of the cervix during labor; aids in cervical dilation. Synthetic oxytocin is sold under the trade name Pitocin, a drug that triggers and augments labor. Oxytocin is also sometimes given after delivery to aid in contraction of the uterus to prevent post-partum bleeding. *See also* pituitary extract, Pituitrin.

paraldehyde   an effective anticonvulsant, hypnotic, and sedative; used to induce sleep. It is administered either rectally or via an intramuscular injection.

parous   having given birth to one or more offspring. *See also* multipara, nullipara, and primipara.

parturient   a woman in labor.

Penthrane   proprietary name for methoxyflurane, an inhalation anesthetic used in the 1960s but withdrawn from the market because of the risk of kidney damage.

pentobarbital   a short-acting barbiturate, used today for preoperative sedation or the treatment of insomnia. It is available in two forms: as a free acid that is only slightly soluble or as a sodium salt that is very soluble. Nembutal is one of the trade names for pentobarbital.

pentobarbital sodium   *see* pentobarbital.

perineum   the region between the vagina and the anus.

pessary   a device inserted into the vagina to support the uterus.

phenazocine   an opioid formerly used as a pre-anesthetic.

phenobarbital   a long-acting barbiturate, used as a sedative, a hypnotic, and an anti-convulsant; administered orally.

Pitocin   *see* oxytocin.

pituitary extract   a hormone produced by the posterior pituitary gland that triggers labor. In modern obstetrics it is used most often to aid in placental expulsion. *See also* oxytocin, Pitocin, and Pituitrin.

Pituitrin   formerly the trademark name for a hormone released by the posterior pi-tuitary. *See also* oxytocin and pituitary extract.

placenta previa   a placenta that develops in the lower part of the uterus and covers part or all of the cervical opening.

pre-eclampsia   one of the most serious complications of pregnancy, symptoms in-clude high blood pressure, unusual swelling of the hands, face, and feet, severe headache, and significant amounts of protein in the urine. When convulsions and coma are also associated with these symptoms, it is called eclampsia.

prep slang employed by doctors and nurses to refer to their ritual preparation for birth of a woman in labor. Most specifically, "the prep" referred to the shaving of pubic hair and administration of an enema.

primary elective cesarean section a cesarean section performed on a first-time mother in the absence of medical indication. *See also* cesarean section and cesarean delivery by maternal request.

primipara a woman who is pregnant and has not previously had a child; a woman who has given birth only once.

promethazine a tranquilizer once used for preoperative sedation; also used as an antihistamine.

pudendal block a local anesthetic injected into the external genitalia to numb the pudendal nerve, the vulva, the perineum, and the vagina.

puerperal sepsis postpartum infection; it usually resulted in death before antibiotics were available; once commonly known as childbed fever.

puerperium the period from the expulsion of the placenta from the uterus until the uterus has returned to its prepregnancy size, usually three to six weeks.

rectal anesthesia general anesthesia following placement of liquid anesthetics in the rectum.

recto-vaginal fistula a connection between the vagina and rectum caused by tears in the vaginal wall due to prolonged labor. Feces leak into the vagina as a result. *See also* vesico-vaginal fistula.

regional anesthesia in obstetrics, anesthesia induced by injection of a local anesthetic near or around a nerve of the spinal cord or some branch of the spinal cord. It creates loss of bodily sensation and sometimes motor function in a specific area without loss of consciousness.

saddle block a spinal anesthetic affecting the area around the perineum and anus. The saddle block was developed by anesthesiologist John Adriani in the 1940s primarily for use in rectal and genital surgery. Adriani later expanded its use to obstetrics. *See also* spinal anesthesia.

scopolamine a central nervous system depressant that causes amnesia and sometimes delirium.

secobarbital a barbiturate (brand name Seconal) used in obstetrics in the 1950s and 1960s but seldom used today because of its depressant effects on the infant. This sedative hypnotic has no analgesic properties and can increase agitation and excitement in patients who are in pain—a common observation and complaint of mothers.

Seconal *see* secobarbital.

second-stage labor the portion of labor occurring after full cervical dilation when the uterine muscle aids the mother in pushing the fetus out of the uterus and through the birth canal.

SOAP *see* Society for Obstetric Anesthesiology and Perinatology.

Society for Obstetric Anesthesiology and Perinatology an organization formed in

1968 by anesthesiologists interested in obstetrics in order to spark interest in the subspecialty and research in the field; now the professional organization for obstetric anesthesiologists.

sodium amytal a barbiturate with sedative-hypnotic properties, also known as "truth serum." Used today mostly for severe insomnia.

spinal anesthesia anesthesia resulting from the injection of local anesthetic into cerebro-spinal fluid to induce lack of feeling in a specified area. Also called spinal block. *See also* saddle block.

spinal block *see* spinal anesthesia.

subcutaneous beneath the skin.

synergistic method an anesthetic method invented by James Tayloe Gwathmey in 1921, in which assorted drugs and techniques are combined to produce the desired effects.

thalidomide a drug manufactured by a German pharmaceutical company and sold as a safe, nonaddictive sedative in almost fifty countries in the late 1950s and early 1960s; thalidomide causes severe fetal deformities if ingested in the first trimester of pregnancy. Almost ten thousand babies were born between 1956 and 1962 with thalidomide-induced malformations, including stunted or missing limbs.

Thorazine a tranquilizer. Thorazine, used today for the treatment of schizophrenia, has been described as giving patients a "chemical lobotomy."

tranquilizer a drug with a calming effect.

transition the shortest portion of first-stage labor, occurring at the very end of first-stage labor, as the cervix fully dilates from eight to ten centimeters. Transition customarily lasts for 10 to 20 minutes. Women customarily describe transition as the most difficult portion of labor to weather. *See also* first-stage labor.

trichloroethylene an anesthetic first used in the United States in the 1930s; it is synthesized from hexachlorethane with zinc and hydrochloric acid.

twilight sleep a mixture of a narcotic and scopolamine given by hypodermic injection to laboring women and, in the first decades of its use in the early twentieth century, accompanied by elaborate medical ritual. Twilight sleep reduced women's pain, erased their memory of birth, and often caused undesirable side effects such as delirium.

uterus the pear-shaped, hollow muscle organ in human females in which the fetus implants and grows.

VBAC vaginal birth after a previous birth by cesarean section (vaginal birth after cesarean).

version the forcible, external, manual movement of the fetus, usually from breech to cephalic position.

vesico-vaginal fistula a connection between the vagina and the bladder caused by tears in the vaginal wall due to prolonged labor. Urine leaks into the vagina as a result. *See also* recto-vaginal fistula.

Introduction · *"Terrible Torture"* or *"The Nicest Sensation I've Ever Had"?*

1. For more on the discovery and use of ether and chloroform, see Martin S. Pernick, *A Calculus of Suffering: Pain, Professionalism, and Anesthesia in Nineteenth-Century America* (Columbia University Press, 1985); Julie M. Fenster, *Ether Day: The Strange Tale of America's Greatest Medical Discovery and the Haunted Men Who Made It* (HarperCollins, 2001); and Linda Stratmann, *Chloroform: The Quest for Oblivion* (Sutton, 2003).

2. The phrases "cheerfulness and gayety" and "terrible torture, hopeless of relief" are in Charles D. Meigs, *Obstetrics: The Science and the Art* (Blanchard and Lear, 1852), 366; and Bedford Brown, "The Therapeutic Action of Chloroform in Parturition," *Journal of the American Medical Association* 25 (August 31, 1895): 354–58, respectively. These types of phrases were not aberrant in the nineteenth century. One sentiment or the other appeared in virtually every obstetric text and article about obstetric anesthesia written in that era. The more recent statements are from Betsy Marvin McKinney, "The Pleasure of Childbirth," *Ladies' Home Journal*, April 1949, 116, 118–21; and Christopher Snowbeck, "Is Elective C-Section Delivery a Good Idea?" *Pittsburgh Post-Gazette*, March 18, 2003, D1.

3. David Bogod, "Advances in Epidural Analgesia for Labour: Progress versus Prudence," *Lancet* 345 (May 6, 1995): 1129; Committee on Obstetrics: Maternal and Fetal Medicine, "Pain Relief during Labor," *ACOG Committee Opinion*, no. 118 (January 1993).

4. Studies indicating that anxiety, expectations, and prior belief increase labor pain include U. Waldenström, V. Bergman, and G. Vasell, "The Complexity of Labor Pain: Experiences of 278 Women," *Journal of Psychosomatic Obstetrics and Gynecology* 17 (1996): 215–28; U. Waldenström, I. M. Borg, B. Olsson, M. Skold, and S. Wall, "The Childbirth Experience: A Study of 295 New Mothers," *Birth* 23 (1996): 144–53.

5. For discussions of how pain differs across cultures and individual experience, see Arthur Kleinman, Paul E. Brodwin, Byron J. Good, and Mary-Jo DelVecchio Good, "Pain as Human Experience: An Introduction," in *Pain as Human Experience: An Anthropological Perspective*, ed. Mary-Jo DelVecchio Good, Paul E. Brodwin,

Byron J. Good, and Arthur Kleinman (University of California Press, 1994), 1–28; David B. Morris, *The Culture of Pain* (University of California Press, 1991), esp. chap. 2, "The Meanings of Pain." For a specific discussion of labor pain across cultures, see Lynn Clark Callister, Inaam Khalaf, Sonia Semenic, Robin Kartchner, and Katri Vehvilainen-Julkunen, "The Pain of Childbirth: Perceptions of Culturally Diverse Women," *Pain Management Nursing* 4 (2003): 145–54. For more on changing perceptions of pain over time, see Roselyne Rey, *The History of Pain* (Harvard University Press, 1995).

6. For discussions of how birth practices differ across cultures, see Louise W. Hedstrom and Niles Newton, "Touch in Labor: A Comparison of Cultures and Eras," *Birth* 13 (September 1986): 181–86; Betsy Lozoff, Brigitte Jordan, and Stephen Malone, "Childbirth in Cross-Cultural Perspective," *Marriage and Family Review* 12 (1988): 35–60; Janice M. Morse and Caroline Park, "Differences in Cultural Expectations of the Perceived Painfulness of Childbirth," in *Childbirth in America: Anthropological Perspectives,* ed. Karen L. Michaelson (Bergin and Garvey, 1988); Russel A. Judkins and Ann B. Judkins, "Commentary: Cultural Dimensions of Hmong Birth," *Birth* 19 (September 1992): 148–50; P. Mancino, J. Melluso, M. Monti, and E. Onorati, "Preparation for Childbirth in Different Cultures," *Clinical and Experimental Obstetrics and Gynecology* 32 (2005): 89–91.

7. For typical textbook descriptions of labor, see Nicholson J. Eastman, *Williams Obstetrics* (Appleton-Century-Crofts, 1950), 324–39; Jack A. Pritchard, Paul C. MacDonald, and Norman F. Gant, *Williams Obstetrics* (Appleton-Century-Crofts, 1985), 306–7; and Neville F. Hacker and J. George Moore, *Essentials of Obstetrics and Gynecology* (W. B. Saunders, 1998), 150–54.

8. "Easily handled," "the part of labor," "joyful, not painful," and "the fun part" are found in Boston Women's Health Book Collective, *Our Bodies, Ourselves: A Book by and for Women* (Simon and Schuster, 1976), 271; "no pain at all" is in Mary Thomas, *Post-War Mothers: Childbirth Letters to Grantly Dick-Read, 1946–1956* (University of Rochester Press, 1997), 171.

9. Robert A. Bradley, "Fathers' Presence in Delivery Rooms," *Psychosomatics* 3 (November–December 1962): 474–79. Bradley eventually formulated the Bradley Method, now touted by the American Academy of Husband-Coached Childbirth. The Bradley Method advocates relaxation exercises, enabled by a coach, during labor. Bradley advocates claim that over 90% of women trained in the Bradley Method enjoy natural childbirth. For more information on the Bradley Method, see Susan McCutcheon-Rosegg and Peter Rosegg, *Natural Childbirth the Bradley Way* (E. P. Dutton, 1984).

10. Practicing family physician, interview by author, tape recording, September 15, 2004, Athens, OH; Barbara Katz Rothman, *In Labor: Women and Power in the Birthplace* (W. W. Norton, 1991), 20–21.

11. For a thorough discussion of this phenomenon, see Jacqueline H. Wolf, "'Mighty Glad to Gasp in the Gas': Perceptions of Pain and the Traditional Timing of Obstetric Anesthesia," *Health* 6 (2002): 365–87.

12. J. Y. Simpson, *Remarks on the Superinduction of Anaesthesia in Natural and Morbid Parturition: With Cases Illustrative of the Use and Effects of Chloroform in Ob-*

stetric Practice (William B. Little, 1848), 11; Joseph B. DeLee, *The Principles and Practice of Obstetrics* (W. B. Saunders, 1925), 137.

13. DeLee, *The Principles and Practice of Obstetrics,* 122–23.

14. Scholars have long noted the indifference exhibited by Western medicine toward pain. See, for example, Isabelle Baszanger, *Inventing Pain Medicine: From the Laboratory to the Clinic* (Rutgers University Press, 1998). Like Baszanger, Eric Cassell argues in *The Nature of Suffering* (Oxford University Press, 1991) that when it comes to the treatment of suffering, Western medicine has consistently failed. Unlike Baszanger, however, Cassell distinguishes between suffering and pain by defining suffering as pain with a temporal element, as in, "If the pain cannot be controlled, I will not be able to take it." Cassell's notion of pain as suffering with a temporal element is especially relevant to childbirth. Women fear that labor pain will last hours, even days, growing in intensity to eventually become unbearable. Lay publications have also taken note of the medical community's longtime disinterest in patients' complaints of pain. See, for example, Mary Carmichael, "The Changing Science of Pain," *Newsweek,* June 4, 2007, 40–47.

15. Morris, *The Culture of Pain,* 278.

16. Cassell, *The Nature of Suffering.*

17. Retired obstetrician, interview by author, tape recording, July 19, 2004, Chicago.

18. For an example of mothers' charges in the 1950s, see Gladys Denny Shultz, "Journal Mothers Report on Cruelty in Maternity Wards," *Ladies' Home Journal,* May 1958, 44–45; and Gladys Denny Shultz, "Journal Mothers Testify to Cruelty in Maternity Wards," *Ladies' Home Journal,* December 1958, 58–59, 135, 137–39.

19. Joan Jacobs Brumberg discusses this phenomenon in *The Body Project: An Intimate History of American Girls* (Random House, 1997), 29–55.

20. Judith Walzer Leavitt first posited the argument that women controlled birthing practices until birth moved to the hospital. Leavitt argues that even as the primary birth attendant changed from midwife to physician, women were able to accept or reject all treatments offered by doctors, to choose who was present at their births, and to select any comforts to be employed as they labored. See Judith Walzer Leavitt, *Brought to Bed: Childbearing in America, 1750–1950* (Oxford University Press, 1986). Also see Charlotte G. Borst, *Catching Babies: The Professionalization of Childbirth, 1870–1920* (Harvard University Press, 1995). For a complete discussion of my findings that physicians shaped key birth practices before the move of birth from home to hospital, see Wolf, " 'Mighty Glad to Gasp in the Gas.' "

Chapter 1 · Ether and Chloroform

1. Edward Wagenknecht, *Mrs. Longfellow: Selected Letters and Journals of Fanny Appleton Longfellow (1817–1861)* (Longmans, Green, 1956), 113. Although Fanny Longfellow was the first woman in the United States to receive obstetric anesthesia from a physician, she might not have been the first American woman to enjoy ether's anesthetic qualities during birth. In 1852 Walter Channing described a patient who told him that her husband, a chemist, had performed experiments with sulfuric ether

nineteen years earlier. Subsequently, during her first labor in 1833, she was in such distress that, in desperation, her husband wiped ether all over her face. Channing reported that, according to the woman, "Her labor was now easy, was soon completed, and a stout living boy born." See Walter Channing, "Notes of Difficult Labors, in the Second of Which Etherization by Sulphuric Ether Was Successfully Employed Nineteen Years Ago," *Boston Medical and Surgical Journal* 46 (1852): 113–15.

2. N. C. Keep, "The Letheon Administered in a Case of Labor," *Boston Medical and Surgical Journal* 36 (1847): 226. This was not Keep's first use of ether; previously he had administered ether to dental patients. N. C. Keep, "Inhalation of Ethereal Vapor for Mitigating Human Suffering in Surgical Operations and Acute Diseases," *Boston Medical and Surgical Journal* 36 (1847): 199–201. For more on Keep's adventure with the Longfellows, see C. B. Pittinger, "The Anesthetization of Fanny Longfellow for Childbirth on April 7, 1847," *Anesthesia and Analgesia* 66 (1987): 368–69; Herschel H. Reynolds, "A Courageous Lady—Mrs. Henry Wadsworth Longfellow," *Journal of the American Dental Association* 55 (December 1957): 840–42; and P. Keep, "Nathan Keep—William Morton's Salieri?" *Anaesthesia* 50 (1995): 233–38.

3. Keep, "The Letheon"; Edward Wagenknecht, *Longfellow: A Full-Length Portrait* (Longmans, Green, 1955), 113, 129, 243.

4. Wagenknecht, *Mrs. Longfellow*, 113.

5. Catherine Esther Beecher quoted in Ann Douglas Wood, "'The Fashionable Diseases': Women's Complaints and Their Treatment in Nineteenth-Century America," *Journal of Interdisciplinary History* 4 (Summer 1973): 25–52, quote at 26. Scholars who have written about the tendency of middle- and upper-class urban women to exhibit weakness in this era offer myriad explanations. Sarah Stage, in writing about women's infatuation with patent medicines in the nineteenth century, argues that men exhibited a false confidence in the face of the uncertainties prompted by rapid industrialization and urbanization. They soon projected their anxieties onto women, idealizing them as vulnerable, weak, and in need of protection. See Sarah Stage, *Female Complaints: Lydia Pinkham and the Business of Women's Medicine* (W. W. Norton, 1979). Others have argued that the nature of Victorian culture encouraged women to complain of physical distress as a sign of femininity and breeding, and so female frailty became fashionable. In writing about the emergence of anorexia nervosa in nineteenth-century America, Joan Jacobs Brumberg argues that self-starvation became one way for daughters to imitate their chic, fragile mothers. Joan Jacobs Brumberg, *Fasting Girls: The History of Anorexia Nervosa* (Plume, 1988), 164–72.

6. Joan Jacobs Brumberg makes this point about vulnerable social audiences specifically in regard to anorexia nervosa, arguing that it became a "communicable" disease in the 1980s after being paraded endlessly in magazines and on television before "a reservoir of susceptible young women." Joan Jacobs Brumberg, "From Psychiatric Syndrome to 'Communicable' Disease: The Case of Anorexia Nervosa," in *Framing Disease: Studies in Cultural History,* ed. Charles E. Rosenberg and Janet Golden (Rutgers University Press, 1992), 141.

7. Cyrus Edson, "American Life and Physical Deterioration," *North American Review* 157 (October 1893): 440–52.

8. Henry Parker Newman, "The Gynecological and Obstetrical Significance of Girlhood," *Chicago Medical Recorder* 20 (May 1901): 458–62, "structural disease" and "juvenile cervix" at 460; "Discussion on Henry Parker Newman, The Gynecological and Obstetrical Significance of Girlhood," *Chicago Medical Recorder* 20 (May 1901): 496–503, "mental labor" at 501.

9. George M. Beard, *American Nervousness: Its Causes and Consequences* (G. P. Putnam's, 1881), vi, 7–8, 20, 65–66; Carl Henry Davis, *Painless Childbirth: Eutocia and Nitrous Oxid-Oxygen Analgesia* (Forbes, 1916), description of birth as "natural" at 9, "hot-house product" at 18. For more on nineteenth-century women and their experience of nervousness and neurasthenia, see Janet Oppenheim, *"Shattered Nerves": Doctors, Patients, and Depression in Victorian England* (Oxford University Press, 1991), 79–109.

10. John H. Dye, *Painless Childbirth; or, Healthy Mothers, and Healthy Children. A Book for All Women* (Baker, Jones, 1889), 53–54. Physician J. H. Kellogg echoed this belief when he lauded the "simple minded, primitive people, in a savage state" who gave birth with remarkable ease. J. H. Kellogg, *Ladies' Guide in Health and Disease: Girlhood, Maidenhood, Wifehood, Motherhood* (Modern Medicine, 1893), 447. For more on slaves and childbirth, see Deborah Gray White, *Ar'n't I a Woman? Female Slaves in the Plantation South* (W. W. Norton, 1985), 96–97, 111–12; and Marie Jenkins Schwartz, *Birthing a Slave: Motherhood and Medicine in the Antebellum South* (Harvard University Press, 2006).

11. The phrase "living mother of a living child" is seen in the letters and diaries of many women in this era. See, for example, Laurel Thatcher Ulrich, "'The Living Mother of a Living Child': Midwifery and Mortality in Post-Revolutionary New England," *William and Mary Quarterly*, 3rd ser., 46 (1989): 27–48; and Caroline G. Curtis, ed., *The Cary Letters* (Riverside Press, 1891), 335.

12. Laurel Thatcher Ulrich, *A Midwife's Tale: The Life of Martha Ballard, Based on Her Diary, 1785–1812* (Vintage Books, 1990), 170. Irvine Loudon discusses maternal death rates in *Death in Childbirth: An International Study of Maternal Care and Maternal Mortality, 1800–1950* (Oxford University Press, 1992). For more on women's fear of death during birth, see Judith Walzer Leavitt, *Brought to Bed: Childbearing in America, 1750–1950* (Oxford University Press, 1986), 13–35. See also Daniel Scott Smith and J. David Hacker, "Cultural Demography: New England Deaths and the Puritan Perception of Risk," *Journal of Interdisciplinary History* 26 (1996): 367–92. Paul Berman argues that descriptions of births in medical journals highlighted tragic outcomes and so contributed to the "dismal and false picture" of childbirth that was prevalent in the culture at large. Paul Berman, "The Practice of Obstetrics in Rural America, 1800–1850," *Journal of the History of Medicine and Allied Sciences* 50 (1995): 175–93.

13. Diary, May 1, 1872 entry, Nettie Fowler McCormick Papers, Manuscripts Library, State Historical Society of Wisconsin, Madison, WI.

14. Richard W. Wertz and Dorothy C. Wertz, *Lying-In: A History of Childbirth in America* (Yale University Press, 1989), "agony which is akin" at 118; Mary Putnam Jacobi, "The Grandmother, 1902," Mary Putnam Jacobi Papers, Schlesinger Library, Radcliffe College, Cambridge, MA; Judith Walzer Leavitt, "Birthing and Anesthesia:

The Debate over Twilight Sleep," *Signs* 6 (Autumn 1980): 147–64, "bursts your brain" at 149; Judith Walzer Leavitt, "Under the Shadow of Maternity: American Women's Responses to Death and Debility Fears in Nineteenth-Century Childbirth," *Feminist Studies* 12 (1986): 129–54, "I have seen" at 133.

15. Linda Gordon discusses the history of the fertility rate in the United States in *Woman's Body, Woman's Right: Birth Control in America* (Penguin Books, 1990), 150. Marion Harland, *Eve's Daughters; or, Common Sense for Maid, Wife, and Mother* (John R. Anderson and Henry S. Allen, 1882), 419–20; "Dogs Better than Baby. American Women Dislike to Bear Children," *Chicago Tribune*, February 4, 1903, 1.

16. E. T. Rulison, "The Use of Chloroform in Labor," *Medical and Surgical Reporter* 65 (1891): 851. For more on the history of attitudes toward abortion and contraception in nineteenth-century America, see Leslie J. Reagan, *When Abortion Was a Crime: Women, Medicine, and Law in the United States, 1867–1973* (University of California Press, 1997); Gordon, *Woman's Body, Woman's Right;* and Janet Farrell Brodie, *Contraception and Abortion in 19th-Century America* (Cornell University Press, 1994).

17. Judith Walzer Leavitt uses the term "social birth" in her book *Brought to Bed.* For vivid descriptions of these births, see *Brought to Bed*, 87–115.

18. Nellie Brown to Polly Brown, April 26, 1858, Nellie Brown Letters, Minnesota Historical Society, St. Paul, MN. For more on childbirth attendants in slaves' quarters, see White, *Ar'n't I a Woman?* 96–97, 111–12; Sally G. McMillen, *Motherhood in the Old South: Pregnancy, Childbirth, and Infant Rearing* (Louisiana State University Press, 1990), 57–78; and Schwartz, *Birthing a Slave.*

19. Josephine Baker quoted in Leavitt, *Brought to Bed,* 110. The physician's description of how birth attendants should behave is in John D. West, *Maidenhood and Motherhood; or, Ten Phases of Woman's Life* (Law, King, and Law, 1887), 481. In some areas of the southern United States, lay midwifery remained an established institution through the 1960s. Alabama ceased issuing permits to "granny" midwives only in the late 1970s, which was effectively the first time that women descended from slave midwives in Alabama could not continue their family's traditional work. See Margaret Charles Smith and Linda Janet Holmes, *Listen to Me Good: The Life Story of an Alabama Midwife* (Ohio State University Press, 1996). Midwives' stories are also in Penfield Chester, *Sisters on a Journey: Portraits of American Midwives* (Rutgers University Press, 1997). Charlotte G. Borst discusses the slow transition from midwife-attended home birth to physician-attended home birth in *Catching Babies: The Professionalization of Childbirth, 1870–1920* (Harvard University Press, 1995).

20. See Nancy M. Theriot, *Mothers and Daughters in Nineteenth-Century America: The Biosocial Construction of Femininity* (University Press of Kentucky, 1996), 58–59. Contemporary studies of this phenomenon include John Kennell, Marshall Klaus, S. McGrath, S. Robertson, and C. Hinkley, "Continuous Emotional Support during Labor in a US Hospital," *Journal of the American Medical Association* 265 (1991): 2197–2201; Marshall Klaus, John Kennell, Gale Berkowitz, and Phyllis Klaus, "Maternal Assistance and Support in Labor: Father, Nurse, Midwife, or Doula?" *Clinical Consultations in Obstetrics and Gynecology* 4 (December 1992): 211–17; Sandy E. Weber, "Cultural Aspects of Pain in Childbearing Women," *Journal of Obstetric, Gy-*

necologic, and Neonatal Nursing 25 (January 1996): 67–72; M. H. Klaus and J. H. Kennell, "The Doula: An Essential Ingredient of Childbirth Rediscovered," *Acta Paediatrica* 86 (1997): 1034–36; and Banyana Cecilia Madi, Jane Sandall, Ruth Bennett, and Christina MacLeod, "Effects of Female Relative Support in Labor: A Randomized Controlled Trial," *Birth* 26 (March 1999): 4–8.

21. Anita McCormick Blaine to Sweetest Mother in the World, August 24, 1890, Nettie Fowler McCormick Papers.

22. For a historical discussion of mothers, daughters, and menstruation, see Joan Jacobs Brumberg, *The Body Project: An Intimate History of American Girls* (Random House, 1997), 29–55. The advice book quotation is from Harland, *Eve's Daughters,* 79–83. Martha G. Ripley, "President's Address," "Report of Maternity Hospital from Nov. 30th 1889 to Nov. 30th 1891," Maternity Hospital Papers, Minnesota Historical Society.

23. Lottie to Myra, February 13, May 29, 1890; May 14, 1891; January 18, 1893, Lottie Isabella Kerr Tubbs papers, 1884–97, Schlesinger Library; Edward Howard Griggs, "On the Education of a Child from Eleven to Eighteen When a Child First Awakens to Manhood or Womanhood," *Ladies' Home Journal,* November 1901, 18. As women's magazines proliferated, they became extremely influential. The *Ladies' Home Journal* was the best-selling magazine in the United States within a few years of its initial appearance in 1883. By 1910, 20% of American women read the *Journal.* See Helen Damon-Moore, *Magazines for the Millions: Gender and Commerce in the "Ladies' Home Journal" and the "Saturday Evening Post," 1880–1910* (State University of New York Press, 1994). See also Cynthia L. White, *Women's Magazines, 1693–1968* (Michael Joseph, 1970), 58–92; and Mary Ellen Zuckerman, *A History of Popular Women's Magazines in the United States, 1792–1995* (Greenwood Press, 1998), 1–23.

24. White, *Ar'n't I a Woman?* 96–97, 111–12.

25. Charles Edward Ziegler, "The Teaching of Obstetrics," *American Journal of Obstetrics and Diseases of Women and Children* 73 (1916): 50–57; Discussion of Joseph DeLee, "The Early Recognition of Impending Obstetric Accidents," *Chicago Medical Recorder* 24 (June 1903): 440–42.

26. Joseph B. DeLee, "Motherhood: An Address before the Women's Society of Isaiah Temple January 4th 1898," Joseph B. DeLee Papers, Northwestern Memorial Hospital Archives, Chicago; D. W. Prentiss, "A Report of Five Hundred Consecutive Cases of Labor in Private Practice, in the District of Columbia, between the Years 1864 and 1888," *American Journal of Obstetrics and Diseases of Women and Children* 21 (1888): 956–70.

27. J. Whitridge Williams, "The Introduction of Clinical Teaching of Obstetrics in the United States," *American Journal of Obstetrics and Diseases of Women and Children* 50 (1904): 302–21, *"gross outrage"* at 308, "utterly incompetent" at 319, "No practitioner" at 318; J. Whitridge Williams, "Why Is the Art of Obstetrics So Poorly Practised?" *Long Island Medical Journal* 11 (May 1917): 169–78.

28. Williams, "The Introduction of Clinical Teaching of Obstetrics"; "The Responsibility of the Obstetrician: Discussion," *American Journal of Obstetrics and Diseases of Women and Children* 64 (1911): 1057–63.

29. DeLee quote in "The Chicago Lying-In Hospital Dispensary First Annual Report, 1895–96," 5, Northwestern Memorial Hospital Archives; Franklin S. Newell, "The Responsibility of the Obstetrician," *American Journal of Obstetrics and Diseases of Women and Children* 64 (1911): 966–77, quote at 971.

30. "The Chicago Lying-In Hospital Dispensary Second Annual Report, 1896–97," 5–6, Northwestern Memorial Hospital Archives; Beatrice E. Tucker and Harry B. Benaron, "Maternal Mortality of the Chicago Maternity Center," *American Journal of Public Health* 27 (January 1937): 33–36; "The Chicago Lying-In Hospital Dispensary First Annual Report."

31. "The Chicago Lying-In Hospital Dispensary Second Annual Report," 5–6; Tucker and Benaron, "Maternal Mortality of the Chicago Maternity Center"; "Report of the Board of Directors," "The Chicago Lying-In Hospital and Dispensary Thirteenth Annual Report, 1906–1907, 1907–1908," Northwestern Memorial Hospital Archives.

32. E. B. Cragin, J. C. Edgar, C. M. Green, E. P. Davis, J. W. Williams, J. C. Webster, and B. C. Hirst, "Report of the Committee of the American Gynecological Society on the Present Status of Obstetrical Education in Europe and America and on Recommendations for the Improvement of Obstetrical Teaching," ca. 1910, Rush University Medical Center Archives, Chicago; George J. Engelmann, "Birth- and Death-Rate as Influenced by Obstetric and Gynecic Progress," *Boston Medical and Surgical Journal* 146 (May 15, 1920): 505–8.

33. Jno. Herbert Claiborne, "Use of Chloroform in Labor," *Journal of the American Medical Association* 3 (October 1884): 401–6, "benefaction" at 402; "insane ethereal furor" in F. Willis Fisher, "Letter from Paris—Ethereal Inhalation in Insanity and Obstetrics," *Boston Medical and Surgical Journal* 36 (1847): 172–74; Charles D. Meigs, *Obstetrics: The Science and the Art* (Blanchard and Lear, 1856), "scene of cheerfulness" at 366; "terrible torture" in Bedford Brown, "The Therapeutic Action of Chloroform in Parturition," *Journal of the American Medical Association* 25 (August 31, 1895): 354–58.

34. Prentiss, "A Report of Five Hundred Consecutive Cases of Labor."

35. Amalie M. Kass, *Midwifery and Medicine in Boston: Walter Channing, M.D., 1786–1876* (Northeastern University Press, 2002), 64–68, 148–52; "imperfect harmony" in Walter Channing, *A Treatise on Etherization in Childbirth* (William D. Ticknor, 1848), 20; "unyielding organs" and "rise to the agony" in Walter Channing, "Painless Delivery, Haemorrhage, Turning, Recovery," *Boston Medical and Surgical Journal* (October 20, 1864): 229–32.

36. Kass, *Midwifery and Medicine in Boston*, 176; Channing, *A Treatise on Etherization*, 135–57. For more on the first use of ether in surgery, see Julie M. Fenster, *Ether Day: The Strange Tale of America's Greatest Medical Discovery and the Haunted Men Who Made It* (HarperCollins, 2001), 5–6, 77–80.

37. Fenster, *Ether Day*, 97–98; H. Laing Gordon, *Sir James Young Simpson and Chloroform (1811–1870)* (T. Fisher Unwin, 1897), 104; J. Y. Simpson, *Notice of a New Anaesthetic Agent, as a Substitute for Sulphuric Ether in Surgery and Midwifery* (Sutherland and Knox, 1847), 5–13, "chloride of hydro-carbon" at 6. The "beds of as-

phodel" quote appears in W. C. Van Bibber, "A New Suggestion concerning the Use of Chloroform and Ammonia in Labor," *Maryland Medical Journal* 10 (October 27, 1883): 401–2.

38. "Fearful sufferings" in J. Y. Simpson, *Remarks on the Superinduction of Anaesthesia in Natural and Morbid Parturition: With Cases Illustrative of the Use and Effects of Chloroform in Obstetric Practice* (William B. Little, 1848), 10–11; "professional cruelty" in Channing, *A Treatise on Etherization*, 11.

39. Samuel Ashwell, "Observations on the Use of Chloroform in Natural Labour," *Lancet* 1 (1848): 291–92. For further details of Simpson's pioneering work with chloroform, see Donald Caton, *What a Blessing She Had Chloroform: The Medical and Social Response to the Pain of Childbirth from 1800 to the Present* (Yale University Press, 1999), 4–19; and Linda Stratmann, *Chloroform: The Quest for Oblivion* (Sutton, 2003), 31–48, 73–77.

40. Stratmann, *Chloroform*, 74; Richard H. Ellis, ed., *The Case Books of Dr. John Snow* (Wellcome Institute for the History of Medicine, 1994), 471. For more on Snow, see Thomas E. Keys, "John Snow, M.D., Anesthetist," *Journal of the History of Medicine and Allied Sciences* 1 (October 1946): 551–66.

41. Meigs, *Obstetrics*, 289–90, 365–66. The medical historian Judith Walzer Leavitt, who has studied women's accounts of birth in diaries, letters, and autobiographies, argues that birthing chambers were most often cheerful places. Women looked forward to being birth attendants, and birthing chambers, when all was going well, were bustling, happy social scenes. Leavitt, *Brought to Bed*.

42. Meigs, *Obstetrics*, 291–92. Meigs's description of labor in this context provides an example of how physicians used the word *pain* in two ways when discussing birth: to describe both the physical action—the cervix opening or the uterus pushing—and the sensation caused by the physical action. Vocabulary shapes perception, and in this case doctors clearly believed a contraction was tantamount to pain; the two were synonymous. "Notes of Lectures delivered by Henry N. Guernsey M.D., Professor of Obstetrics and Diseases of Women and Children in the Homeopathic Medical College of Pennsylvania, Session [18]'64 and [18]'65 by Jacob G. Street," National Library of Medicine, History of Medicine Division, Bethesda, MD. For an observation similar to Guernsey's, see West, *Maidenhood and Motherhood*, 484. West notes of first-stage labor (as opposed to women rallying during the second stage), "Women generally say that it is impossible for them to survive."

43. Simpson, *Remarks on the Superinduction of Anaesthesia*, 11; Claiborne, "Use of Chloroform in Labor," 403.

44. Simpson, *Remarks on the Superinduction of Anaesthesia*, 22–23; Brown, "The Therapeutic Action of Chloroform in Parturition."

45. Meigs, *Obstetrics*, 371–75. The exchange between Meigs and Simpson is described in B. P. Watson, "American Gynecological Society Sixty-first Annual Meeting President's Address," *American Journal of Obstetrics and Gynecology* 32 (October 1936): 547–60. Meigs said in a letter to Simpson dated February 18, 1848: "And here, allow me to say, I have been accustomed to look upon the sensation of labor as a phys-

iological relation of the power, or force; and notwithstanding I have seen so many women in the throes of labor, I have always regarded a labor-pain as a most desirable, salutary, and conservative manifestation of life-force." Meigs, *Obstetrics*, 373.

46. J. Y. Simpson to My Dear Doctor, February 26, May 1, 1847, Francis Henry Ramsbotham–James Young Simpson Correspondence, 1844–53, National Library of Medicine, History of Medicine Division, Bethesda, MD. Ramsbotham was the author of multiple editions of *The Principles and Practice of Obstetric Medicine and Surgery, in Reference to the Process of Parturition* (Blanchard and Lea). A brief biography of Ramsbotham appears in the *Oxford Dictionary of National Biography: From the Earliest Times to the Year 2000* (Oxford University Press, 2004), 45:958–59.

47. J. Y. Simpson to My Dear Doctor, January 14, October 10, 1851; Frances Henry Ramsbotham to My Dear Dr. Simpson, January 23, 1852; J. Y. Simpson to My Dear Doctor, September 15, 1853, Francis Henry Ramsbotham–James Young Simpson Correspondence, 1844–53.

48. Channing, *A Treatise on Etherization*, 21.

49. Ibid, 144–45; "Dr. Simpson surely forgets" in Ashwell, "Observations on the Use of Chloroform, 291–92. A. D. Farr argues that religious opposition to obstetric anesthesia was never so significant as to affect medical practice. See A. D. Farr, "Religious Opposition to Obstetric Anaesthesia: A Myth?" *Annals of Science* 40 (1983): 159–77.

50. Ziegler, "The Teaching of Obstetrics"; J. C. Hoag, "Progress in Obstetric Practice," *Chicago Medical Recorder* 19 (July 1900): 1–9.

51. Simpson, *Remarks on the Superinduction of Anaesthesia*, 22–23; Channing, *A Treatise on Etherization*, 20, 135–56, "as if a miracle" at 20; Channing, "Notes of Difficult Labors," 113–15; Thomas Edward Beatty, *Observations on the Use of Chloroform in Conjunction with Ergot of Rye in Parturition* (Hodges and Smith, 1850), Rare Books and Special Collections, Francis A. Countway Library of Medicine, Boston.

52. Channing, *A Treatise on Etherization*, 1–2, 332–64, "birthplace of etherization" at 2, "the happiest results" at 355, "preferred to trust" at 349. In later years physicians discovered that chloroform did indeed cause hemorrhage, but when this physician made and dismissed his casual observation, the medical community was decades away from acknowledging this side effect.

53. S. William J. Merriman, *Arguments against the Indiscriminate Use of Chloroform in Midwifery* (John Churchill, 1848), 22, Rare Books and Special Collections, Francis A. Countway Library of Medicine; Baron Paul Dubois, "On the Inhalation of Ether Applied to Cases of Midwifery," *Lancet* 1 (1847): 246–49; B. H. Ogden, "Experience with Hyoscine-Morphine Anesthesia, with Special Reference to Its Use in Obstetrics," *Saint Paul Medical Journal* 10 (1908): 388–91.

54. Harland, *Eve's Daughters*, 439; Mrs. P. B. Saur, *Maternity: A Book for Every Wife and Mother* (L. P. Miller, 1889), 216–20, 223, 227, 228–30, "one of the greatest" at 228.

55. Claiborne, "Use of Chloroform in Labor," 401–6.

56. Emily Foster, ed., *American Grit: A Woman's Letters from the Ohio Frontier* (University Press of Kentucky, 2002), 157, 178.

57. Pocket Diary for 1856, March 20, 1856, entry; Folder Diary, 1857, October 12, 1857, entry, James Peet Papers, 1846–71, Minnesota Historical Society.

58. Virginia Ingraham Burr, ed., *The Secret Eye: The Journal of Ella Gertrude Clanton Thomas, 1848–1889* (University of North Carolina Press, 1990), 119.

59. Ibid., 215.

60. Ibid., 161–62, 258.

61. Boston doctor George Snow's obstetric logs indicate that his missing a birth was an event he and his patients viewed calmly; birth occurring before the physician arrived was apparently common and uneventful. George William Snow Obstetrical Case Records, 1865–75, October 27, 1869, and May 1, 1872, entries, Rare Books and Special Collections, Francis A. Countway Library of Medicine. Christopher Graham, who practiced in Rochester, MN, reported similar nonchalance when he arrived after a woman had already given birth. Christopher Graham Obstetric Record and Related Papers, 1888–1904, 1914, 1955, Minnesota Historical Society. Lottie to Myra, May 14, 1891, Lottie Isabella Kerr Tubbs papers, 1884–97; Bertha Van Hoosen, *Petticoat Surgeon* (Pellegrini and Cudahy, 1947), quote at 3; see also 193.

62. Josephine K. Laflin Diary, January–May 1898, March 20–21 entries, Laflin Family Papers, Chicago Historical Society, Chicago; "First Annual Report Augusta Memorial Visiting Nurses" (1888), 10, Visiting Nurses Association of Chicago Papers, Chicago Historical Society.

63. *Annual Report of the New-England Hospital for Women and Children for the Year Ending Nov. 10, 1864* (Prentiss and Deland, 1865); Marie E. Zakrzewska, "Report of the Attending Physician," *Annual Report of the New-England Hospital for Women and Children for the Year Ending Nov. 14, 1865* (Prentiss and Deland, 1865), 13; Marie E. Zakrzewska, "Report of the Attending Physician," *Annual Report of the New-England Hospital for Women and Children for the Year Ending Nov. 1, 1868* (Prentiss and Deland, 1868), 10, all in New England Hospital Papers, Sophia Smith Collection, Neilson Library, Smith College, Northampton, MA. For more on Zakrzewska's life and work, see Arleen Marcia Tuchman, *Science Has No Sex: The Life of Maria E. Zakrzewska, M.D.* (University of North Carolina Press, 2006).

64. Zakrzewska, "Report of the Attending Physician" (1868), 15–16; "Report of Maternity Hospital 1889," Maternity Hospital Papers, Minnesota Historical Society.

65. George F. Jelby to Dr. Pope, no date; F. Minot to Dr. Pope, February 17, 1888; A. T. Cabot, MD, to Dr. Pope, February 17, 1888; George G. Turbell to Dr. Pope, February 17, 1888; Henry I. Bowditch to Dr. Pope, February 18, 1888; Henry O. March to Dr. Bowditch, February 21, 1888, New England Hospital Papers; Boston Lying-in Hospital Casebooks, vol. 34, July 1 to October 5, 1886, July 4 and July 19 entries; vol. 70, March 23 to June 5, 1895; and vol. 100, November 21, 1900, to February 8, 1901, Rare Books and Special Collections, Francis A. Countway Library of Medicine.

66. "67th Annual Report and Announcement Philadelphia Lying-In Charity," 1895; Philadelphia Lying-In Charity, Patient Charts, vol. 1, 1891, all housed at Pennsylvania Hospital Historic Collections, Philadelphia, PA. See, for example, May 30, June 11, and June 15, 1891, entries.

67. Philadelphia Lying-In Charity, Patient Charts, vol. 1, June 7 and June 13, 1891, entries; vol. 15, June 29, 1898, entry; vol. 1, December 24, June 22, and August 4, 1891, entries; vol. 9, May 6, 1895, entry, Pennsylvania Hospital Historic Collections. The pa-

tient complaining of "headache and dizziness of vision" died shortly after giving birth, probably of eclampsia.

68. Ibid., vol. 9, June 12, 1895, entry.

69. Ibid., vol. 40 (1907). Joel D. Howell argues that newly introduced hospital technologies and paperwork reflect historical change rather than prompt change. See Joel D. Howell, *Technology in the Hospital: Transforming Patient Care in the Early Twentieth Century* (Johns Hopkins University Press, 1995).

70. Missy Hammond to Nettie Fowler McCormick, August 29, 1890, Anita McCormick Blaine Papers, State Historical Society of Wisconsin, Madison, WI.

71. Katharine Kerr Moore to May Walden Kerr, June 6, 1921, May Walden Kerr Papers, Newberry Library, Chicago.

72. For a more detailed discussion of the traditional timing of obstetric anesthesia and its effect on women's and physicians' perceptions of labor and birth, see Jacqueline H. Wolf, "'Mighty Glad to Gasp in the Gas': Perceptions of Pain and the Traditional Timing of Obstetric Anesthesia," *Health* 6 (July 2002): 365–87.

73. George William Snow Obstetrical Case Records, 1865–75, October 26, 1865, May 22, 1866, February 14, 1867, and October 27, 1869, entries, Rare Books and Special Collections, Francis A. Countway Library of Medicine; Ellis, *The Case Books of Dr. John Snow,* 21.

74. Ellis, *The Case Books of Dr. John Snow,* 18.

75. William Thornton Parker Obstetrical Cases, 1848–49, March 1, 1848, entry, Rare Books and Special Collections, Francis A. Countway Library of Medicine.

76. Christopher Graham, Obstetric Record and Related Papers, 1888–1904, 1914, 1955, Minnesota Historical Society.

77. Walter Channing, "Cases of Inhalation of Ether in Labor," *Boston Medical and Surgical Journal* 36 (1847): 415–19; "It was heaven" in Beatty, *Observations on the Use of Chloroform,* 11; Geo. N. Burwell, "Statement of Twenty-three Cases of Midwifery in Which Chloroform Was Administered," *Buffalo Medical Journal and Monthly Review of Medical and Surgical Science* 5 (1850): 7–29.

78. A. R. Thompson, MD, to Walter Channing, MD, January 28, 1848, in Channing, *A Treatise on Etherization,* 334–35.

79. Van Bibber, "A New Suggestion concerning the Use of Chloroform and Ammonia in Labor," 401–2; Palmer Findley, "Nitrous Oxid and Oxygen Analgesia in Obstetrics," *International Journal of Surgery* 29 (January 1916): 1–2.

80. Channing, *A Treatise on Etherization,* 10; J. Y. Simpson to My Dear Sir, July 23, 1848, Francis Henry Ramsbotham–James Young Simpson Correspondence, 1844–53.

81. There appears to have been no uniformity in physicians' use of obstetric anesthesia. Some used it only in the event of a highly unusual situation, such as a shoulder presentation. Others used it every time they applied forceps. Others used it routinely with first-time mothers, because those labors lasted longest. For varied examples of anesthesia use, see John George Metcalf, "A Case of Midwifery Shoulder Presentation," handwritten talk, 1856, Union Medical Association Papers, University of Massachusetts Medical School Library, Worcester, MA; George William Snow

ual physicians, is discussed in detail in the previous section of this chapter.indiNotes to Pages 39–43   217
Obstetrical Case Records, 1865–75, October 29, 1867, entry, Rare Books and Special Collections, Francis A. Countway Library of Medicine; Charles Edward Fawcett, Obstetrical Chart, 1894–1939, Minnesota Historical Society; Van Hoosen, *Petticoat Surgeon,* 99–101; Christopher Graham, Obstetric Record and Related Papers, 1888–1904, 1914, 1955, November 6, 1888, November 9, 1889, November 29, 1890, August 25, 1895, May 24, 1896, September 11, 1900, entries, Minnesota Historical Society. The pattern of anesthesia use in these early years at lying-in charity hospitals, as opposed to among individual physicians, is discussed in detail in the previous section of this chapter.

82. Keep, "Inhalation of Ethereal Vapor"; and Simpson, *Notice of a New Anaesthetic Agent,* 17.

83. Beatty, Observations on the Use of Chloroform; "Discussion of the Bromide of Ethyl as an Anesthetic in Labor," *American Journal of Obstetrics and Diseases of Women and Children* 18 (1885): 958–59.

84. Joseph B. DeLee, *The Principles and Practice of Obstetrics* (W. B. Saunders, 1918), 303.

85. Russell Kelso Carter, *The Sleeping Car 'Twilight' or Motherhood without Pain* (Chapple, 1915), 43–44.

86. Findley, "Nitrous Oxid and Oxygen Analgesia in Obstetrics," 1–2; DeLee, *The Principles and Practice of Obstetrics,* 303.

87. T. W. Parkinson, "A Plea for the More Frequent Use of Chloroform in Labour," *Lancet* 2 (September 20, 1902): 835–36.

88. J. S. Hammond, "A Resume of One Thousand Cases of Labor," *American Journal of Obstetrics and Diseases of Women and Children* 38 (1898): 855–62, quotes at 857.

89. J. F. Ford, "Use of Drugs in Labor," *Wisconsin Medical Journal* 3 (1904–5): 257–65, "a case of confinement" and "you get that doctor" at 264; H. M. Clarkson, "Chloroform and Chloral in Childbirth," *Virginia Medical Monthly* 13 (1886–87): 680–89, "do something" at 682; Henry Bixby Hemenway, "Abnormal Labor," *Chicago Recorder* 26 (December 1904): 795–803.

90. Examples of women's descriptions of second-stage labor after experiencing an unmedicated birth are in Robert A. Bradley, "Fathers' Presence in Delivery Rooms," *Psychosomatics* 3 (November–December 1962): 474–79; Boston Women's Health Book Collective, *Our Bodies, Ourselves: A Book by and for Women* (Simon and Schuster, 1976), 271; Barbara Katz Rothman, *In Labor: Women and Power in the Birthplace* (W. W. Norton, 1991), 20–21; and Mary Thomas, ed., *Post-War Mothers: Childbirth Letters to Grantly Dick-Read, 1946–1956* (University of Rochester Press, 1997).

91. Judith Walzer Leavitt first posited the argument that women controlled birthing practices until birth moved to the hospital. Leavitt, *Brought to Bed.* Also see Borst, *Catching Babies.*

92. For a more detailed investigation of this phenomenon and its effect on childbirth, see Wolf, "'Mighty Glad to Gasp in the Gas.'"

93. Clarkson, "Chloroform and Chloral in Childbirth," 687.

94. Simpson, *Notice of a New Anaesthetic Agent,* 17; John Snow, *On Chloroform and Other Anaesthetics: Their Action and Administration* (John Churchill, 1858), 322.

Chapter 2 · Twilight Sleep

1. Marguerite Tracy and Mary Boyd, *Painless Childbirth: A General Survey of All Painless Methods with Special Stress on 'Twilight Sleep' and Its Extension to America* (Frederick A. Stokes, 1915), xxxii, 185–91.

2. Ibid., 190.

3. Marguerite Tracy and Constance Leupp, "Painless Childbirth," *McClure's Magazine*, June 1914, 37–51, quote at 38. Although Tracy and Leupp do not acknowledge this birth as Stewart's, her picture accompanies the article, and the story is identical to the one ascribed to Stewart in Tracy and Boyd, *Painless Childbirth*, 189–91.

4. Other articles published by lay magazines and newspapers in the aftermath of the *McClure's* article include Marguerite Tracy, "Bringing Babies into the World," *Ladies' World*, September 1914, 9–10; Van Buren Thorne, "'Twilight Sleep' Is Successful in 120 Cases Here," *New York Times*, magazine section, August 30, 1914, 8; Sam Schmalhauer, "The Twilight Sleep for Women," *International Socialist Review* 15 (1914): 232–35; "The 'Twilight Sleep' Dispute," *Literary Digest*, September 19, 1914, 50, 60–61; Mrs. Hanna Rion Ver Beck, "The Painless Childbirth: Testimony of American Mothers Who Have Tried 'The Twilight Sleep,'" *Ladies' Home Journal*, September 1914, 9–10; Dr. William H. W. Knipe, "The Truth about Twilight Sleep," *Delineator*, November 1914, 9.

5. "Labor with Scopolamin-Morphine," *American Journal of Obstetrics and Diseases of Women and Children* 54 (1906): 886–87. For previous accounts of twilight sleep written by historians, see Lawrence G. Miller, "Pain, Parturition, and the Profession: Twilight Sleep in America," in *Health Care in America: Essays in Social History*, ed. Susan Reverby and David Rosner (Temple University Press, 1979), 19–44; and Judith Walzer Leavitt, "Birthing and Anesthesia: The Debate over Twilight Sleep," *Signs* 6 (Autumn 1980): 147–64.

6. William L. Holt, "Scopolamine-Morphine in Obstetrics," *American Journal of Clinical Medicine* (May 1907): 565–77.

7. A. J. Rongy, "The Use of Scopolamine in Obstetrics," *Transactions of the American Association of Obstetricians and Gynecologists* 27 (1914): 364–71; A. M. Hilkowich, "Further Observations on Scopolamine-Narcophin Anesthesia during Labor with Report of Two Hundred (200) Cases," *American Medicine* 20 (December 1914): 786–94; Wm. H. Wellington Knipe, "The Freiburg Method of Dämmerschlaf or Twilight Sleep," *American Journal of Obstetrics and Diseases of Women and Children* 70 (1914): 884–909; Hanna Rion, *The Truth about Twilight Sleep* (McBride, Nast, 1915), 249–51.

8. Charlotte Teller, "The Neglected Psychology of the 'Twilight Sleep,'" *Good Housekeeping*, July 1915, 17–24, quote at 23; Franklin S. Newell, "Anaesthesia in the First Stage of Labor," *Surgery, Gynecology, and Obstetrics* 3 (1906): 126–30.

9. Teller, "The Neglected Psychology of the 'Twilight Sleep'"; Professor Bernhard Krönig, "Scopolamine-Morphine Narcosis in Labour," *British Medical Journal* (September 19, 1908): 805–8.

10. Albert S. Barnes, "'Twilight Sleep': A Discussion of the Question with Timely

Comments by American Observers," *Ohio State Medical Journal* (October 1914): 623–25; Joseph B. DeLee, *The Principles and Practice of Obstetrics* (W. B. Saunders, 1918), 306; George F. Butler, "Hyoscine Anesthesia in Obstetrics," *American Journal of Obstetrics and Diseases of Women and Children* 56 (1907): 171–77; "The 'Twilight Sleep': A Sensational Resurrection of the Discredited and Dangerous Scopolamin-Morphin Anesthesia in Labor," pamphlet published by the American Medical Association, 1914, AMA Health Fraud and Alternative Medicine Collection, box 867, folder 0867-05, American Medical Association Archives, Chicago.

11. Stella Lehr, "A Possible Explanation of the Conflicting Reports on Twilight Sleep," *California State Journal of Medicine* 13 (1915): 220–23; the first two quoted phrases are in Tracy and Leupp, "Painless Childbirth," 208; Tracy, "Bringing Babies into the World"; Rion, *The Truth about Twilight Sleep*, 326; Mary Boyd, "The Story of Dämmerschlaf: An American Woman's Personal Experience and Study at Freiburg," *Survey* 33 (1914–15): 125–29, "quick peasant births" at 127.

12. Philadelphia Lying-In Charity, Patient Charts, vols. 42 (1908) and 43 (1908), Pennsylvania Hospital Historic Collections, Philadelphia, PA.

13. Ibid., vol. 43 (1908), March 30, April 30, May 26, and June 1 entries.

14. Bertha Van Hoosen, *Scopolamine-Morphine Anaesthesia* (House of Manz, 1915), 15.

15. Bertha Van Hoosen, *Petticoat Surgeon* (Pellegrini and Cudahy, 1947), 275.

16. Van Hoosen, *Scopolamine-Morphine Anaesthesia*, 86; Bertha Van Hoosen, "A Fixed Dosage in Scopolamine-Morphine Anaesthesia," *Woman's Medical Journal* 26 (March 1916): 57–58.

17. In a systematic sampling of Philadelphia Lying-In Charity patient charts through 1922, I could find no use of twilight sleep after 1908.

18. Mary Boyd and Marguerite Tracy, "More about Painless Childbirth," *McClure's Magazine*, October 1914, 56–69.

19. Tracy and Leupp, "Painless Childbirth," 38–39; "the new gospel" in "Painless Childbirth Bureau," McClure Publications leaflet, undated, ca. 1914, box 867, folder 0867-05, AMA Health Fraud and Alternative Medicine Collection.

20. Charles B. Reed, "A Contribution to the Study of 'Twilight Sleep,'" *Surgery, Gynecology, and Obstetrics* 22 (1916): 656–59.

21. M. A. Lee, Wisconsin physician, to *Journal of the American Medical Association*, May 20, 1914; letter from Dr. Guy Hale McKinstry, Pennsylvania physician, July 27, 1914, box 867, folder 0867-05, AMA Health Fraud and Alternative Medicine Collection; Barnes, "Twilight Sleep."

22. S. Josephine Baker, "The High Cost of Babies," *Ladies' Home Journal*, October 1923, 13.

23. Quoted in Linda Gordon, *Woman's Body, Woman's Right: Birth Control in America* (Penguin Books, 1990), 133. For more on the history of the eugenic movement and eugenic thought in the United States, see Martin Pernick, *The Black Stork: Eugenics and the Death of "Defective" Babies in American Medicine and Motion Pictures since 1915* (Oxford University Press, 1996); Martin Pernick, "Eugenics and Public Health in American History," *American Journal of Public Health* 87 (November 1997):

167–72; Wendy Kline, *Building a Better Race: Gender, Sexuality, and Eugenics from the Turn of the Century to the Baby Boom* (University of California Press, 2001); and Alexandra Minna Stern, *Eugenic Nation: Faults and Frontiers of Better Breeding in Modern America* (University of California Press, 2005). Publications reflecting physicians' eugenic-inspired hopes for scopolamine include Holt, "Scopolamine-Morphine in Obstetrics"; Butler, "Hyoscine Anesthesia in Obstetrics"; Henry Smith Williams, *Twilight Sleep: A Simple Account of New Discoveries in Painless Childbirth* (Harper, 1914), 29–42; A. J. Rongy, "The Use of Scopolamine in Labor," *American Medicine* 21 (January 1915): 45–57.

24. Bertha Van Hoosen, "The New Movement in Obstetrics," *Woman's Medical Journal* 25 (June 1915): 121–23.

25. Thorne, "'Twilight Sleep' Is Successful," 8; "The Motherhood Educational Society Announces Science's Greatest Triumph Twilight Sleep (Dämmerschlaf)," leaflet dated May 9, 1916, box 867, folder 0867-05, AMA Health Fraud and Alternative Medicine Collection.

26. See, for example, the photographs accompanying the original *McClure's* article, Tracy and Leupp, "Painless Childbirth." For more on the infant mortality rate at the turn of the twentieth century and attempts to mitigate it, see Richard A. Meckel, *Save the Babies: American Public Health Reform and the Prevention of Infant Mortality, 1850–1929* (Johns Hopkins University Press, 1990); Samuel H. Preston and Michael R. Haines, *Fatal Years: Child Mortality in Late Nineteenth-Century America* (Princeton University Press, 1991); Kriste Lindenmeyer, *"A Right to Childhood": The U.S. Children's Bureau and Child Welfare, 1912–46* (University of Illinois Press, 1997); Jacqueline H. Wolf, *Don't Kill Your Baby: Public Health and the Decline of Breastfeeding in the 19th and 20th Centuries* (Ohio State University Press, 2001), 42–73; and Eilidh Garrett, Chris Galley, Nicola Shelton, and Robert Woods, eds., *Infant Mortality: A Continuing Social Problem* (Ashgate, 2006). For more on the movement for "better babies," see Annette K. Vance Dorey, *Better Baby Contests: The Scientific Quest for Perfect Childhood Health in the Early Twentieth Century* (McFarland, 1999).

27. Tracy, "Bringing Babies into the World," 9–10; Schmalhauer, "The Twilight Sleep for Women"; Tracy and Boyd, *Painless Childbirth*, 203; Geo. C. Mosher, "Scopolamin Semi-Narcosis or Twilight Sleep in Labor," *Journal of the Kansas Medical Society* 14 (December 1914): 441–53.

28. Rion, *The Truth about Twilight Sleep.*

29. Van Hoosen, "The New Movement in Obstetrics."

30. Tracy and Boyd, *Painless Childbirth*, 200–204; "Holds West Leads in Twilight Sleep," *New York Times*, May 10, 1915, 24. For information on women's activism and the sheer variety of women's organizations during the Progressive Era, see Kathleen D. McCarthy, *Noblesse Oblige: Charity and Cultural Philanthropy in Chicago, 1849–1929* (University of Chicago Press, 1982); Molly Ladd-Taylor, *Mother-Work: Women, Child Welfare, and the State, 1890–1930* (University of Illinois Press, 1994); Kathryn Kish Sklar, *Florence Kelley and the Nation's Work: The Rise of Women's Political Culture, 1830–1900* (Yale University Press, 1995); Kathryn Kish Sklar, "Florence Kelley and Women's Activism in the Progressive Era," in *Women's America: Refocusing the Past,*

ed. Linda K. Kerber and Jane Sherron De Hart (Oxford University Press, 2000), 312–24. For more information on women's clubs in this era, what they aimed to do, and their umbrella organization, the General Federation of Women's Clubs, see also a contemporary book, Rheta Childe Dorr, *What Eight Million Women Want* (1910; Kraus Reprint, 1971).

31. "Mothers Discuss 'Twilight Sleep,'" *New York Times,* November 18, 1914, 18.

32. Advertisement in *Old Colony Memorial* newspaper, Plymouth, MA, January 19, 1917; "The Motherhood Educational Society Announces Science's Greatest Triumph Twilight Sleep (Dämmerschlaf)," leaflet dated May 9, 1916, box 867, folder 0867-05, AMA Health Fraud and Alternative Medicine Collection; Tracy, "Bringing Babies into the World."

33. Boyd and Tracy, "More about Painless Childbirth," 65; James A. Harrar and Ross McPherson, "Scopolamine-Narcophin Seminarcosis in Labor," *Transactions of the American Association of Obstetricians and Gynecologists* 27 (1914): 372–89.

34. "Accusing the Medical Profession," *New York Times,* September 17, 1914, 8. For the story of Ignác Semmelweis and childbed fever, see Sherwin B. Nuland, *The Doctors' Plague: Germs, Childbed Fever, and the Strange Story of Ignác Semmelweis* (W. W. Norton, 2003). See also Irvine Loudon, *The Tragedy of Childbed Fever* (Oxford University Press, 2000).

35. For more on the popularization in the lay press of health and healthy habits, see Harvey Green, *Fit for America: Health, Fitness, Sport, and American Society* (Johns Hopkins University Press, 1986); and Nancy Tomes, *The Gospel of Germs: Men, Women, and the Microbe in American Life* (Harvard University Press, 1998).

36. "Twilight Sleep Again," *American Medicine* 21 (March 1915): 149; "Painless Labor," undated memo, box 867, folder 0867-05, AMA Health Fraud and Alternative Medicine Collection; William Gillespie, "Analgesics and Anaesthetics in Labor: Their Indications and Contra-Indications," *Ohio State Medical Journal* 11 (October 1915): 611–15; Knipe, "The Truth about Twilight Sleep." For another prediction of the dangers of untrained physicians rushing to use twilight sleep, also see E. M. Lazard, "The Twilight Sleep Propaganda in the Lay Press," *Southern California Practitioner* 30 (1915): 13–22.

37. Ross McPherson, "Technic of the Scopolamine-Narcophine Narcosis, with Notes in Its Adaptation and Use," *Ohio State Medical Journal* 11 (1915): 7–11, "flanked on the one side" at 7; "'Authority' Spoke Too Soon!" *New York Times,* August 24, 1914, 8; "Is the Twilight Sleep Safe—*For Me?*" *Woman's Home Companion,* January 1915, 10, 43; Chas. A. Ferris, "Scopolamin Amnesia, or Twilight Sleep," *Colorado Medicine* (March 1916): 88–92, "the honest practitioner" at 88; "the latest appeal" in "Medical Experts on the Claims Made for the Painless Childbirth," *Current Opinion* 57 (September 1914): 185.

38. "'Twilight Sleep' in the Light for Day," *Scientific American,* February 13, 1915, 112.

39. *Official Bulletin of the Medical Women's Club of Chicago,* November 1915, Rush University Medical Center Archives, Chicago.

40. Harrar and McPherson, "Scopolamine-Narcophin Seminarcosis in Labor,"

372–89; "unstable and deteriorated" in McPherson, "Technic of the Scopolamine-Narcophine Narcosis," 8; Hilkowich, "Further Observations on Scopolamine-Narcophin Anesthesia"; Rongy, "The Use of Scopolamine in Obstetrics"; Alfred M. Hellman, *Amnesia and Analgesia in Parturition (Twilight Sleep)* (Paul B. Hoeber, 1915), 104–6.

41. "Twilight Sleep Vindicated," *New York Times,* October 20, 1914, 12. Knipe was one of the physicians who began to dismiss criticism of twilight sleep as imperfect implementation of the Krönig-Gauss technique. See Wm. H. W. Knipe, "Twilight Sleep: Its Future and Relation to the General Practitioner," *American Medicine* 21 (January 1915): 29–32.

42. Ralph M. Beach, "Twilight Sleep," *American Medicine* 21 (January 1915): 37–43; Ralph M. Beach, "'Twilight Sleep' Report of One Thousand Cases," *American Journal of Obstetrics and Diseases of Women and Children* 71 (1915): 727–41; the quotes are in Boyd, "The Story of Dämmerschlaf," 129.

43. Tracy and Leupp, "Painless Childbirth"; McPherson, "Technic of the Scopolamine-Narcophine Narcosis"; quotes in Beach, "'Twilight Sleep' Report of One Thousand Cases," 732–33; W. Francis B. Wakefield, "Scopolamin Amnesia in Labor," *American Journal of Obstetrics and Diseases of Women and Children* 71 (1915): 422–28. Use of the phrase "better babies" was deliberate; better-baby contests were especially popular at the time. See Vance Dorey, *Better Baby Contests.*

44. James R. Freeland, "Scopolamin-Morphin Anesthesia in Labor: A Report of Seven Year's Experience," *Pennsylvania Medical Journal* 19 (July 1916): 768–75, quotes at 775.

45. Eleanor Early, "Unusual Party of 200 Twilight Sleep Babies," 1930 broadside, a blow-up of an *EveryWeek Magazine* page, September 13–14, 1930, Eliza Taylor Ransom Papers, Schlesinger Library, Radcliffe College, Cambridge, MA.

46. Ibid.

47. "Twilight Sleep Babes Exhibited. Demonstrate Lungs Are O. K. at Cort Theatre Meeting," *Boston Herald,* May 25, 1915.

48. Early, "Unusual Party of 200 Twilight Sleep Babies," Eliza Taylor Ransom Papers.

49. The quotations are in Eliza Taylor Ransom, "Gymnastics Following Childbirth," *Monthly Journal of Homeopathic Medicine* (May 1916): 250–52; "Book Review of *Painless Childbirth: A General Survey of All Painless Methods with Special Stress on 'Twilight Sleep' and Its Extension to America,* by Marguerite Tracy and Mary Boyd," *Lancet-Clinic* 114 (August 28, 1915): 199–200.

50. C. E. Ziegler, "How Can We Best Solve the Midwifery Problem," *American Journal of Public Health* 12 (1922): 409.

51. Frederick Leavitt, "More about 'Twilight Sleep' in Labor," *American Journal of Clinical Medicine* 22 (1915): 309–15, quotes at 314.

52. Joseph DeLee to Ogden T. McClurg, August 8, 1922, Joseph B. DeLee Papers, Northwestern Memorial Hospital Archives, Chicago. Despite his ongoing enthusiasm for the aseptic, nonintrusive obstetrics performed so successfully by his Maxwell Street Dispensary physicians, DeLee also offered a host of medical interventions to

Chicago's wealthy mothers. Providing this treatment to that clientele appeared to be part of DeLee's strategy to make obstetrics a well-respected specialty. For more on DeLee and the dichotomy in his obstetric practice, see Judith Walzer Leavitt, "Joseph B. DeLee and the Practice of Preventive Obstetrics," *American Journal of Public Health* 78 (October 1988): 1353–60. As the administration of anesthesia became more common during birth, obstetricians' insistence on proper payment and respect became particularly emphatic whenever anesthesia was mentioned. See, for example, "Discussion of W. C. Danforth and C. Henry Davis, Obstetric Analgesia and Anesthesia," *Journal of the American Medical Association* 81 (September 29, 1923): 1093–96.

53. Paul Starr, *The Social Transformation of American Medicine: The Rise of a Sovereign Profession and the Making of a Vast Industry* (Basic Books, 1982), 117–20.

54. Abraham Flexner, *Medical Education in the United States and Canada: A Report to the Carnegie Foundation for the Advancement of Teaching* (Carnegie Foundation for the Advancement of Teaching, 1910), 117–18.

55. Quotes relating to the survey are in J. Whitridge Williams, "Medical Education and the Midwife Problem in the United States," *Journal of the American Medical Association* 58 (January 6, 1912): 1–7, at 2 and 5; the other quotes are in J. Whitridge Williams, "Why Is the Art of Obstetrics So Poorly Practised?" *Long Island Medical Journal* 11 (May 1917): 169–78, at 171 and 177.

56. Knipe, "Twilight Sleep."

57. Tracy and Leupp, "Painless Childbirth"; quote in Teller, "The Neglected Psychology of the 'Twilight Sleep,'" 17–24, at 21.

58. Oliver Paul Humpstone, "Twilight Sleep," *Long Island Medical Journal* 8 (1914): 461–65, "isles of memory" at 463; Rongy, "The Use of Scopolamine in Obstetrics"; Hilkowich, "Further Observations on Scopolamine-Narcophin Anesthesia."

59. A. J. Rongy and S. S. Arluck, "The Use of Scopolamine-Morphine in Labor," *New York Medical Journal* 100 (1914): 619–21; McPherson, "Technic of the Scopolamine-Narcophine Narcosis"; quote in J. Clarence Webster, "Nitrous Oxid Gas Analgesia in Obstetrics," *Journal of the American Medical Association* 64 (1915): 812–13.

60. "Book Review of *Painless Childbirth*."

61. Quoted in Ira Berkow, *Maxwell Street: Survival in a Bazaar* (Doubleday, 1977), 178; George L. Brodhead, "Progress of the Year in Obstetrics," *American Journal of Obstetrics and Diseases of Women and Children* 62 (1910): 1037–41.

62. Charles B. Reed, "Twilight Sleep," *Wesley Memorial Hospital Twenty-sixth Annual Report, 1914–1915,* 11, Northwestern Memorial Hospital Archives.

63. Advertisement, *Southwestern Stockman-Farmer,* October 9, 1914, 12, box 867, folder 0867-05, AMA Health Fraud and Alternative Medicine Collection. Rosemary Stevens discusses the contribution of obstetrics to the rise of hospitals in *In Sickness and in Wealth: American Hospitals in the Twentieth Century* (Basic Books, 1989), 105–7, 173–74.

64. Phillips J. Carter, "Twilight Sleep," *New Orleans Medical and Surgical Journal* 67 (1914–15): 618–24; Ferris, "Scopolamin Amnesia, or Twilight Sleep," 88–92; Elizabeth R. Miner, "Letter and Report of Nineteen Cases in Which 'Twilight' Was Used," *Woman's Medical Journal* 26 (May 1916): 131; Bertha Van Hoosen, "Twilight Sleep in

the Home," *Woman's Medical Journal* 26 (May 1916): 132; C. E. Boys, "Scopolamine-Morphine in Labor: A Study of Twenty-one Consecutive Cases," *Journal of the Michigan State Medical Society* 15 (1916): 282–85.

65. Frank B. Gilbreth Jr. and Ernestine Gilbreth Carey, *Cheaper by the Dozen* (T. Y. Crowell, 1948), 145–54, quotes at 147 and 153.

66. Katharine Kerr Moore to May Walden Kerr, January 20, February 20, 1914; January 13, 1921, May Walden Kerr Papers, Special Collections, Newberry Library, Chicago.

67. " 'Twilight Sleep' in the Light for Day," 112; Mosher, "Scopolamin Semi-Narcosis or Twilight Sleep in Labor," 441–53, quote at 442.

68. Ross McPherson and James A. Harrar, "Report of a Series of Cases in Which the 'Twilight Sleep' Was Used," *Medical Record* 86 (December 5, 1914): 988–90.

69. McPherson, "Technic of the Scopolamine-Narcophine Narcosis"; quote in J. W. Brandau, "Morphin-Hyoscin Analgesia in Labor, with Report of Cases," *Journal of the Tennessee State Medical Association* 8 (December 1915): 350–55, at 354; Lazard, "The Twilight Sleep Propaganda in the Lay Press," 13–22.

70. Joseph Louis Baer, "Scopolamin-Morphin Treatment in Labor," *Journal of the American Medical Association* 64 (1915): 1723–28, quotes at 1726.

71. Ibid.; Andrew M. Claye, *The Evolution of Obstetric Analgesia* (Oxford University Press, 1939), 67.

72. Philadelphia Lying-In Charity Patient Charts, 1908 to 1922, Pennsylvania Hospital, Pennsylvania Hospital Historic Collections; "Safeguarding against Scopolamin Casualties," *Journal of the American Medical Association* 64 (1915): 598; "Drops Twilight Sleep," *New York Times*, May 29, 1915, 20; "Gives Up Twilight Sleep," *New York Times*, August 16, 1916, 7.

73. "Mothers Exhibit 'Twilight' Babies," *New York Times*, April 30, 1915, 8.

74. Holt, "Scopolamine-Morphine in Obstetrics"; Carter, "Twilight Sleep."

75. Rongy, "The Use of Scopolamine in Labor"; Van Hoosen, *Scopolamine-Morphine Anaesthesia*, 93; Boyd and Tracy, "More about Painless Childbirth."

76. "Mrs. Francis X. Carmody Buried," *New York Times*, August 25, 1915, 11; Tracy and Boyd, *Painless Childbirth*, 200–204.

77. "To Fight Twilight Sleep. Brooklyn Woman to Start Association to Oppose the Treatment," *New York Times*, August 31, 1915, 5.

78. "Doctors Disagree on Twilight Sleep. Death of First American Patient Renews Discussion of Painless Childbirth," *New York Times*, August 24, 1915, 7. Rongy's own previous strong advocacy for twilight sleep can be seen in Rongy, "The Use of Scopolamine in Obstetrics." In this article, Rongy details his work with a Freiburg physician, after which he found that "this mode of treatment deserved all that Krönig and Gauss claimed for it" (367).

79. As evidence of ongoing use of scopolamine, if not the specific twilight sleep protocol, see "Twilight Sleep," *Hygeia* 5 (October 1927): 538; Harry M. Kirschbaum, "Scopolamine in Obstetrics," *American Journal of Obstetrics and Gynecology* 44 (1942): 664–72; G. G. Passmore and Edgar W. Santa Cruz, "The Use of Intravenous and Intramuscular Injections of Demerol and Scopolamine in Labor and Delivery,"

American Journal of Obstetrics and Gynecology 68 (1954): 998–1008; and Samuel S. Rosenfeld, Bernard Lapan, Martin Kurzner, and Morton S. Weinstein, "The Relief of the Pains of Labor by the Continuous Intravenous Drop of Meperidine and Scopolamine," *American Journal of Obstetrics and Gynecology* 67 (1954): 1067–73.

80. James A. Harrar, "Rectal Ether Analgesia in Labor," *American Journal of Obstetrics and Gynecology* 13 (1927): 486–94, "as definite as" at 490; Clifford B. Lull, "A Preliminary Report on the Use of Barbiturates with Ether by Rectum," *American Journal of Obstetrics and Gynecology* 24 (1932): 888–91; Kirschbaum, "Scopolamine in Obstetrics," 664–72; Discussion of William F. Mengert, "Morphine Sulfate as an Obstetric Analgesic," *American Journal of Obstetrics and Gynecology* 44 (1942): 895–96; retired obstetrician, interview by author, tape recording, Winnetka, IL, July 12, 1996. Nicholson J. Eastman, professor of obstetrics at Johns Hopkins University, observed after World War II that twilight sleep was still used by a number of physicians and that obstetricians prided themselves on ensuring that women would remember nothing about their labors. See Nicholson J. Eastman, *Expectant Motherhood* (Little, Brown, 1946), 132, 134.

81. James R. Bloss, "Modern Obstetrics in the Home," *American Journal of Obstetrics and Gynecology* 15 (1928): 424–31, quote at 424.

82. I. H. Adams, "Dämmerschlaf, or Twilight Sleep," *Journal of the Medical Association of Georgia* 5 (1915–16): 163–66.

83. Butler, "Hyoscine Anesthesia in Obstetrics"; "Doctors Disagree on Twilight Sleep," 7.

84. Holt, "Scopolamine-Morphine in Obstetrics," 574; Tracy, "Bringing Babies into the World."

85. Sylvia Plath, *The Bell Jar* (New York: Harper and Row, 1971), 53.

Chapter 3 · Developing the Obstetric Anesthesia Arsenal

1. Dorothy Reed Mendenhall, "Dorothy Reed Mendenhall's Autobiography," typed manuscript, Dorothy Reed Mendenhall Papers, Sophia Smith Collection, Neilson Library, Smith College, Northampton, MA. The manuscript does not explicitly say that Mendenhall received anesthesia at Margaret's birth, but she clearly implies that she did. She also notes elsewhere that before a visit to Denmark in 1926 she had never been to an unanesthetized birth: see D. R. Mendenhall to Miss Abbott, June 7, 1926, from Göttingen, Germany, Dorothy Reed Mendenhall Papers.

2. Gena Corea, "Dorothy Reed Mendenhall: 'Childbirth Is Not a Disease,'" *Ms.*, April 1974, 98–104; quoted in Molly Ladd-Taylor, *Mother-Work: Women, Child Welfare, and the State, 1890–1930* (University of Illinois Press, 1994), 82.

3. Grace L. Meigs, *Maternal Mortality from All Conditions Connected with Childbirth in the United States and Certain Other Countries* (Government Printing Office, 1917); Kriste Lindenmeyer, *"A Right to Childhood": The U.S. Children's Bureau and Child Welfare, 1912–46* (University of Illinois Press, 1997), 1–7. George Newman, a British physician and pioneer in the fields of public and child health who was influential on both sides of the Atlantic, made the connection between mothers' and babies'

health explicit in his 1906 book *Infant Mortality: A Social Problem*, the first book-length publication to address infant mortality. Newman argued that infants' health was largely dependent on their mothers' ability to properly care for them. See Eilidh Garrett, Chris Galley, Nicola Shelton, and Robert Woods, eds., *Infant Mortality: A Continuing Social Problem* (Ashgate, 2006).

4. Meigs, *Maternal Mortality*.

5. Matthias Nicoll, "Maternity as a Public Health Problem," *American Journal of Public Health* 19 (September 1929): 961–68, quote at 963; Helena Huntington Smith, "Death at Birth: Our High Maternal Mortality," *Outlook and Independent*, November 13, 1929, 405–8.

6. Between 1900 and 1920, infant deaths dropped from 130 to 76 per 1,000 live births, while deaths from maternity-related causes rose from 13.3 to 16.9 per 100,000 population, peaking in 1918 and 1920 with rates of 22.3 and 19 deaths (some of the deaths in those years, of course, were caused by the influenza pandemic). For more detailed statistics on infant mortality in the early twentieth century, see Samuel H. Preston and Michael R. Haines, *Fatal Years: Child Mortality in Late Nineteenth-Century America* (Princeton University Press, 1991), 77; Richard A. Meckel, *Save the Babies: American Public Health Reform and the Prevention of Infant Mortality, 1850–1929* (Johns Hopkins University Press, 1990), 238; and Jacqueline H. Wolf, *Don't Kill Your Baby: Public Health and the Decline of Breastfeeding in the 19th and 20th Centuries* (Ohio State University Press, 2001), 205–11. For maternal death statistics in this era, see Robert Morse Woodbury, *Infant Mortality and Its Causes with an Appendix on the Trend of Maternal Mortality Rates in the United States* (Williams and Wilkins, 1926), 180–92.

7. S. Josephine Baker, "Maternal Mortality in the United States," *Journal of the American Medical Association* 89 (1927): 2016–17; Dorothy Dunbar Bromley, "What Risk Motherhood?" *Harper's Magazine*, June 1929, 11–22, quote at 14; Nicoll, "Maternity as a Public Health Problem," 966; John Osborn Polak, "What Is the Matter with American Obstetrics?" *American Journal of Obstetrics and Gynecology* 19 (1930): 598–99. The geographical area of the United States in which deaths were recorded was slowly expanded from 40.5% of the population in 1900 to 82.2% in 1920. This expansion does not explain the increase in maternal deaths, however. In most of the added states, the maternal rate was higher in 1921 than in the year of admission to the death registration area. See Woodbury, *Infant Mortality*, 180–92.

8. Dorothy Reed Mendenhall, "Prenatal and Natal Conditions in Wisconsin," *Wisconsin Medical Journal* 15 (March 1917): 363–64; Joseph B. DeLee, "Meddlesome Midwifery in Renaissance," *Journal of the American Medical Association* 67 (October 14, 1916): 1126–29. Deaths due to anesthesia were most often indirectly caused by anesthesia, prompted by the increase in forceps use due to uterine inertia and groggy women. Deaths directly attributable to anesthesia were relatively few, especially by the 1940s and 1950s. In North Carolina, for example, from August 1946 through December 1954, only 2.6% of the 1,733 maternal deaths were due primarily to anesthesia. Frank R. Lock and Frank C. Greiss, "The Anesthetic Hazards in Obstetrics," *American Journal of Obstetrics and Gynecology* 70 (1955): 861–75. As deaths due to infection and

hemorrhage decreased, however (owing to blood banking and the availability of antibiotics after World War II), the relative number of maternal deaths from anesthesia increased. In Michigan from 1950 through 1953, researchers blamed 9.8% of 346 maternal deaths on anesthesia. Charles S. Stevenson, Harold A. Ott, Palmer E. Sutton, and Mary Lou Byrd, "Maternal Deaths from Obstetric Anesthesia and Analgesia: Can They Be Eliminated?" *Obstetrics and Gynecology* 8 (1956): 88–97.

9. Dorothy Reed Mendenhall, *Midwifery in Denmark* (Government Printing Office, 1929), n.p.

10. New York Academy of Medicine Committee on Public Health Relations, *Maternal Mortality in New York City: A Study of All Puerperal Deaths, 1930–1932* (Commonwealth Fund, 1933), 113–16; "Maternity Death Rate: Mortality Survey Finds 65.8% Preventable," *Newsweek*, November 25, 1933, 27. Physicians consistently complained that anesthesia necessitated forceps for many reasons. Spinal anesthesia dulled mothers' urge and ability to push, and morphine seemed to have the same effect. Pharmacologically, both ether and chloroform depress the frequency and strength of spontaneous smooth muscle contractions; the uterus is a smooth muscle. And since inhalation anesthesia also renders women either groggy or unconscious, doctors explained that "instrumental aid at the perineal stage is practically always necessary." Howard F. Kane and George B. Roth, "The Use of Paraldehyde in Obtaining Obstetric Analgesia and Amnesia," *American Journal of Obstetrics and Gynecology* 29 (1935): 366–69, quote at 368. See also Discussion of William F. Mengert, "Morphine Sulfate as an Obstetric Analgesic," *American Journal of Obstetrics and Gynecology* 44 (1942): 895–96.

11. Charles D. Meigs, *Obstetrics: The Science and the Art* (Blanchard and Lea, 1856), 529, 542; Edgar L. Engel Sr., interview by Chad Berry, June 14, 1993, Indiana University Center for the History of Medicine Oral History Project, Indiana Historical Society, Indianapolis, IN. For more on the history of forceps, see Bryan Hibbard, *The Obstetrician's Armamentarium* (Norman, 2000).

12. Rates of forceps use are in James Young, "Maternal Mortality and Maternal Mortality Rates," *American Journal of Obstetrics and Gynecology* 31 (1936): 198–212, "the surgical stream" at 207. Rates of maternal mortality are in Irvine Loudon, *Death in Childbirth: An International Study of Maternal Care and Maternal Mortality, 1800–1950* (Oxford University Press, 1992), 366, 451. For an analysis of maternal death rates over time in Western countries, see Vincent De Brouwere, "The Comparative Study of Maternal Mortality over Time: The Role of the Professionalisation of Childbirth," *Social History of Medicine* 20 (December 2007): 541–62.

13. Mary Sumner Boyd, "Why Mothers Die," *Nation*, March 18, 1931, 293–95, quotes at 295.

14. Diaries, April 2–November 21, 1946, November 17, 1946, entry, Neal Heywood Papers, Arizona Historical Society, Tucson, AZ.

15. Judith Walzer Leavitt, *Brought to Bed: Childbearing in America, 1750–1950* (Oxford University Press, 1986), 268–69; William G. Rothstein, *American Medical Schools and the Practice of Medicine: A History* (Oxford University Press, 1987), 127; Joseph B. DeLee, "How Should the Maternity Be Isolated?" *Modern Hospital* 29 (September

1927): 65–72; Joseph B. DeLee and Heinz Siedentopf, "The Maternity Ward of the General Hospital," *Journal of the American Medical Association* 100 (January 7, 1933): 6–14.

16. Anthony Ruppersberg, "Maternal Mortality Studies in Ohio," *Obstetrics and Gynecology* 10 (1957): 77–83. A review of maternal mortality at the Pennsylvania Hospital from 1929 through 1953 reflected the effect of blood banking and antibiotics on women's ability to survive childbirth. During the first 8.5-year period of the study, there was 1 maternal death for every 179 live births; in the second 8-year period, there was 1 maternal death for every 549 live births; and in the last 8-year period, there was 1 maternal death for every 1,374 live births. Robert McNair Mitchell, "Maternal Mortality in the Pennsylvania Hospital," *Obstetrics and Gynecology* 5 (February 1955): 123–36. Otto C. Phillips, George H. Davis, Todd M. Frazier, and Alfred T. Nelson, "The Role of Anesthesia in Obstetric Mortality," *Anesthesia and Analgesia* 40 (September–October 1961): 557–66; Otto C. Phillips, Todd M. Frazier, and George H. Davis, "Factors in Obstetric Mortality," *American Journal of Obstetrics and Gynecology* (September 1, 1963): 71–76. These two articles are a study of 455,553 live births and 694 maternal deaths from 1936 to 1958 in Baltimore. Experts noted at the time, however, that inferences for the entire country could be made from the Baltimore study. Indeed, Chester W. White, anesthesiologist-in-chief at the Boston Lying-in Hospital, noted at the time that the obstetric situation in Baltimore was probably better than the national average. For more on the history of the maternal death rate in the United States, see Loudon, *Death in Childbirth,* 365–97.

17. See, for example, Dorothy Dunbar Bromley, "Lifting the Curse of Eve," *Woman Citizen,* October 1927, 8–10+; Constance L. Todd, "Easier Motherhood," *Ladies' Home Journal,* March 1930, 9, 204, 207, 209; "Better Care for Mothers in Childbirth," *New Republic,* May 13, 1931, 339; Constance L. Todd, "You, Too, Should Have Your Babies without Pain," *Good Housekeeping,* November 1937, 78–79+; J. P. McEvoy, "Our Streamlined Baby," *Reader's Digest,* May 1938, 18; "I Had a Baby, Too: A Symposium," *Atlantic Monthly,* June 1939, 764–72; Marguerite Ball, "Without Pain," *Woman's Home Companion,* May 1943, 16, 85.

18. Quote appears in Charles B. Reed, "Hospital Maternity," *39th Annual Report of the Wesley Memorial Hospital (January 1, 1927 to January 1928),* 37, Northwestern Memorial Hospital Archives, Chicago. Some of the earliest articles about epidural anesthesia include Charles B. Odom, "A Review of Page's Epidural Anesthesia with a Report of 100 Cases," *New Orleans Medical and Surgical Journal* 88 (1936): 618–27 (which includes a brief history of the development of epidural anesthesia); P. Graffagnino and Louis W. Seyler, "Epidural Anesthesia in Obstetrics," *American Journal of Obstetrics and Gynecology* 35 (1938): 597–602; and "Childbirth Aids," *Time,* October 31, 1938, 37.

19. S. A. Cosgrove, "Spinal Anesthesia in Obstetrics," *American Journal of Obstetrics and Gynecology* 14 (1927): 751–60, quote at 751.

20. D. R. Mendenhall to Miss Abbott, June 7, 1926, from Göttingen, Germany, Dorothy Reed Mendenhall Papers. Mendenhall wrote about her experience in Denmark, when her perception of birth and women's ability to tolerate labor changed, in

Mendenhall, *Midwifery in Denmark*. Clifford B. Lull and Robert A. Hingson, *Control of Pain in Childbirth: Anesthesia, Analgesia, Amnesia* (J. B. Lippincott, 1948), 131–32.

21. Constance L. Todd, *Easier Motherhood: A Discussion of the Abolition of Needless Pain* (John Day, 1931), 108; E. D. Colvin and R. A. Bartholomew, "Improvements in the Paraldehyde Method of Relief of Pain in Labor," *American Journal of Obstetrics and Gynecology* 35 (1938): 589–97.

22. For examples of the language physicians used to describe childbirth in this era, see "Discussion of W. C. Danforth and C. Henry Davis, Obstetric Analgesia and Anesthesia," *Journal of the American Medical Association* 81 (September 29, 1923): 1093–96. Examples of similar language used by laypeople are in Todd, *Easier Motherhood*, 3; and Dorothy Smith Dushkin Diary, October 8, 1932, entry, Dorothy Smith Dushkin Papers, Sophia Smith Collection, Neilson Library, Smith College, Northampton, MA.

23. Roy P. Finney, *The Story of Motherhood* (Liveright, 1937), 3, 12, 6–7; Bernard DeVoto, "Maternity Floor," *Harper's Magazine*, April 1940, 559.

24. Diaries, April 2–November 21, 1946, September 20, 1946, entry, Neal Heywood Papers.

25. "I Had a Baby, Too," 765, 767.

26. "Obstetrics Class Lecture Notes," October 31, 1931, Stanton A. Friedberg, MD, Papers, Rush–Presbyterian–St. Luke's Medical Center Archives, Chicago.

27. Cecilia Hennel Hendricks, *Letters from Honeyhill: A Woman's View of Homesteading, 1914–1931*, Cecilia Hendricks Wahl, ed. (Pruett, 1986), 174, 192–93, 340, 423, quotes at 192–93.

28. Maxwell E. Lapham, *Maternity Care in a Rural Community: Pike County, Mississippi, 1931–1936* (Commonwealth Fund, 1938).

29. Thaddeus L. Montgomery, "Analgesia with the Barbituric and Derivatives and Its Relationship to Sudden Death in Labor," *American Journal of Obstetrics and Gynecology* 33 (1937): 745–50, quote at 745.

30. B. P. Watson, "American Gynecological Society Sixty-first Annual Meeting President's Address," *American Journal of Obstetrics and Gynecology* 32 (October 1936): 547–60; J. T. Gwathmey, "Modified Rectal Analgesia in Obstetrics," *American Journal of Obstetrics and Gynecology* 9 (1925): 401–8. Hirst made these comments after Gwathmey presented his paper. Robert A. Hingson, "The Control of Pain and Fear in the Management of Labor and Delivery," *Surgical Clinics of North America* 25 (December 1945): 1352–81.

31. Purvis L. Martin and Steward H. Smith, "Public Relations in Our Maternity Wards," *American Journal of Obstetrics and Gynecology* 81 (June 1961): 1079–85, quote at 1082; Betsy Marvin McKinney, "The Pleasure of Childbirth," *Ladies' Home Journal*, April 1949, 116, 118–21.

32. A mother, interview by author, tape recording, November 1, 2005, Glencoe, IL.

33. Since a few charity hospitals scattered throughout the country had long served as a midwifery training ground for both medical students and physicians via their "ward cases," hospital-based training in obstetrics was not a wholly new concept. Charles E. Rosenberg discusses the inception of hospital-based obstetric training in

The Care of Strangers: The Rise of America's Hospital System (Basic Books, 1987; paperback ed., Johns Hopkins University Press, 1995), 170–71. The medical historian Charlotte Borst argues that the popularization of hospital birth was instrumental in making obstetrics a prestigious specialty. She contends that because obstetrics initially adopted a public health focus to build its authority, rather than following the example of surgeons who embraced the more prestigious goals of the laboratory and the hospital, obstetrics long remained a specialty held in low esteem. Not until birth and the training of obstetricians moved from homes to hospitals in the 1930s and 1940s and obstetrics became a surgical specialty, with all the impressive accoutrements that surgery implies, did the public and the medical community begin to view obstetrics as a respectable and necessary discipline. See Charlotte G. Borst, *Catching Babies: The Professionalization of Childbirth, 1870–1920* (Harvard University Press, 1995).

34. Clyde L. Randall, *Developments in the Certification of Obstetricians and Gynecologists in the United States, 1930–1980: The American Board of Obstetrics and Gynecology* (American Board of Obstetrics and Gynecology, 1989); Paul Starr, *The Social Transformation of American Medicine: The Rise of a Sovereign Profession and the Making of a Vast Industry* (Basic Books, 1982), 356–57.

35. Starr, *The Social Transformation of American Medicine,* 356–57; Rosemary Stevens, *American Medicine and the Public Interest* (Yale University Press, 1971), 202. General practitioners did fight back in many areas of the country. Before World War II, for example, a physician helped form the Indiana Academy of General Practitioners after general practitioners found themselves subject to new rules: although they could continue attending home births, unless they were certified in obstetrics they could not deliver babies in hospitals. The battle waged by the Indiana Academy of General Practitioners eventually led to a new specialty in family practice. Family practitioners, after a family-practice residency, were allowed to attend hospital births. Frank P. Albertson, interview by Patrick Ettinger, October 28, 1993, Indiana University Center for the History of Medicine Oral History Project.

36. "Hospitals Approved for Residencies in Specialties," *Journal of the American Medical Association* 197 (August 29, 1936): 703–15; "Approved Residencies and Fellowships for Veteran and Civilian Physicians," *Journal of the American Medical Association* 131 (August 17, 1946): 1322–54.

37. "Hospital Grows in Popularity as Family Birthplace," *Presbyterian Hospital of the City of Chicago Bulletin* 32 (May 1940): 3; "Maternity Department Shows a Great Increase," *Presbyterian Hospital of the City of Chicago Bulletin* 35 (June–July 1943): 1, 3, Rush University Medical Center Archives, Chicago; American College of Obstetricians and Gynecologists, "Trends in Out-of-Hospital Births," in *Manpower Planning in Obstetrics and Gynecology* (American College of Obstetricians and Gynecologists, 1991).

38. William Ray Arney, *Power and the Profession of Obstetrics* (University of Chicago Press, 1982), 51.

39. H. J. Stander, "Undergraduate and Graduate Instruction in Obstetrics and Gynecology," *American Journal of Obstetrics and Gynecology* 51 (1946): 771–79; Deborah Kuhn McGregor, *From Midwives to Medicine: The Birth of American Gynecology* (Rutgers University Press, 1998), 6, 33, 55, 110, "accidents of childbirth" at 6.

40. J. B. DeLee, "The Prophylactic Forceps Operation," *American Journal of Obstetrics and Gynecology* 1 (October 1920): 34–44, quotes at 40–43.

41. Marsden Wagner, *Born in the USA: How a Broken Maternity System Must Be Fixed to Put Women and Children First* (University of California Press, 2006), 15–17; resident quoted in Robbie E. Davis-Floyd, *Birth as an American Rite of Passage* (University of California Press, 2003), 226.

42. Retired obstetrician, interview by author, tape recording, Glenview, IL, June 29, 2006.

43. "Discussion of W. C. Danforth and C. Henry Davis, Obstetric Analgesia and Anesthesia," *Journal of the American Medical Association* 81 (September 29, 1923): 1093–96. As late as 1940, two physicians at the University of Wisconsin, one an anesthesiologist and the other an obstetrician, wrote, "Opinion regarding pain relief in labor is in a chaotic state." R. M. Waters and J. W. Harris, "Factors Influencing the Safety of Pain Relief in Labor," *American Journal of Surgery* 48 (1940): 129–34. Woman quoted in Todd, *Easier Motherhood*, 128.

44. James R. Freeland, "Scopolamin-Morphin Anesthesia in Labor: A Report of Seven Years' Experience," *Pennsylvania Medical Journal* 19 (July 1916): 768–75, quotes at 773–74.

45. Arthur Dean Bevan, "The Choice of Anesthetic Methods," typed manuscript dated October 16, 1931, Arthur Dean Bevan, MD, papers, Rush University Medical Center Archives; Arthur E. Guedel, "Nitrous Oxid Anesthesia in Obstetrics," *Journal of the Indiana State Medical Association* 8 (March 15, 1915): 113–16; "Discussion of Arthur E. Guedel, Nitrous Oxid Anesthesia in Obstetrics," *Journal of the Indiana State Medical Association* 8 (March 15, 1915): 116–19; L. Stanley James, "Fond Memories of Virginia Apgar," *Pediatrics* 55 (January 1975): 1–4; John Adriani to Mr. Bernard Jensen, C.R.N.A., Department of Anesthesia, Swain County Hospital, Bryson City, NC, May 11, 1981, John Adriani Papers, 1925–88, National Library of Medicine, History of Medicine Division, Bethesda, MD.

46. James T. Gwathmey and James Greenough, "Clinical Experience with Synergistic Analgesia," *Annals of Surgery* 74 (1921): 185–95.

47. J. Y. Simpson to Dr. Storer, April 25, 1870, Horatio Robinson Storer Papers, 1859–1911, National Library of Medicine, History of Medicine Division. Storer, a physician at the Boston Lying-In Hospital, greatly admired Simpson and edited a collection of his works. See W. O. Priestley and Horatio R. Storer, eds., *The Obstetric Memoirs and Contributions of James Y. Simpson, M.D., F.R.S.E.* (J. B. Lippincott, 1855).

48. Florence Slown Hyde, "Anesthesia Important Factor in Surgery: Ethylene-Oxygen First Used in Presbyterian Hospital Now Widely Accepted," *Presbyterian Hospital of the City of Chicago Bulletin*, April 1936, Presbyterian Hospital Papers, Rush University Medical Center Archives.

49. Todd, *Easier Motherhood*, 12, 30, 113, 123, 129–44; Colvin and Bartholomew, "Improvements in the Paraldehyde Method"; "Relief for Childbirth Pain," *Science News Letter* 51 (May 31, 1947): 341.

50. Doris K. Cope, "James Tayloe Gwathmey: Seeds of a Developing Specialty," *Anesthesia and Analgesia* 76 (1993): 642–47; and Richard Foregger, "Gwathmey," *Anes-*

thesiology 5 (1944): 296–99. For more on Gwathmey's life and work, see Charles B. Pittinger, *James Tayloe Gwathmey, M.D.: American Pioneer Anesthesiologist* (Vanderbilt University School of Medicine, 1989). This text contains a short biography of Gwathmey, a complete bibliography of his work, and copies of his articles. The American Board of Anesthesiology was formed in 1937 to certify physicians practicing anesthesiology.

51. J. T. Gwathmey, "Oil-Ether Anaesthesia," *Lancet* (December 20, 1913): 1756–58; J. T. Gwathmey, "Five Hundred Cases of Oil-Ether Colonic Anesthesia," *American Journal of Surgery* 28 (July 1914): 268–74; James T. Gwathmey, "Oil-Ether Anaesthesia: An Attempt to Abolish Inhalation Anaesthesia," *Anaesthesia* (1914): 163–66; Harry M. Kirschbaum, "Scopolamine in Obstetrics," *American Journal of Obstetrics and Gynecology* 44 (1942): 664–72.

52. Gwathmey and Greenough, "Clinical Experience with Synergistic Analgesia," 185–95; James T. Gwathmey, "Synergistic Colonic Analgesia," *Journal of the American Medical Association* 76 (1921): 222–25; James Tayloe Gwathmey, *Anesthesia* (Macmillan, 1924): 732–48; James T. Gwathmey, "Obstetrical Analgesia: A Further Study, Based on More than Twenty Thousand Cases," *Surgery, Gynecology, and Obstetrics* 51 (1930): 190–95.

53. Todd, *Easier Motherhood*, quotes at 9, 204, 207, 209.

54. Ibid., 12, 30, 113, 123, 129–44, "large, fat" at 113.

55. Henry Rosenberg and Jean K. Axelrod, "Robert Andrew Hingson: His Unique Contributions to World Health as Well as to Anesthesiology," *American Journal of Anesthesiology* 25 (March–April 1998): 90–93, quote at 90. See also Hingson's obituary: Wolfgang Saxon, "Robert Andrew Hingson, 83, a Pioneer in Public Health," *New York Times*, October 13, 1996, 36. Robert A. Hingson and James L. Southworth, "Continuous Caudal Anesthesia," *American Journal of Surgery* 38 (January 1942): 93–96.

56. Waldo B. Edwards and Robert A. Hingson, "Continuous Caudal Anesthesia in Obstetrics," *American Journal of Surgery* 57 (September 1942): 459–64; Nathan Block and Samuel Rochberg, "Continuous Caudal Anesthesia in Obstetrics," *American Journal of Obstetrics and Gynecology* 45 (1943): 645–50.

57. Cosgrove, "Spinal Anesthesia in Obstetrics," 751–60; Herbert E. Schmitz and George Baba, "Low Spinal Nupercaine Anesthesia in Obstetrics," *American Journal of Obstetrics and Gynecology* 54 (1947): 838–47; American Society of Anesthesiologists, "Men of Anesthesia," videotaped interview of Robert Hingson by Frank Grabill, no date, ca. 1960s, Wood Library and Museum, film archive, American Society of Anesthesiologists, Park Ridge, IL.

58. Peter Y. Sussman, ed., *Decca: The Letters of Jessica Mitford* (Alfred A. Knopf, 2006), 117.

59. "New Anesthetic for Childbirth," *Time*, September 14, 1942, 66; "Painless Childbirth," *Time*, February 1, 1943, 38, 40; "Childbirth without Pain," *Newsweek*, February 1, 1943, 65–66; Ball, "Without Pain," 16, 85; "An Interview with Dr. Robert Hingson by Dr. Ralph Hingson," videotape, Living History Series, March 31, 1989, film archive, Wood Library, American Society of Anesthesiologists.

60. Thaddeus L. Montgomery, Heath Bumgardner, Frank S. Deming, and Elsie

Reed, "A Comparison of the Value and Applicability of Caudal and Spinal Anesthesia in Obstetric Practice," *Pennsylvania Medical Journal* (February 1945): 1–7; Roy E. Nicodemus, LeRoy F. Ritmiller, and Lewis J. Ledden, "Continuous Caudal Analgesia in Obstetrics on Trial," *American Journal of Obstetrics and Gynecology* 50 (1945): 312–16; "Discussion of Roy E. Nicodemus, LeRoy F. Ritmiller, and Lewis J. Ledden, "Continuous Caudal Analgesia in Obstetrics on Trial," *American Journal of Obstetrics and Gynecology* 50 (1945): 316–18; Francis R. Irving, C. Albertson Lippincott, and Frank C. Meyer, "Continuous Caudal Anesthesia in Obstetrics," *New York State Journal of Medicine* 43 (June 1, 1943): 1023–29.

61. Sol M. Shnider, "Training in Obstetric Anesthesia in the United States," *American Journal of Obstetrics and Gynecology* 93 (September 15, 1963): 243–52; J. Garrott Allen, MD, to Dr. Sarah H. Hardwicke, secretary, Council on Professional Practice, American Hospital Association, April 22, 1957, John Adriani Papers, 1925–88, National Library of Medicine, History of Medicine Division. The joint statement of the two organizations is included with this letter.

62. John J. Bonica and George H. Mix, "Twenty-four Hour Medical Anesthesia Coverage for Obstetric Patients," *Journal of the American Medical Association* 159 (October 8, 1955): 551–54; retired obstetrician, interview by author, tape recording, September 16, 1999, St. Paul, MN.

63. John Adriani, MD, to Coy L. Lay, MD, medical editor, International Correspondence Society of Obstetricians and Gynecologists, March 12, 1965, John Adriani Papers, 1925–88, National Library of Medicine, History of Medicine Division.

64. Retired obstetrician, interview by author, tape recording, July 19, 2004, Chicago; Phillips, Davis, Frazier, and Nelson, "The Role of Anesthesia in Obstetric Mortality," 557–66.

65. Oral history interview of John J. Bonica by John C. Liebeskind, tape recording, typed transcript, pp. 49–58, quotes at 45–46, John C. Liebeskind History of Pain Collection, John J. Bonica Papers, UCLA Biomedical Library, History and Special Collections Division, Los Angeles.

66. Ibid.; Bonica and Mix, "Twenty-four Hour Medical Anesthesia Coverage"; "An Interview with Dr. Robert Hingson by Dr. Ralph Hingson."

67. Bonica and Mix, "Twenty-four Hour Medical Anesthesia Coverage."

68. Retired obstetrician, interview by author, tape recording, July 19, 2004, Chicago; W. F. Windle and R. F. Becker, "Role of Carbon Dioxide in Resuscitation at Birth after Asphyxia and after Nembutal Anesthesia," *American Journal of Obstetrics and Gynecology* 42 (1941): 852, 854.

69. Thaddeus L. Montgomery, "Obstetric Amnesia, Analgesia, and Anesthesia: Their Relationship to Sudden Death in Labor," *Journal of the American Medical Association* 108 (May 15, 1937): 1679–83, "treatment of drug confusion" at 1683; Nicholson J. Eastman, "Clinic of Dr. Nicholson J. Eastman, The Johns Hopkins Hospital: Monday Afternoon Obstetrical Clinic," *Surgical Clinics of North America* 16 (October 1936): 1337–62.

70. Eastman, "Clinic of Dr. Nicholson J. Eastman," 1351.

71. Bedford Brown, "The Therapeutic Action of Chloroform in Parturition," *Jour-*

nal of the American Medical Association 25 (August 31, 1895): 354–58; L. C. Bacon, "The Indications for Chloroform during Labor," *Northwestern Lancet* 19 (1899): 104–7. As early as the 1850s, physicians expressed concern about the risks of anesthesia in surgery. For more on medical and public concerns about these risks, see Stephanie J. Snow, *Operations without Pain: The Practice and Science of Anaesthesia in Victorian Britain* (Palgrave Macmillan, 2006), 93–112. For examples of insistent statements that laboring women were not immune to the dangers of anesthesia, see "On the Necessity of Caution in the Employment of Chloroform during Labor," *American Journal of Obstetrics and Diseases of Women and Children* 10 (1877): 538–39; "Discussion of the Bromide of Ethyl as an Anesthetic in Labor," *American Journal of Obstetrics and Diseases of Women and Children* 18 (1885): 958.

72. J. Y. Simpson, *Notice of a New Anaesthetic Agent, as a Substitute for Sulphuric Ether in Surgery and Midwifery* (Sutherland and Knox, 1847), 5–13. For more on the history of chloroform, see Linda Stratmann, *Chloroform: The Quest for Oblivion* (Sutton, 2003).

73. Geo. N. Burwell, "Statement of Twenty-three Cases of Midwifery in Which Chloroform Was Administered," *Buffalo Medical Journal and Monthly Review of Medical and Surgical Science* 5 (1850): 7–29; J. N. Upshur, "The Therapeutic Application of Chloroform in Labor," *American Journal of Obstetrics and Diseases of Women and Children* 28 (1893): 718–19.

74. J. Whitridge Williams, *Obstetrics: A Text-Book for the Use of Students and Practitioners* (D. Appleton, 1904), 292; Discussion of Joseph DeLee, "The Early Recognition of Impending Obstetric Accidents," *Chicago Medical Recorder* 24 (June 1903): 440–42.

75. John Adriani, MD, to Anthony J. J. Rourke, MD, November 7, 1960; Adriani to Carla Jordan, Harris Hospital, Fort Worth, TX, December 19, 1960, John Adriani Papers, 1925–88, National Library of Medicine, History of Medicine Division; Martin M. Shir and Isidore Daichman, "The Use of Sodium Amytal in Labor," *American Journal of Obstetrics and Gynecology* 24 (1932): 115–17; Edwin J. DeCosta and Ralph A. Reis, "The Oral Administration of Paraldehyde for Relief of Pain during Labor," *American Journal of Obstetrics and Gynecology* 34 (1937): 448–55; Harold F. Burkons, "Rapid Obstetric Analgesia by Means of Intravenous Vinbarbital Sodium," *American Journal of Obstetrics and Gynecology* 56 (1948): 549–52; Robert A. Hingson, "Comparative Negro and White Mortality during Anesthesia, Obstetrics, and Surgery," *Journal of the American Medical Association* 49 (July 1957): 203–11. For the customary litany of complaints about a variety of anesthetics and analgesics, see Kane and Roth, "The Use of Paraldehyde"; Thomas R. Turino and Harold R. Merwarth, "Anoxia following Nitrous Oxide Anesthesia for Labor," *American Journal of Obstetrics and Gynecology* 41 (1941): 843–49; Henry S. Ruth and Newlin F. Paxson, "Obstetric Anesthesia and Analgesia with Sodium-Iso-Amyl-Ethyl-Barbiturate and Nitrous-Oxide-Oxygen," *American Journal of Obstetrics and Gynecology* 23 (1932): 90–96; Discussion of William F. Mengert, "Morphine Sulfate as an Obstetric Analgesic," 895–96; C. O. McCormick, "The Effects of Analgesia on the Newborn Infant," *American Journal of Obstetrics and Gynecology* 41 (1941): 391–402; N. Sproat Heaney, "Ethylene and Oxygen Anesthesia for Gyneco-

logical and Obstetrical Work," *American Journal of Obstetrics and Gynecology* 8 (1924): 416–19; Montgomery, "Analgesia with the Barbituric and Derivatives," 745–50; Waters and Harris, "Factors Influencing the Safety of Pain Relief," 129–34; "Obstetrics Class Lecture Notes."

76. Isadore Hill, "The Use of Chloroform in the First Stages of Labor," *Journal of the American Medical Association* 67 (August 19, 1916): 559–64, quote at 563. Rural physicians who attended births had long pointed out that they could not follow all the dictates of modern obstetric practice. See, for example, J. F. Ford, "Use of Drugs in Labor," *Wisconsin Medical Journal* 3 (1904–5): 257–65.

77. Joseph DeLee to J. Whitridge Williams, January 23, 1925; "Case of Mrs. Nicholas Longworth July 1924," Joseph B. DeLee, MD, papers, Northwestern Memorial Hospital Archives; retired obstetrician, interview by author, tape recording, November 1, 2005, Northbrook, IL.

78. Kane and Roth, "The Use of Paraldehyde"; Sylvan M. Shane, D. Frank Kaltreider, and Harry M. Cohen, "Dilute Solution, Catheter, Continuous Spinal Analgesia for Labor and Delivery," *American Journal of Obstetrics and Gynecology* 54 (1947): 488–95; Leonard Averett, Walter Sussman, and David Zimring, "Spinal Anesthesia," *American Journal of Obstetrics and Gynecology* 24 (1932): 339–47; McCormick, "The Effects of Analgesia on the Newborn," 391–402; Norris W. Vaux, Clifford B. Lull, Robert A. Hingson, and Selwyn D. Collins, "A Further Evaluation of Continuous Caudal Analgesia," in Lull and Hingson, *Control of Pain in Childbirth*; William Ridgely Stone, "Cocainization of the Spinal Cord by Means of Lumbar Puncture during Labor," *American Journal of Obstetrics and Diseases of Women and Children* 43 (February 1901): 145–54. Physicians first employed spinal anesthesia at the very end of the nineteenth century. Some of the first articles in American medical journals about spinal anesthesia in obstetrics include S. Marx, "My Failures and Successes with Spinal Anesthesia," *American Journal of Obstetrics and Diseases of Women and Children* 43 (1901): 102–6; and Samuel L. Weber, "Spinal Anesthesia," *American Journal of Obstetrics and Diseases of Women and Children* 46 (1902): 297–304.

79. M. Pierce Rucker, "The Use of Novocaine in Obstetrics," *American Journal of Obstetrics and Gynecology* 35 (1925): 35–47, quotes at 46.

80. Mahlon C. Hinebaugh and Warren R. Lang, "Continuous Spinal Anesthesia for Labor and Delivery," *Annals of Surgery* 120 (August 1944): 143–51, quote at 148; Montgomery, Bumgardner, Deming, and Reed, "A Comparison of the Value and Applicability of Caudal and Spinal Anesthesia," 1–7.

81. Waters and Harris, "Factors Influencing the Safety of Pain Relief," 129–34, "reciprocally incompatible" at 134. Representative general assessments of the potential dangers of obstetric anesthesia are in Clifford B. Lull, "A Preliminary Report on the Use of Barbiturates with Ether by Rectum," *American Journal of Obstetrics and Gynecology* 24 (1932): 888–91, "enthusiastically endorsed" at 888; and Harold C. Ingraham and James Alan Rosen, "Obstetric Analgesia with Acid Alurate in Rectal Ether Oil," *American Journal of Obstetrics and Gynecology* 34 (1937): 672–75.

82. Ruth and Paxson, "Obstetric Anesthesia and Analgesia," 90–96, "A patient" at

94; Colvin and Bartholomew, "Improvements in the Paraldehyde Method," "most pronounced" at 591.

83. William G. Cullen and Harold R. Griffith, "Postpartum Results of Spinal Anesthesia in Obstetrics," *Anesthesia and Analgesia* 26 (May–June 1947): 114–21, quote at 115–16; Todd, "Easier Motherhood," quote at 204.

84. J. T. Gwathmey, Robert Abbe McKenzie, and F. J. Hudson, "Painless Childbirth by Synergistic Methods," *American Journal of Obstetrics and Gynecology* 8 (1924): 154–63; DeCosta and Reis, "The Oral Administration of Paraldehyde."

85. Todd, *Easier Motherhood*, 110.

86. "Regulations of the Out-Patient Obstetrical Department of the Rush Medical College, Presbyterian Hospital, and the Central Free Dispensary," 1931, Presbyterian Hospital Papers, Rush University Medical Center Archives; Frank P. Albertson, interview by Patrick Ettinger, October 28, 1993, Indiana University Center for the History of Medicine Oral History Project. Lack of supervision of medical students was common in many areas of the country. Although medical students in the 1930s attended considerably more births than earlier in the twentieth century, they consistently attested to how little oversight they received at those births. See Naomi Dalton, interview by Steven Stowe, March 25, 1993; Frank P. Albertson, interview by Patrick Ettinger, October 28, 1993; Frank H. Green, interview by Steven Stowe, July 7, 1992; William M. Sholty, interview by Patrick Ettinger, June 30, 1993, Indiana University Center for the History of Medicine Oral History Project; Clarence W. Monroe, MD, Oral History, conducted by Stuart W. Campbell, June 20, 1994, Rush University Medical Center Archives; "Regulations of the Out-Patient Obstetrical Department of the Rush Medical College, Presbyterian Hospital, and the Central Free Dispensary."

87. Saddle block anesthesia cases, John Adriani Papers, 1925–88, National Library of Medicine, History of Medicine Division; "Proceedings," *American Society of Anesthesiologists Obstetric Anesthesia Committee Seminar on Obstetric Anesthesia Coverage*, Magee-Women's Hospital, Pittsburgh, PA, June 10, 1966. Carolyn Leonard Carson offers statistics from an unnamed hospital showing how few black patients received obstetric anesthesia compared to white patients. Carolyn Leonard Carson, "And the Results Showed Promise . . . Physicians, Childbirth, and Southern Black Migrant Women, 1916–1930: Pittsburgh as a Case Study," in *Women and Health in America,* ed. Judith Walzer Leavitt (University of Wisconsin Press, 1999), 363.

88. Nicholson J. Eastman, "Fetal Blood Studies: The Role of Anesthesia in the Production of Asphyxia Neonatorum," *American Journal of Obstetrics and Gynecology* 31 (1936): 563–72; Curtis J. Lund, "The Relation of Inhalation Analgesia and Anesthesia to Asphyxia Neonatorum," *American Journal of Obstetrics and Gynecology* 43 (March 1942): 375; quote in Harold Henderson, Bruce Foster, and L. S. Eno, "The Relative Effect of Analgesia and Anesthesia in the Production of Asphyxia Neonatorum," *American Journal of Obstetrics and Gynecology* 41 (1941): 605. For examples of articles that effectively dismissed side effects in newborns, see Mathia F. F. Kohl, "Intravenous Vinbarbital Sodium for Obstetric Analgesia," *American Journal of Obstetrics and Gynecology* 56 (1948): 811–14; Jacob Kotz and Morton S. Kaufman, "The Effects of Ob-

stetric Analgesia on the Newborn Infant," *Journal of the American Medical Association* 113 (December 2, 1939): 2035–38.

89. Henderson, Foster, and Eno, "The Relative Effect of Analgesia and Anesthesia," 596–606; McCormick, "The Effects of Analgesia on the Newborn Infant," "what percentage" at 400; "all the obstetricians" quote from Karen Dolby, interview by Regina Morantz, April 1, 1978, Medical College of Pennsylvania Oral History Collection on Women in Medicine, Schlesinger Library, Radcliffe College, Cambridge, MA; Daniel D. Backner, Francis F. Foldes, and Elizabeth H. Gordon, "The Combined Use of Alphaprodine (Nisentil) Hydrochloride and Levallorphan (Lorfan) Tartrate for Analgesia in Obstetrics," *American Journal of Obstetrics and Gynecology* 74 (August 1957): 271–82; retired obstetrician, interview by author, tape recording, July 12, 1996, Winnetka, IL.

90. Retired obstetrician, interview by author, tape recording, June 29, 2006, Glenview, IL.

91. Virginia Apgar, "A Proposal for a New Method of Evaluation of the Newborn Infant," *Current Researches in Anesthesia and Analgesia* 32 (July–August 1953): 260–67; Virginia Apgar, Duncan A. Holaday, L. Stanley James, and Irvin M. Weisbrot, "Evaluation of the Newborn Infant—Second Report," *Journal of the American Medical Association* 168 (December 13, 1958): 1985–88; J. S. Drage, C. Kennedy, and B. K. Schwarz, "The Apgar Score as an Index of Neonatal Mortality," *Obstetrics and Gynecology* 24 (August 1964): 222–30; *Apgar on Apgar*, part of the training film series *Pediatric Basics*, undated, ca. 1950s, produced with a grant from Gerber Baby Foods, available at Wood Library, film archives, American Society of Anesthesiologists. Short biographies of Virginia Apgar's life and work are James, "Fond Memories of Virginia Apgar," 1–4; and Selma Harrison Calmes, "Virginia Apgar: A Woman Physician's Career in a Developing Specialty," *Journal of the American Medical Women's Association* 39 (November–December 1984): 184–88. While Apgar was the first American physician to prove that drugs received by the mother during labor cross the placenta, Swiss physician Paul Zweifel offered irreconcilable proof of this phenomenon in 1877 with chloroform. See Donald Caton, *What a Blessing She Had Chloroform: The Medical and Social Response to the Pain of Childbirth from 1800 to the Present* (Yale University Press, 1999), 78–79. Apgar offered her proof first with Demerol and later with cyclopropane. See Virginia Apgar, J. J. Burns, Bernard B. Brodie, and E. M. Papper, "The Transmission of Meperidine across the Human Placenta," *American Journal of Obstetrics and Gynecology* 64 (December 1952): 1368–70; Virginia Apgar, Duncan A. Holaday, Stanley James, C. Edward Prince, and Irwin M. Weisbrot, "Comparison of Regional and General Anesthesia in Obstetrics," *Journal of the American Medical Association* 165 (December 28, 1957): 2155–61. Today, calculating and recording one- and five-minute Apgar Scores continue to be a routine culmination of births around the world. The scores have proved to be reliable predictors not only of neuromuscular deficit at ages two and three but also of whether a newborn will survive.

92. John W. Scanlon, "Perinatal Pharmacology and Evaluation of the Newborn," *International Anesthesiology Clinics* 11 (Summer 1973): 163–74; Esther Conway and

Yvonne Brackbill, "Delivery Medication and Infant Outcome: An Empirical Study," *Monographs of the Society for Research in Child Development* 35 (June 1970): 24–34, quote at 24.

93. Bailey Patterson Sweeny Diary, November 2, 1933, entry, Schlesinger Library. Sweeny lived for almost sixty more years; she died in 1992 at age eighty-two.

94. Dorothy Smith Dushkin Diary, March 31, 1940, entry, Dorothy Smith Dushkin Papers.

95. DeLee often used the phrase "modern advances" when discussing progress in obstetrics. See, for example, *The Chicago Lying-In Hospital and Dispensary Twentieth Report,* July 1, 1926, to June 30, 1930, p. 3, Northwestern Memorial Hospital Archives. Dorothy Smith Dushkin Diary, October 8, 1932, entry, Dorothy Smith Dushkin Papers.

Chapter 4 · Giving Birth to the Baby Boomers

1. Alice Munro Isaacs, "Saddle Block and Forceps," in *Birth Stories: The Experience Remembered,* ed. Janet Isaacs Ashford (Crossing Press, 1984), 24–28.

2. Linda Gordon, *Woman's Body, Woman's Right: Birth Control in America* (Penguin Books, 1990), 150; and Elaine Tyler May, *Homeward Bound: American Families in the Cold War Era* (Basic Books, 1999), xii–xv, 120–21. The figures from 1800, 1880, and 1900 are the reproductive rate of white women of childbearing age; those for 1930 and the 1950s are the reproductive rate of all women of childbearing age.

3. May, *Homeward Bound,* 120–21.

4. Ibid. May writes, "The postwar consensus was nowhere more evident than in the matter of having children."

5. Irvine Loudon, *Death in Childbirth* (Oxford University Press, 1992), 366.

6. Esther Bridgman Clark, interview by Regina Morantz, December 18, 1977, Medical College of Pennsylvania Oral History Collection on Women in Medicine, Schlesinger Library, Radcliffe College, Cambridge, MA. For more on how penicillin contributed to attitudes toward modern medicine, see Eric Lax, *The Mold in Dr. Florey's Coat: The Story of the Penicillin Miracle* (Henry Holt, 2004). See also Nancy Tomes, *The Gospel of Germs: Men, Women, and the Microbe in American Life* (Harvard University Press, 1998), 252–55.

7. Paul Starr, *The Social Transformation of American Medicine: The Rise of a Sovereign Profession and the Making of a Vast Industry* (Basic Books, 1982), 79–144, quote at 127.

8. Arthur H. Bill, "The Newer Obstetrics," *American Journal of Obstetrics and Gynecology* 23 (February 1932): 155–64, quote at 160–61.

9. Bailey Patterson Sweeny Diary, December 11, 1933, entry, Schlesinger Library.

10. "I Had a Baby, Too: A Symposium," *Atlantic Monthly,* June 1939, 766–67.

11. Stork Club Fathers' Book, March 15, 1949, and February 9, 1950, entries, Northwestern Memorial Hospital Archives, Chicago.

12. James R. Bloss, "The Ideals, Responsibilities, and Reward of the Obstetrician," *American Journal of Obstetrics and Gynecology* 59 (June 1950): 1183–88, quote at 1187.

13. Mr. and Mrs. A. P. Albrecht, Los Angeles, to Dr. John Adriani, July 6, 1946, telegram; Mrs. Elmo Collins Jr., Gainesville, FL, to Dear Sirs, July 1946; Mrs. R. McDonald, Detroit, MI, to Adriani, October 13, 1946; Mrs. Andrew Moore, Stockton, CA, to Adriani, November 21, 1946; Mrs. T. K. Kelly, Biloxi, MS, to Adriani, July 1946; Adriani to Mrs. Thomas K. Kelly, Biloxi, MS, July 29, 1946; James G. Smith, Shuler-Womack Clinic, Carlsbad, NM, to Obstetrical Department, Charity Hospital, New Orleans, LA, June 30, 1946; P. Woodward, MD, Bryan, TX, to Adriani, August 13, 1946, John Adriani Papers, 1925–88, National Library of Medicine, History of Medicine Division, Bethesda, MD.

14. Quote from a mother, interview by author, tape recording, October 29, 2005, Northfield, IL. The number of requisite prenatal visits in the United States has remained static since the 1940s and contrasts with the number of visits in European countries with lower infant mortality rates: Danish women on average have 8 prenatal visits, French women 6, German women 9, and Swiss women 5. See Thomas H. Strong, *Expecting Trouble: The Myth of Prenatal Care in America* (New York University Press, 2000), 6–7. Breast cancer treatment is another example of paternalism in women's medicine. What today are five separate steps in the diagnosis and treatment of breast cancer (biopsy, diagnosis, discussion of treatment options with the patient, choosing an appropriate treatment, and finally treatment) used to be one step, performed wholly at the discretion of the physician immediately after the biopsy, while the patient was anesthetized. For a history of breast cancer treatment, see Ellen Leopold, *A Darker Ribbon: Breast Cancer, Women, and Their Doctors in the Twentieth Century* (Beacon Press, 1999); and Barron H. Lerner, *The Breast Cancer Wars: Hope, Fear, and the Pursuit of a Cure in Twentieth-Century America* (Oxford University Press, 2001).

15. Bailey Patterson Sweeny Diary, May 3, 1933, entry, Schlesinger Library.

16. Only three states, Connecticut, Illinois, and Massachusetts, refused Sheppard-Towner funds. For more on the implementation and effect of the Sheppard-Towner Act, see Kriste Lindenmeyer, *"A Right to Childhood": The U.S. Children's Bureau and Child Welfare, 1912–46* (University of Illinois Press, 1997), 76–108; Molly Ladd-Taylor, "'Grannies' and 'Spinsters': Midwife Education under the Sheppard-Towner Act," *Journal of Social History* 22 (Winter 1988): 255–75; Molly Ladd-Taylor, "'My Work Came out of My Agony and Grief': Mothers and the Making of the Sheppard-Towner Act," in *Mothers of a New World: Maternalist Politics and the Origins of Welfare States,* ed. Seth Koven and Sonya Michel (Routledge, 1993), 321–42; Molly Ladd-Taylor, *Mother-Work: Women, Child Welfare, and the State, 1890–1930* (University of Illinois Press, 1994), 167–90.

17. "Close of the EMIC Program," *American Journal of Public Health* 39 (December 1949): 1579–81; Lindenmeyer, *"A Right to Childhood,"* 237–47.

18. Constance J. Foster, "New Techniques in Childbirth," *Parents Magazine* 15 (May 1940): 24–25, 41, 83–84. For a timeline of pregnancy testing development, see *A Thin Blue Line: The History of the Pregnancy Test Kit,* at the Office of National Institute of Health History Web site, http://history.nih.gov/exhibits/thinblueline/timeline.html. Sarah A. Leavitt points out in her article "'A Private Little Revolution': The

Home Pregnancy Test in American Culture," *Bulletin of the History of Medicine* 80 (Summer 2006): 317–45 that the home pregnancy test, first marketed in the late 1970s, "is an example of the reversing of the medicalization of pregnancy." The test returned to women a diagnosis that had earlier been in women's hands. Definition of obstetrics in Maude M. Gerdes, "Newer Concepts and Procedures of Maternal Care," *American Journal of Public Health* 29 (September 1939): 1029–33, quote at 1029.

19. John C. Donovan, "Some Psychosomatic Aspects of Obstetrics and Gynecology," *American Journal of Obstetrics and Gynecology* 75 (January 1958): 72–81, quotes at 76 and 75.

20. Advertisement for Dexedrine, *Obstetrics and Gynecology* 15 (1960). Advertisement for Equanil, *Obstetrics and Gynecology* 15 (1960). For more on the postwar penchant for controlling mood through medication, see Andrea Tone and Elizabeth Siegel Watkins, eds., *Medicating Modern America: Prescription Drugs in History* (New York University Press, 2007), particularly the chapters by David Healy ("Folie to Folly: The Modern Mania for Bipolar Disorders and Mood Stabilizers," 42–62), Ilina Singh ("Not Just Naughty: 50 Years of Stimulant Drug Advertising," 131–55), and Andrea Tone ("Tranquilizers on Trial: Psychopharmacology in the Age of Anxiety," 156–81).

21. Stork Club Fathers' Book 1, 1949–1950, August 21, 1950, entry, Northwestern Memorial Hospital Archives; William G. Cullen and Harold R. Griffith, "Postpartum Results of Spinal Anesthesia in Obstetrics," *Anesthesia and Analgesia* 26 (May–June 1947): 114–21.

22. Retired obstetrician, interview by author, tape recording, July 19, 2004, Winnetka, IL.

23. Mary Thomas, ed., *Post-War Mothers: Childbirth Letters to Grantly Dick-Read, 1946–1956* (University of Rochester Press, 1997), 190.

24. Howard S. Becker, Everett C. Hughes, Blanche Geer, and Anselm L. Strauss, *Boys in White: Student Culture in Medical School* (University of Chicago Press, 1961), 337.

25. Robert A. Hingson, "The Control of Pain and Fear in the Management of Labor and Delivery," *Surgical Clinics of North America* 25 (December 1945): 1352–81.

26. For examples of doctors' contending that analgesia elicited women's cooperation, see Celso Ramon Garcia, Richard Waltman, and Samuel Lubin, "Continuous Intravenous Infusion of Demerol in Labor," *American Journal of Obstetrics and Gynecology* 66 (1953): 312–18; Marion E. Black, "Psychorelaxation Management for Labor and Delivery," *Clinical Obstetrics and Gynecology* 4 (March 1961): 108–16, quote at 110.

27. William M. Kane, "The Results of Nisentil in 1,000 Obstetrical Cases," *American Journal of Obstetrics and Gynecology* 65 (1953): 1020–26; John P. Emich, "Nisentil—An Obstetric Analgesic," *American Journal of Obstetrics and Gynecology* 69 (1955): 124–27; Daniel D. Backner, Francis F. Foldes, and Elizabeth H. Gordon, "The Combined Use of Alphaprodine (Nisentil) Hydrochloride and Levallorphan (Lorfan) Tartrate for Analgesia in Obstetrics," *American Journal of Obstetrics and Gynecology* 74 (August 1957): 271–82; "nice 'n still" in Robbie E. Davis-Floyd, *Birth as an American Rite of Passage* (University of California Press, 1992), 102.

28. Garcia, Waltman, and Lubin, "Continuous Intravenous Infusion of Demerol in Labor," 312–18, "fairly quiet" at 316; Backner, Foldes, and Gordon, "The Combined

Use," 271–82; Robert O. Olson, H. L. Riva, "Evaluation of Phenazocine with Meperidine as an Analgesic Agent during Labor, by the Double Blind Method," *American Journal of Obstetrics and Gynecology* 88 (1964): 601–5, "produced" at 604.

29. Mothers, interviews by author, tape recordings, July 17, 2004, Chicago; October 29, 2005, Northfield, IL; and November 1, 2005, Glencoe, IL; Arthur J. Mandy, Theodore E. Mandy, Robert Farkas, and Ernest Scher, "Is Natural Childbirth Natural?" *Psychosomatic Medicine* 14 (November 1958): 431–38, quote at 432.

30. Joseph B. DeLee, *Principles and Practice of Obstetrics* (W. B. Saunders, 1918), 652, 666–68, 675–96; Nicholson J. Eastman, *Williams Obstetrics* (Appleton-Century-Crofts, 1950), 778–85.

31. Friedman originally revealed his curve in E. A. Friedman, "Primigravid Labor: A Graphicostatistical Analysis," *Obstetrics and Gynecology* 6 (1955): 567–89. Some now criticize the curve as "too stringent." One study indicates a substantially slower active phase of cervical dilation—5.5 hours from four to ten centimeters (with more than 2 hours of no perceivable change in cervical dilation not uncommon)—instead of Friedman's 2.5 hours. See Jun Zhang, James F. Troendle, and Michael K. Yancey, "Reassessing the Labor Curve in Nulliparous Women," *American Journal of Obstetrics and Gynecology* 187 (October 2002): 824–28. Friedman quoted in Davis-Floyd, *Birth as an American Rite of Passage*, 269–70.

32. Diane J. Macunovich, *Birth Quake: The Baby Boom and Its Aftershocks* (University of Chicago Press, 2002), 63.

33. For more on the history of efficiency, see Jennifer Karns Alexander, *The Mantra of Efficiency: From Waterwheel to Social Control* (Johns Hopkins University Press, 2008).

34. Daniel A. Wren and Ronald G. Greenwood, *Management Innovators: The People and Ideas That Have Shaped Modern Business* (Oxford University Press, 1998), 134–48, quote at 146.

35. Jno. G. Metcalf, "Obstetrical Statistics," handwritten notes, May 7, 1838, Union Medical Association Papers, University of Massachusetts Medical School Library, Worcester, MA; Julius Levy, "Maternal Mortality and Mortality in the First Month of Life in Relation to Attendant at Birth," *American Journal of Public Health* 13 (February 1923): 88–95.

36. Bruce Gould and Beatrice Blackmar Gould, "A Country Doctor Writes a Letter," *Ladies' Home Journal*, May 1937, 4.

37. Lyman Niles, "Right Up from Childbirth," *Parents Magazine*, February 1947, 22–23, 138.

38. Retired obstetrician, interview by author, July 12, 1996, Winnetka. IL.

39. Retired obstetrician, interview by author, tape recording, July 19, 2004, Chicago.

40. Peter Y. Sussman, ed., *Decca: The Letters of Jessica Mitford* (Alfred A. Knopf, 2006), 126–27.

41. J. B. DeLee, "The Prophylactic Forceps Operation," *American Journal of Obstetrics and Gynecology* 1 (October 1920): 34–44.

42. "Discussion," *American Journal of Obstetrics and Gynecology* 1 (1920): 77–80.

DeLee eventually regretted some of the practices he fostered. Shortly before his death in 1942, he assured a lay audience that 95% of pregnancies required "only good obstetric treatment," which he defined simply as prenatal care, treatment of complications before they endangered mother or baby, aseptic practice, and the presence of a skilled physician who did not attempt to "streamline" birth. He told his lay listeners: "Mother nature's methods of bringing babies are still the best." J. B. DeLee, Mother's Day Address, May 12, 1940, Joseph B. DeLee, MD, Papers, Northwestern Memorial Hospital Archives.

43. William F. Mengert, "Obstetrics and Gynecology Today: President's Address," *American Journal of Obstetrics and Gynecology* 77 (April 1959): 697–705; "The Doctor Talks about Babies by Appointment," *McCall's*, January 1957, 4, 81.

44. Foster, "New Techniques in Childbirth," "muscles continue" at 41, "I'd much rather" at 83–84.

45. George H. Ryder, "Some Observations on Nitrous Oxide Gas as an Analgesic in Labor, with Report of 135 Cases," *American Journal of Obstetrics and Diseases of Women and Children* 75 (1917): 981–88.

46. Joseph B. DeLee, "The Use of Solution of Posterior Pituitary in Modern Obstetrics," *Journal of the American Medical Association* 115 (October 19, 1940): 1320–26; Charles B. Reed, "The Induction of Labor at Term," *American Journal of Obstetrics and Gynecology* 1 (1920): 24–33.

47. Richard C. Norris, "The Ultimate Results of Induced labor for Minor Degrees of Pelvic Contractions," *American Journal of Obstetrics and Diseases of Women and Children* 50 (September 1904): 289–301; J. Whitridge Williams, *Obstetrics: A Text-Book for the Use of Students and Practitioners* (D. Appleton, 1904), 341–49; and J. Whitridge Williams, *Obstetrics: A Text-Book for the Use of Students and Practitioners* (D. Appleton, 1909), 377–82; Clifford R. Taylor, "The Intrauterine Bougie and Voorhees Bag Today," *American Journal of Obstetrics and Gynecology* 76 (September 1958): 553–57.

48. Katherine Shedd Bradley Diaries, Diary 1918–22, March 31, 1920, to April 30, 1920, entries, Newberry Library Special Collections, Chicago. The doctor told Bradley that David, unlike her first child, had to be breastfed because he did not have the strength to survive the inherent dangers of artificial feeding. In ensuing days, Bradley marveled at how her tiny son thrived on breast milk; she methodically recorded his steady weight gain in her diary.

49. Reed, "The Induction of Labor at Term," 24–33; Foster, "New Techniques in Childbirth," 24–25, 41, 83–84, "have to huff" at 25. This new theory likely caused numerous tragedies. Chicago doctor Rudolph W. Holmes recalled one woman who was about to be induced because her baby was "over large." Holmes intervened and urged her to continue the pregnancy. Almost three months later she gave birth spontaneously. Holmes warned that if induction for "postmaturity" became the norm, similar miscalculations would be common. "Discussion on Papers of Drs. Watson and Reed," *American Journal of Obstetrics and Gynecology* 1 (1920): 72–76.

50. DeLee, "The Use of Solution of Posterior Pituitary," 1320–24. Just how many physicians embraced elective induction in the 1930s is unclear, but one study published in 1939 found that a comparatively small number of physicians were probably responsible for the majority of the nation's elective inductions. R. S. Cron, L. M. Ran-

dall, N. R. Kretzschmar, "A Report of the Committee on the Induction of Labor," *American Journal of Obstetrics and Gynecology* 37 (1939): 873–77.

51. Retired obstetrician, interview by author, tape recording, June 29, 2006, Glenview, IL; retired obstetrician, interview by author, tape recording, July 19, 2004, Chicago.

52. "Abstract of Discussion on Papers of Drs. Sharkey, Pendleton, and DeLee," *Journal of the American Medical Association* 115 (October 19, 1940): 1324–26.

53. J. P. McEvoy, "Our Streamlined Baby," *Reader's Digest*, May 1938, 15–18.

54. "Birth by Appointment," *Newsweek*, July 20, 1970, 87.

55. By 1949 doctors reported seeing a marked rise in inductions. Edwin L. Hukill, "Elective Induction of Labor Using Pituitrin," *American Journal of Obstetrics and Gynecology* 70 (1955): 972–82. The rate varied by region; in 1957 Dr. J. Edward Hall of the State University of New York found that 10% of American babies were being delivered by appointment, although the practice was far more predominant than that in certain areas. See "Babies by Appointment Bring Many Conveniences," *Science Digest*, June 1957, 52; Charles Ronald Straghan MacKenzie, "Induction of Labor," *American Journal of Obstetrics and Gynecology* 68 (1954): 981–87.

56. Edward L. Cornell, "Objections to Induction of Labor in Normal Pregnant Women," *American Journal of Obstetrics and Gynecology* 41 (1941): 438–42; J. Robert Willson, "Elective Induction of Labor: Is It Justifiable in Normally Pregnant Women," *American Journal of Obstetrics and Gynecology* 65 (April 1953): 848–58, "some patients" at 855–56.

57. Robert Landesman, "New Promise of Easier Childbirth," *Woman's Home Companion*, August 1955, 38–39.

58. Stork Club Fathers' Book, June 12, 1950-January 9, 1953, January 27, 1951, entry, Northwestern Memorial Hospital Archives.

59. R. M. Grier, "Elective Induction of Labor," *American Journal of Obstetrics and Gynecology* 54 (1947): 511–16, quotes at 512.

60. John Adriani, MD, to Irene Evans, RN, May 6, 1970, John Adriani Papers, 1925–88, National Library of Medicine, History of Medicine Division; M. J. Wizenberg, I. A. Siegel, W. Korman, and H. N. Rosenthal, "The Use of Anileridine in Labor for the Control of Pain," *American Journal of Obstetrics and Gynecology* 78 (August 1959): 405–10; Bert B. Hershenson, Claude H. Koons, and Duncan E. Reid, "Chlorpromazine as a Sedative in Labor," *American Journal of Obstetrics and Gynecology* 72 (November 1956): 1007–14.

61. Isidore Daichman, George Kornfeld, and Martin M. Shir, "Obstetric Analgesia: A Comparative Study of Sodium Amytal, Sodium Amytal and Scopolamine, Gwathmey (ether in oil), and Avertin," *American Journal of Obstetrics and Gynecology* 28 (1934): 101–6, quote at 102; E. D. Colvin and R. A. Bartholomew, "Improvements in the Paraldehyde Method of Relief of Pain in Labor," *American Journal of Obstetrics and Gynecology* 35 (1938): 589–97.

62. Charles Iverson Bryans Jr. and Charles McL. Mulherin, "The Use of Chlorpromazine in Obstetrical Analgesia," *American Journal of Obstetrics and Gynecology* 77 (February 1959): 406–11, "maniacal excitement" at 406; Hershenson, Koons, and Reid, "Chlorpromazine as a Sedative in Labor," 1007–14, "various states" at 1007; advertise-

ments for Thorazine, *Obstetrics and Gynecology* 10 (1957); 15 (1960), "one of the fundamental" in the 1960 ad.

63. Mary Karp, Verner E. Lamb, and Harry B. W. Benaron, "The Use of Chlorpromazine in the Obstetric Patient: A Preliminary Report," *American Journal of Obstetrics and Gynecology* 69 (1955): 780–85, quotes at 785 and 783. R. Caldeyro-Barcia, J. J. Poseiro, H. Alvarez, and P. Tost, "The Action of Chlorpromazine on Uterine Contractility and Arterial Pressure in Normal and Toxemic Pregnant Women," *American Journal of Obstetrics and Gynecology* 75 (May 1958): 1088–95; Bryans and Mulherin, "The Use of Chlorpromazine in Obstetrical Analgesia"; Harry I. Norton, Maxwell Weingarten, and Edward T. McDonough, "The Use of Chlorpromazine in Obstetrical Sedation," *American Journal of Obstetrics and Gynecology* 71 (1956): 1251–57; Jack D. Pressman, *Last Resort: Psychosurgery and the Limits of Medicine* (Cambridge University Press, 1998), 401.

64. Retired obstetrician, interview by author, tape recording, July 19, 2004, Chicago; Virginia Apgar, "Anesthesia for Vaginal Delivery," *Journal of the American Medical Women's Association* 11 (March 1956): 83–86, "for apprehension" at 83; Gordon Gilbert and Alfred B. Dinon, "Observations on Demerol as an Obstetric Analgesic," *American Journal of Obstetrics and Gynecology* 45 (1943): 320–26; E. Stewart Taylor and William W. Jack, "A Critical Analysis of Local Anesthesia as an Agent for the Relief of Pain in Vaginal Delivery," *American Journal of Obstetrics and Gynecology* 58 (1949): 281.

65. Retired obstetrician, interview by author, tape recording, July 19, 2004, Chicago.

66. Richard L. Miller, "An Analysis of Generalists' Obstetrics," *American Journal of Obstetrics and Gynecology* 80 (October 1960): 813–22, quotes at 815–16. The routine use of multiple drugs during labor, particularly in urban areas, was in place early in the baby boom. Thus neither Medicaid (instituted in 1965) nor employer-funded insurance coverage of maternity care seems to have had much impact on this particular use of obstetric analgesia and anesthesia. Although laws governing health insurance have always varied from state to state, before the early 1960s pregnancy was considered a voluntary condition not automatically covered by health insurance. The American Society of Anesthesiologists did not even issue its first guide for relative costs of obstetric anesthesia for insurance company usage until 1962. *ASA Relative Value Guide* (American Society of Anesthesiologists, 1962). Not until 1978 did the U.S. Congress pass the Pregnancy Discrimination Act, requiring all employers in all states to cover maternity care as they would any other medical condition if they offered health insurance to their employees. Yet even this legislation had loopholes leaving many women without maternity coverage: it did not apply to individually purchased policies; it did not apply to employers with fifteen or fewer employees; and it covered only the employee and spouse, not pregnant teenage daughters. Rachel Benson Gold, Asta M. Kenney, and Susheela Singh, "Paying for Maternity Care in the United States," *Family Planning Perspectives* 19 (September–October 1987): 190–93, 195–206.

67. Lawrence E. Gordon and Clarence L. Ruffin, "Promethazine as an Adjunct to Obstetrical Analgesia and Sedation," *American Journal of Obstetrics and Gynecology* 76 (July 1958): 147–51, quote at 147.

68. Ibid.

69. Hingson, "The Control of Pain and Fear," 1352–81, quote at 1355–57; Bloss, "The Ideals, Responsibilities, and Reward," 1183–88, "Carefully trained" at 1184–85; Black, "Psychorelaxation Management," 108–16, "offered confidence" at 110.

70. Philip C. Williams and Tanner B. McMahon, "Intravenous Pitocin Infusion in Obstetrics," *American Journal of Obstetrics and Gynecology* 71 (1956): 1264–73, "propelling" at 1273; Bill Davidson, "The Case for and against Induced Labor," *Good Housekeeping*, January 1964, 58–59, 114–15, "a significant price" at 114.

71. "The Doctor Talks about Babies by Appointment," 4, 81; "Childbirth: When Labor Is Induced," *Good Housekeeping*, September 1961, 147; "Babies by Appointment," 48–50.

72. Davidson, "The Case for and against Induced Labor," 58–59, 114–15. In 1964 obstetrician Edward H. Bishop mitigated much of the criticism of elective inductions when he invented a scoring system to judge when inducing labor was unlikely to result in iatrogenic prematurity. Bishop's system, similar to the Apgar Score, awarded 0 to 2 points for each of five cervical signs indicating preparedness for labor: dilation, effacement, station, consistency, and position. Edward H. Bishop, "Pelvic Scoring for Elective Induction," *Obstetrics and Gynecology* 24 (August 1964): 266–68.

73. C. H. Peckham and R. W. King, "Study of Intercurrent Conditions Observed during Pregnancy," *American Journal of Obstetrics and Gynecology* 87 (November 1, 1963): 609–20. For more on the history of thalidomide and its effect on attitudes toward medicine, see Rock Brynner and Trent Stephens, *Dark Remedy: The Impact of Thalidomide and Its Revival as a Vital Medicine* (Perseus, 2001).

74. Virginia Apgar, "Drugs in Pregnancy," *Journal of the American Medical Association* 190 (November 30, 1964): 840–41.

75. See, for example, arguably the most influential article of that era to charge "inhumane" treatment, Gladys Denny Shultz, "*Journal* Mothers Report on Cruelty in Maternity Wards," *Ladies' Home Journal*, May 1958, 44–45, 152–55.

76. William A. Nolen, "Induced Labor: When Is It a Good Idea?" *McCall's*, July 1971, 24–25.

77. Eastman, *Williams Obstetrics*, 410; Barbara Katz Rothman, *In Labor: Women and Power in the Birthplace* (W. W. Norton, 1991), 277.

78. Lena H. Fletcher to Dr. Joseph DeLee, Forks, WA, October 21, 1938, Joseph B. DeLee Papers, Northwestern Memorial Hospital Archives; Constance L. Todd, *Easier Motherhood: A Discussion of the Abolition of Needless Pain* (John Day, 1931), 107.

79. Sussman, *Decca*, 69–73.

80. Davis-Floyd, *Birth as an American Rite of Passage*, 268.

Chapter 5 · Natural Childbirth and Birth Reform

1. Ina May Gaskin, *Babies, Breastfeeding, and Bonding* (Bergin and Garvey, 1987), 16–19.

2. Ina May Gaskin, *Spiritual Midwifery* (Book Publishing, 1980), 8–23.

3. See, for example, Lenore Pelham Friedrich, "I Had a Baby," *Atlantic Monthly*, April 1939, 461–65. Articles critical of obstetric practice became increasingly numer-

ous in the 1940s and 1950s, long before mainstream medicine acknowledged that natural childbirth and demand for birth reform were potent forces. These articles include "I Had My Baby without an Anesthetic," *Parents Magazine*, January 1948, 18–19, 86; Gretta Palmer, "Having Your Baby the New Way," *Collier's*, November 13, 1948, 26–27, 61; Morton Sontheimer, "Miracle in the Delivery Room," *Woman's Home Companion*, December 1948, 4, 164; Betsy Marvin McKinney, "The Pleasure of Childbirth," *Ladies' Home Journal*, April 1949, 116, 118–21; "Painless Childbirth at Yale," *Newsweek*, November 7, 1949, 51; "Natural Childbirth," *Life*, January 30, 1950, 71–77; ·Dorothy Barclay, "'Natural Childbirth': A Progress Report," *New York Times Magazine*, July 29, 1950, 34; Nicholson J. Eastman, "The Middle Road in Obstetrics," *Ladies' Home Journal*, May 1952, 11, 91; "Natural or Unnatural?" *Time*, January 19, 1953, 52–53; Jack Harrison Pollack, "The Case for Natural Childbirth," *Cosmopolitan*, July 1953, 38–43; "Painless Childbirth," *Look*, May 1, 1956, 74; Jennette H. Fernn, "Training for Childbirth: Mothers Who've Had Babies by Natural Childbirth Almost Always Say That's the Way They'd Do It Again," *Today's Health*, September 1957, 36–38.

4. Joan Haggerty, "Childbirth Made Difficult," *Ms.*, January 1973, 16–17.

5. Gaskin, *Spiritual Midwifery*, 8–23, quotes at 11; A. Mark Durand, "The Safety of Home Birth: The Farm Study," *American Journal of Public Health* 82 (March 1992): 450–53. Gaskin was president of the influential Midwives Alliance of North America from 1996 through 2002. For more on Gaskin, see Katie Allison Granju, "The Midwife of Modern Midwifery," Salon.com (June 1, 1999), available at www.salon.com/people/bc/1999/06/01/gaskin/ (accessed May 31, 2008).

6. Laura E. Ettinger, "Mission to Mothers: Nuns, Latino Families, and the Founding of Santa Fe's Catholic Maternity Institute," in *Women, Health, and Nation: Canada and the United States since 1945*, ed. Georgina Feldberg, Molly Ladd-Taylor, Alison Li, and Kathryn McPherson (McGill–Queen's University Press, 2003), 144–60; Kaye Lowman, *The LLLove Story* (La Leche League International, 1978); Lynn Y. Weiner, "Reconstructing Motherhood: The La Leche League in Postwar America," *Journal of American History* 80 (March 1994): 1357–81.

7. Pope Pius XII, "Natural Painless Childbirth: Address of Pope Pius XII to a Group of Catholic Obstetricians and Gynecologists," *Pope Speaks*, January 8, 1956, 25–34, quotes at 34 and 33; Mary Louise Grossman, "Natural Childbirth Was Easy for Me," *Parents' Magazine*, January 1959, 36–37. The first childbirth preparation classes in the United States were held at Grace–New Haven Community Hospital in conjunction with the Yale University School of Medicine. For more information on that program, see Herbert Thoms, *Training for Childbirth: A Program of Natural Childbirth with Rooming-in* (McGraw-Hill, 1950); Herbert Thoms and Robert H. Wyatt, "A Natural Childbirth Program," *American Journal of Public Health* 40 (July 1950): 787–91; and Herbert Thoms and Robert H. Wyatt, "One Thousand Consecutive Deliveries under a Training for Childbirth Program," *American Journal of Obstetrics and Gynecology* 61 (January 1951): 205–9.

8. Helen Wessel, *Natural Childbirth and the Christian Family* (Harper and Row, 1973), xiii–xx, quote at xx.

9. Stork Club Fathers' Book, May 5, 1949, entry, Northwestern Memorial Hospital Archives, Chicago.

10. "I Had My 3rd Baby without an Anesthetic," *Parents Magazine,* January 1948, 18–19, 86.

11. Pollack, "The Case for Natural Childbirth," 38–43, quote at 39.

12. Registered nurse, Chicago, "Sadism in Delivery Rooms?" *Ladies' Home Journal,* November 1957, 4.

13. Gladys Denny Shultz, "*Journal* Mothers Report on Cruelty in Maternity Wards," *Ladies' Home Journal,* May 1958, 44–45, 152–55.

14. Gladys Denny Shultz, "*Journal* Mothers Testify to Cruelty in Maternity Wards," *Ladies' Home Journal,* December 1958, 58–59, 135, 137–39.

15. For a description of the transformation of medical decision-making between 1966 and 1976 and an explanation of how lawyers, judges, legislators, academics, and patients became as integral to medical decisions as doctors, see David J. Rothman, *Strangers at the Bedside: A History of How Law and Bioethics Transformed Medical Decision Making* (Basic Books, 1991).

16. Jacqueline Juhl, "I Had This Baby under Hypnosis," *Better Homes and Gardens,* November 1959, 152B–155.

17. Shultz, "*Journal* Mothers Testify to Cruelty in Maternity Wards," 59. For overviews of developments in late-twentieth-century birth reform, see Margot Edwards and Mary Waldorf, *Reclaiming Birth: History and Heroines of American Childbirth Reform* (Crossing Press, 1984); and Joan J. Mathews and Kathleen Zadak, "The Alternative Birth Movement in the United States: History and Current Status," *Women and Health* 17 (1991): 39–56. Sandra Morgen discusses the broader women's health movement in *Into Our Own Hands: The Women's Health Movement in the United States, 1969–1990* (Rutgers University Press, 2002).

18. William F. Mengert, "Obstetrics and Gynecology Today: President's Address," *American Journal of Obstetrics and Gynecology* 77 (April 1959): 697–705, quote at 699; Shultz, "*Journal* Mothers Testify to Cruelty in Maternity Wards," quotes at 59.

19. Boston Women's Health Book Collective, *Our Bodies, Ourselves: A Book by and for Women* (Simon and Schuster, 1976), 11; Morgen, *Into Our Own Hands,* 5–6, 31–35. For a complete history of the Chicago Women's Liberation Union's abortion collective, see Laura Kaplan, *The Story of Jane* (Pantheon Books, 1995).

20. Boston Women's Health Book Collective, *Our Bodies, Ourselves,* 267, 269. The mainstream medical community did not become aware of the Farm's successes until the 1990s, when an article in the *American Journal of Public Health* compared almost two thousand home births at the Farm with like hospital births. The cesarean section rate at the Farm was 1.46% versus 16.46% in the hospital. Only 2.11% of births at the Farm were assisted deliveries—that is, forceps or vacuum-extraction births—versus 26.60% of hospital births. Yet despite the lack of conventional medical treatment, the article's authors found no differences in fetal and neonatal mortality or five-minute Apgar Scores at the Farm's home births compared to similar hospital births. Durand, "The Safety of Home Birth," 450–53.

21. Barbara Frankel, *Childbirth in the Ghetto: Folk Beliefs of Negro Women in a North Philadelphia Hospital Ward* (R and E Research Associates, 1977), 66–68.

22. Margaret Charles Smith and Linda Janet Holmes, *Listen to Me Good: The Life Story of an Alabama Midwife* (Ohio State University Press, 1996), 1–2, 90.

23. Archie Brodsky, "Midwifery, Public Health, and Infant Mortality," *MANA News* 4 (May 1987): 1–3, Midwives Alliance of North America Records, 1973–97, Sophia Smith Collection, Neilson Library, Smith College, Northampton, MA. An interview with Shafia Monroe is in Penfield Chester, *Sisters on a Journey: Portraits of American Midwives* (Rutgers University Press, 1997), 195–98.

24. Boston Women's Health Book Collective, *Our Bodies, Ourselves*, 11, 267, 271, 278–82.

25. Articles appeared in many magazines during this era about the benefit and safety of home birth. See, for example, M. F. Ashley Montagu, "Babies Should Be Born at Home!" *Ladies' Home Journal*, August 1955, 52–53, 81, 85; Joan Younger, "Our Baby Was Born at Home," *Ladies' Home Journal*, January 1960, 111–14, 116–17; "Home Delivery," *Newsweek*, May 10, 1971, 104; "Have the Baby at Home," *Changing Times*, July 1976, 16; Janet Gardner, "Having Your Baby at Home: A Clear-Headed Report to Help You Make Up Your Mind," *Glamour*, March 1979, 240–42, 244; Angela H. Kinamore, "Childbirth at Home: Doing It My Way," *Essence*, December 1981, 64–66.

26. Family physician, interview by author, tape recording, September 15, 2004, Athens, OH.

27. Ruth Watson Lubic and Eunice K. M. Ernst, "Psychological Analgesia (Natural Childbirth and Psychoprophylaxis)," *Clinics in Obstetrics and Gynecology* 2 (December 1975): 531–44.

28. Barbara H. Cane, "Home Birth in Perspective," Barbara H. Cane Papers, Schlesinger Library, Radcliffe College, Cambridge, MA; "Procedures for Birth Certificate," undated memo to Gail; "An Important Message from Birth Community Please Help, Subject: Lay Midwifery in Minnesota, August 17, 1988; Birth Community Inc. Board meeting minutes, January 13, 1983, all three in Birth Community Inc. Records, Minnesota Historical Society, St. Paul, MN.

29. Francie Hornstein, letter for WATCH (Women Acting Together to Combat Harassment) members from Feminist Women's Health Center, Los Angeles, July 23, 1977, Boston Association for Childbirth Education papers, Schlesinger Library.

30. "MOTHER Is an Organization to *Demand* Changes in the Hospital," undated, ca. 1970s; *Mothers Of the wHole Earth Revolt*, undated pamphlet, ca. 1970s, both in Women's Community Health Center papers, Schlesinger Library.

31. Willson recalls the burning of his book in J. Robert Willson, typed transcript of Presidential Address at Obstetrical Society of Philadelphia, February 12, 1981, J. Robert Willson Papers, National Library of Medicine, History of Medicine Division, Bethesda, MD. The offending chapter is in J. Robert Willson, Clayton T. Beecham, and Elsie Reid Carrington, *Obstetrics and Gynecology* (C. V. Mosby, 1971), 41. The chapter is heavily revised in subsequent editions of the text. See J. Robert Willson, Clayton T. Beecham, and Elsie Reid Carrington, *Obstetrics and Gynecology* (C. V. Mosby,

1975), 50–51; and J. Robert Willson and Elsie Reid Carrington, *Obstetrics and Gynecology* (C. V. Mosby, 1979), 50.

32. Jack A. Pritchard and Paul C. MacDonald, *Williams Obstetrics,* 15th ed. (Appleton-Century-Crofts, 1976), 940; Jack A. Pritchard and Paul C. MacDonald, *Williams Obstetrics,* 16th ed. (Appleton-Century-Crofts, 1980), 1116; Jack A. Pritchard, Paul C. MacDonald, and Norman F. Gant, *Williams Obstetrics,* 17th ed. (Appleton-Century-Crofts, 1985). I am very grateful to Vicki Elson, a childbirth educator in Northampton, MA, for alerting me to these extraordinary index entries and to Timothy Johnson, chair of the Department of Obstetrics and Gynecology at the University of Michigan and a friend of Jack Pritchard's, for disclosing to me the heretofore mysterious writer of these entries.

33. *The Psychoprophylactic Method of Prepared Childbirth (Lamaze): An Overview for Physicians and Medical Personnel,* pamphlet written by Westchester Chapter, 1974, Elisabeth Bing and Lamaze International Papers, Schlesinger Library; Gertie F. Marx, "Natural Childbirth: A Tempered View," *Birth Defects* 21 (1985): 205–8; Gaskin, *Spiritual Midwifery,* 19; "The sensation" in C. Lee Buxton, *A Study of Psychophysical Methods for Relief of Childbirth Pain* (W. B. Saunders, 1962), 38.

34. Barbara L. Kaiser and Irwin H. Kaiser, "The Challenge of the Women's Movement to American Gynecology," *American Journal of Obstetrics and Gynecology* 120 (November 1, 1974): 652–65, quotes at 652, 653.

35. Ibid., quotes at 663, 665.

36. Morgen, *Into Our Own Hands,* 124–26.

37. "Your Personalized Birth Plan," undated leaflet, The Maternity Center Birth Options List, St. Joseph's Hospital, St. Paul, MN, Birth Community Inc. Records, 1980–1991, Minnesota Historical Society.

38. Sol M. Shnider, "Tie Me Up! Tie Me Down! The Changing Styles of OB Anesthesia 1950–1990," Rovenstine Lecture, December 1990, videotape. A videotape of this lecture is housed at the Wood Library, American Society of Anesthesiologists, Park Ridge, IL. For more on the specific successes of birth reform, see Edwards and Waldorf, *Reclaiming Birth.* Yale University conducted the first rooming-in experiments in a U.S. hospital. See Herbert Thoms, Edith B. Jackson, Lyman M. Stowe, and Frederick W. Goodrich, "The Rooming-In Plan for Mothers and Infants," *American Journal of Obstetrics and Gynecology* 56 (1948): 707–11; Edith B. Jackson, "General Reactions of Mothers and Nurses to Rooming-In," *American Journal of Public Health* 38 (May 1948): 689–95; Edith B. Jackson, "Pediatric and Psychiatric Aspects of the Yale Rooming-In Project," *Connecticut State Medical Journal* 14 (1950): 616–21; Edith Jackson, "New Trends in Maternity Care," *American Journal of Nursing* 55 (May 1955): 584–87.

39. Grossman, "Natural Childbirth Was Easy for Me," 36–37; "Husband's Report on Wife's Delivery, 1947," Edith Banfield Jackson Papers, Schlesinger Library. A spate of articles appeared in the lay press around this time about the wonder of fathers seeing their children being born. See, for example, "A Father Sees His Child Born," *Life,* June 15, 1955, 133–38; Peter Browne, "I Saw My Son Born," *Readers' Digest,* November 1957, 61–64; Muriel and Robert W. Goldfarb, "We Shared Our Baby's Birth," *Ladies'*

Home Journal, December 1958, 140, 142; Robert Spero, "A Father Watches the Birth of His Son," *Redbook,* May 1965, 54, 114–16, 118, 121.

40. Grossman, "Natural Childbirth Was Easy for Me"; retired obstetrician, interview by author, tape recording, July 19, 2004, Chicago; Roy Petty, *Home Birth* (Domus Books, 1979), 102; retired obstetrician, interview by author, tape recording, July 1996, Winnetka, IL; Judith L. Sensibar, "Why We Chose Natural Childbirth," *Redbook,* January 1969, 22–23, 28.

41. Ina May Gaskin and Yvonne Thornton, interview by Ray Suarez, typewritten transcript, *Talk of the Nation,* National Public Radio, March 31, 1999.

42. See Jane Erikson, "New Focus on Women in Hospitals Here," *Arizona Daily Star,* January 3, 2006.

43. A woman describes her discovery of Grantly Dick-Read in Jean Fay Webster, "Something NEW in Childbirth: A Mother Who Has Tried Natural Childbirth Says She Would Never Have a Baby Any Other Way," *Parents' Magazine,* December 1949, 34–35. Women who gave birth in the 1950s also attested in oral history interviews to stumbling onto Dick-Read's books. A mother, interview by author, November 1, 2005, Glencoe, IL. Ina May Gaskin tells of discovering Dick-Read before the birth of her first child in 1966 in Gaskin, *Babies, Breastfeeding, and Bonding,* 16–19. Grantly Dick-Read, *Natural Childbirth* (William Heinemann [Medical Books], 1933), vii–viii, 16–24, 42–45.

44. Dick-Read, *Childbirth without Fear: The Principles and Practice of Natural Childbirth* (Harper, 1953), 6–7.

45. Charles D. Meigs, *Obstetrics: The Science and the Art* (Blanchard and Lear, 1856), 373; Dick-Read, *Childbirth without Fear,* 6–8, 12.

46. Milton J. E. Senn, "Let's Be Sensible about Natural Childbirth," *Woman's Home Companion,* May 1953, 30–31; Jan Ruby, Mary Taylor, Mary S. Foerster, and Mrs. Arnold Brawner, "We Had Our Babies without Fear," *Parents' Magazine,* June 1950, 38, 78, 80–83, "I realized" at 38.

47. Marjorie Karmel, *Thank You, Dr. Lamaze: A Mother's Experience in Painless Childbirth* (J. B. Lippincott, 1959), 13–20, quotes at 18 and 20.

48. Barclay, "Natural Childbirth," 34.

49. Donald Caton, *What a Blessing She Had Chloroform: The Medical and Social Response to the Pain of Childbirth from 1800 to the Present* (Yale University Press, 1999), 173; A. Noyes Thomas, *Doctor Courageous: The Story of Dr. Grantly Dick Read* (Harper, 1957); "magnetic and persuasive personality" in Buxton, *A Study of Psychophysical Methods for Relief of Childbirth Pain,* 36; Arthur J. Mandy, Theodore E. Mandy, Robert Farkas, and Ernest Scher, "Is Natural Childbirth Natural?" *Psychosomatic Medicine* 14 (November 1958): 431–38, "great personal charm" at 433; "patients" from retired obstetrician, interview by author, July 19, 2004, tape recording, Chicago.

50. Thomas, *Post-War Mothers,* 8–20.

51. Dick-Read, *Natural Childbirth,* 59.

52. Ibid., vii–viii, 16–24, 42–45, "eighteen, doctor" at 44.

53. Edmund Jacobson, *Progressive Relaxation: A Physiological and Clinical Investigation of Muscular States and Their Significance in Psychology and Medical Practice* (University of Chicago Press, 1929), 112–26.

54. Buxton, *A Study of Psychophysical Methods for Relief of Childbirth Pain*, 35; Helen Heardman, *A Way to Natural Childbirth: A Manual for Physiotherapists and Parents-to-Be* (E. and S. Livingstone, 1958); Helen Heardman, *Relaxation and Exercise for Natural Childbirth* (E. and S. Livingstone, 1960).

55. Fernand Lamaze, *Painless Childbirth: Psychoprophylactic Method* (Henry Regnery, 1970), 11–15.

56. Karmel, *Thank You, Dr. Lamaze*; Elisabeth Bing, *Six Practical Lessons for an Easier Childbirth* (Grosset and Dunlap, 1967); "Curriculum Vitae Elisabeth Bing," undated, ca. 1967; and Elisabeth D. Bing, "Thoughts on Prepared Childbirth," March 1973, typed manuscript, both in Elisabeth Bing and Lamaze International Papers, Schlesinger Library.

57. In the 1970s, *All in the Family* was one of the first television shows to feature the tenets of Lamaze when Gloria Stivic (played by Sally Struthers), the daughter of Archie Bunker (played by Carroll O'Connor), was pregnant with her first child.

58. Nora Ephron, "Having a Baby after 35," *New York Times*, November 26, 1978, SM17.

59. Sherwin B. Nuland, *The Wisdom of the Body* (Alfred A. Knopf, 1997), 192–94.

60. Susan McCutcheon-Rosegg and Peter Rosegg, *Natural Childbirth the Bradley Way* (E. P. Dutton, 1984), x, 7–13; Maude Longwell, "The Happiest Way to Have a Baby," *Farm Journal*, May 1966, 84–85, 107.

61. "NATURAL CHILDBIRTH" in *The Psychoprophylactic Method of Prepared Childbirth (Lamaze)*; Steven V. Roberts, "We Had a Baby," *Good Housekeeping*, May 1969, 102–3, 162–68, "Lamaze . . . stresses" at 103. An example of the animosity between organizations and proponents of different childbirth methods can be seen in a report written by a representative of the Women's Community Health Center in Cambridge, MA, in which she called Elisabeth Bing "a very silly woman." "NEW YORK TRIP REPORT," November 14, 15, 16, 1976, Women's Community Health Center Papers, Schlesinger Library.

62. McCutcheon-Rosegg and Rosegg, *Natural Childbirth the Bradley Way*, x, 7–13, quotes at x; Marie F. Mongan, *HypnoBirthing®: A Celebration of Life* (Rivertree, 1992), 10–11.

63. For an overview of the evolution of feminist thought in the twentieth century, see Rosemarie Tong, *Feminist Thought: A More Comprehensive Introduction* (Westview Press, 1998).

64. Jean Winchester, "I Shared the Wonder of Birth with My Baby," *Parents' Magazine*, May 1961, 36–37, 80–85, quote at 36–37.

65. Ibid., 80.

66. Ibid., 84.

67. Joni Magee, interview by Regina Morantz, April 1, 1977, Medical College of Pennsylvania Oral History Collection on Women in Medicine, Schlesinger Library.

68. Edith M. Stoney, "Let's Be Reasonable about Natural Childbirth," *Today's Health*, February 1953, 46–52, quotes at 47–48.

69. "Natural—or Unnatural?" *Newsweek*, March 15, 1965, 96–97; Mandy, Mandy, Farkas, and Scher, "Is Natural Childbirth Natural?" 431–38; Jacqueline H. Wolf, *Don't*

Kill Your Baby: Public Health and the Decline of Breastfeeding in the 19th and 20th Centuries (Ohio State University Press, 2001), 191–96; Floyd Sterling Rogers, "Dangers of the Read Method in Patients with Major Personality Problems," *American Journal of Obstetrics and Gynecology* 71 (June 1956): 1236–41, quotes at 1237–38.

70. Suzanne Arms, *Immaculate Deception: A New Look at Women and Childbirth in America* (Bantam Books, 1975), 89.

71. Buxton, *A Study of Psychophysical Methods for Relief of Childbirth Pain*, 36–37.

72. Sloan Wilson, "The American Way of Birth," *Harper's Magazine*, July 1964, 48–54, quote at 48.

73. Milton J. E. Senn, "Storm over Childbirth: The Most Controversial Issue in Modern Medicine," *McCall's*, February 1963, 40, 130; Sontheimer, "Miracle in the Delivery Room," 4, 164; "Painless Childbirth," 74.

74. Marguerite Ball, "Without Pain," *Woman's Home Companion*, May 1943, 16, "five hideous days" at 82; remaining quotes in Senn, "Let's Be Sensible about Natural Childbirth," 30–31. For examples of women who contrasted their anesthetized births with their superior unanesthetized births, see Friedrich, "I Had a Baby," 461–65; and Bimbetta Coats, "The Most Glorious Experience," *Readers' Digest*, May 1950, 23–27.

75. Senn, "Storm over Childbirth"; Laurence G. Roth, "Natural Childbirth in a General Hospital," *American Journal of Obstetrics and Gynecology* 61 (1951): 167–72, quote at 171.

76. Gurney Williams, "Natural Childbirth Comes of Age," *Reader's Digest* 103 (December 1973): 153–56.

77. Herbert Thoms and Robert H. Wyatt, "Management of Normal Pregnancy, Labor and Puerperium," *American Journal of Public Health* 40 (1950): 163–67. Eastman's commentary is appended to the end of this article.

78. Myriam Miedzian Malinovich, "An Opinion: On Natural Childbirth," *Mademoiselle*, March 1977, 30–31+, quotes at 31.

79. Dian G. Smith, "Nothing in My Natural Childbirth Lessons Prepared Me for the Reality," *Glamour*, November 1979, 118. Herbert Thoms and Robert H. Wyatt discuss women's unrealistic expectations of natural birth in "Management of Normal Pregnancy, Labor and Puerperium."

80. Rahima Baldwin, "Whatever Happened to Normal Birth?" undated typed manuscript, Informed Homebirth–Informed Birth and Parenting Papers, Sophia Smith Collection.

81. Joni Magee, interview by Regina Morantz, April 1, 1977, Medical College of Pennsylvania Oral History Collection on Women in Medicine, Schlesinger Library.

82. Niels C. Beck and David Hall, "Natural Childbirth: A Review and Analysis," *Obstetrics and Gynecology* 52 (September 1978): 371–79, quotes at 371.

83. "Babies die" in K. C. Cole, "Can Childbirth Survive Technology?" in National Women's Health Network, *Maternal Health and Childbirth Resource Guide* 4 (1980), 15, National Women's Health Network Papers, Sophia Smith Collection; Kathryn Rose Gertz, "The Truth about Painless Childbirth," *Harper's Bazaar*, February 1978, 128, 149, "utter nonsense" at 154.

84. Don Sloan," To the Editor"; and Clayton T. Beecham, "Dr. Beecham Replies,"

both in *The Female Patient* 15 (March 15, 1990): 14, 16. An example of a single magazine that ran very different articles about natural childbirth in the 1970s, as opposed to the 1990s, is *Parents Magazine.* See, for example, "A Husband and Wife Share the Deeply Satisfying Experience of Natural Childbirth," *Parents Magazine,* March 1971, 56–59; and Laurel Graeber, "How Do You Spell Relief? E-P-I-D-U-R-A-L," *Parents Magazine,* July 1998, 77–78.

85. Purvis L. Martin and Steward H. Smith, "Public Relations in Our Maternity Wards," *American Journal of Obstetrics and Gynecology* 81 (June 1961): 1079–85, quote at 1079.

86. Erikson, in "New Focus on Women in Hospitals Here," referred to a hospital's promotion of birthing facilities to convince patients to come for other treatments.

87. For a critique of Lamaze and its hospital-oriented approach to birth, see Barbara Katz Rothman, *In Labor: Women and Power in the Birthplace* (W. W. Norton, 1991), 170–74. See the foundational philosophy of American Lamaze classes in Bing, "Thoughts on Prepared Childbirth"; and Elizabeth Harlan, "An Experience Is Born with Elisabeth Bing: The Lamaze Method of Psychoprophylactic Childbirth," July 1971, both in Elisabeth Bing and Lamaze International Papers, Schlesinger Library.

88. Sol M. Shnider, "Tie Me Up! Tie Me Down!" A brief biography of Shnider is Samuel C. Hughes, "A Remembrance Sol M. Shnider, M.D.—1929–1994," *CSA Bulletin* (May–June 1994), 24–28. Shnider was president of the Society for Obstetric Anesthesia and Perinatology in 1973.

Chapter 6 · Epidural Anesthesia and Cesarean Section

1. A mother, interview by author, tape recording, November 2, 2005, Lombard, IL. "Anna Dobros," "Mike," and "Julie" are pseudonyms.

2. Julia Kirk Blackwelder, *Now Hiring: The Feminization of Work in the United States, 1900–1995* (Texas A&M University Press, 1997), 195, 225; Barbara Downs, "Fertility of American Women: June 2002," in *Current Population Reports, P20–548* (U.S. Census Bureau, October 2003), www.census.gov/prod/2003pubs/p20–548.pdf.

3. Betty Friedan, *The Feminine Mystique* (W. W. Norton, 1963); Betty Friedan, *The Second Stage* (Summit Books, 1981), 15.

4. Many articles have examined differences between mandated benefits for mothers in the United States and elsewhere in the world. See, for example, Nora V. Demleitner, "Maternity Leave Policies of the United States and Germany: A Comparative Study," *New York Law School Journal of International and Comparative Law* 13 (1992): 229–55; Samuel Issacharoff and Elyse Rosenblum, "Women and the Workplace: Accommodating the Demands of Pregnancy," *Columbia Law Review* 94 (1994): 2154–2221; Fred Deven and Peter Moss, "Leave Arrangements for Parents: Overview and Future Outlook," *Community, Work, and Family* 5 (2002): 237–55. For a list of countries' maternity leave policies, see International Labour Organization, "More than 120 Nations Provide Paid Maternity Leave," February 16, 1998, www.ilo.org/global/About_the_ ILO/Media_and_public_information/Press_releases/lang—en/WCMS_008009.

5. Judith Warner, "Mommy Madness," *Newsweek,* February 21, 2005, 42–49. War-

ner adapted the article from her book *Perfect Madness: Motherhood in the Age of Anxiety* (Riverhead Books, 2005).

6. Kathryn Woodruff, letter in response to "Pay on Delivery," *New York Times Magazine*, November 21, 1999, 21.

7. Examples of articles extolling epidural anesthesia and ridiculing natural childbirth include Margaret Talbot, "Pay on Delivery," *New York Times Magazine*, October 31, 1999, 19–20; Margery Eagan, "Drugs Limiting Childbirth Pain Can Be Every Mother's Gain," *Boston Herald*, October 14, 1999, 14; and Darshak Sanghavi, "The Mother Lode of Pain," *Boston Globe Magazine*, July 23, 2006, 18.

8. L. P. Smith, B. A. Nagourney, F. H. McLean, and R. H. Usher, "Hazards and Benefits of Elective Induction of Labor," *American Journal of Obstetrics and Gynecology* 148 (March 1, 1984): 579–85, quote at 584.

9. Shari Roan, "Inducing Labor for Convenience Gets a Second Look. New Studies Show the Practice Has a Role in Rising Costs and the Risk of Complications," *Los Angeles Times*, August 13, 2007; Richard A. Marini, "Time for Labor—More Women Are Asking for Induced Childbirth," *San Antonio Express-News*, September 3, 2001, 1E; Liz F. Kay, "In Howard, Babies Born to Fit Busy Schedules," *Baltimore Sun*, April 27, 2003. The rate of inductions per 1,000 live births went from 95.3 in 1990 to 206 in 2003. The ACOG Resource Center compiled this data from the annual *National Vital Statistics Reports*. See also Luis Sanchez-Ramos, "Induction of Labor," *Obstetrics and Gynecology Clinics of North America* 32 (2005): 181–200.

10. Practicing obstetrician, interview by author, tape recording, June 26, 2006, Chicago.

11. Talbot, "Pay on Delivery," 19–20. A fascinating and comprehensive study of obstetrics today is Jennifer Block, *Pushed: The Painful Truth about Childbirth and Modern Maternity Care* (Da Capo Press, 2007).

12. Toshio J. Akamatsu and John J. Bonica, "Spinal and Extradural Analgesia-Anesthesia for Parturition," *Clinical Obstetrics and Gynecology* 17 (1974): 183–98; David Zuck, "Epidural Analgesia in Obstetrics," *Nursing Times* 64 (November 15, 1968): 1548–50; J. N. Haug, G. A. Roback, and B. C. Martin, *Distribution of Physicians in the United States, 1970* (American Medical Association, 1971), 25; Catherine M. Bidese and Donald G. Danais, *Physician Characteristics and Distribution in the U.S.* (American Medical Association, 1982), 13; Gene Roback, Lillian Randolph, Bradley Seidman, and Thomas Pasko, *Physician Characteristics and Distribution in the U.S.* (American Medical Association, 1994), 20; Derek R. Smart, *Physician Characteristics and Distribution in the U.S.* (American Medical Association, 2006), 29.

13. Clarissa Dasser and John J. O'Connor, "Continuous Epidural Block for Obstetric Anesthesia," *American Journal of Nursing* 60 (1960): 1296–99; H. Glenn Thompson, Kenneth R. Johnson, and John J. O'Connor, "Epidural Anesthesia in Obstetrics," *Obstetrics and Gynecology* 29 (May 1967): 682–86. Studies indicating the safety of epidural anesthesia contrasted with studies that showed that inhalation anesthesia contributed to maternal mortality. One study in Baltimore found that between 1946 and 1958, anesthesia contributed to about 12% of all maternal deaths, most notably through soft tissue airway obstruction and aspiration of vomitus. See Otto C.

Phillips and George H. Davis, "The Role of Anesthesia in Obstetric Mortality: A Review of 455,443 Live Births from 1936 to 1958 in the City of Baltimore," *Anesthesia and Analgesia* 40 (September–October 1961): 557–66.

14. Sol M. Shnider, "Training in Obstetric Anesthesia in the United States," *American Journal of Obstetrics and Gynecology* 93 (September 15, 1963): 243–52; practicing obstetrician, interview by author, tape recording, October 31, 2005, Highland Park, IL; practicing obstetrician, interview by author, tape recording, November 1, 2005, Northbrook, IL.

15. Retired obstetrician, interview by author, tape recording, July 19, 2004, Chicago. Anesthesiologists often acknowledged the competence of nurse-anesthetists, even putting them in the same category as the physicians who were board-certified in anesthesiology. Robert Hingson, for example, noted at a 1966 meeting on obstetric anesthesia coverage, "Today only 52 percent of obstetric patients in the United States are given anesthesia care by either a trained anesthesiologist or nurse anesthetist." "Proceedings," "American Society of Anesthesiologists Obstetric Anesthesia Committee Seminar on Obstetric Anesthesia Coverage," Magee–Women's Hospital, Pittsburgh, PA, June 10, 1966.

16. A discussion of the attitude of anesthesiologists toward obstetrics is in Charles P. Gibbs, Jeffrey Krischer, Ben M. Peckham, Harry Sharp, and Thomas H. Kirschbaum, "Obstetric Anesthesia: A National Survey," *Anesthesiology* 65 (1986): 298–306. Anesthesiologist Virginia Apgar accused her colleagues of ignoring obstetrics. See Virginia Apgar, "The Role of the Anesthesiologist in Reducing Neonatal Mortality," *New York State Medical Journal* (August 15, 1955): 2365–68. Shnider, "Training in Obstetric Anesthesia in the United States."

17. Carolyn J. Nicholson and Thomas H. Joyce, "Who Administers Obstetrical Anesthesia?" *Journal of the American Association of Nurse Anesthetists* 44 (October 1976): 485–89; Committee on Obstetric Practice, "Obstetric Analgesia and Anesthesia," *ACOG Technical Bulletin* 11, February 1969 (rev. October 1973).

18. Practicing obstetrician, interview by author, tape recording, October 31, 2005, Highland Park, IL; practicing obstetrician, interview by author, tape recording, November 1, 2005, Northbrook, IL; Brenda A. Bucklin, Joy L. Hawkins, James R. Anderson, and Fred A. Ullrich, "Obstetric Anesthesia Workforce Survey," *Anesthesiology* 103 (2005): 645–53.

19. John Adriani, MD, to John J. Bonica, February 28, 1966; Adriani to Benjamin G. Covino, PhD, MD, editor of the periodical *Regional Anesthesia and Pain Medicine*, Brigham and Women's Hospital, September 15, 1983, John Adriani Papers, 1925–88, National Library of Medicine, History of Medicine Division, Bethesda, MD. The *ASA Newsletter* eventually published a version of Adriani's strong opinions about nurse-anesthetists. John Adriani, "The Role of the Nurse Anesthetists in the Health Care Field," *ASA Newsletter* (May 1984): 5–6.

20. J. P. Greenhill, *Analgesia and Anesthesia in Obstetrics* (Charles C. Thomas, 1952); J. P. Greenhill, *Analgesia and Anesthesia in Obstetrics* (Charles C. Thomas, 1962); Dr. J. P. Greenhill, Chicago, to Mr. Charles C. Thomas, publisher, Springfield, IL, February 12, 1964; John Adriani, MD, to Mr. Payne Thomas, Charles C. Thomas, pub-

lisher, Fort Lauderdale, FL, February 25, 1964, John Adriani Papers, 1925–88, National Library of Medicine, History of Medicine Division.

21. S.O.A.P. Newsletters 5 (July 1, 1973), 6 (August 1, 1974), 8 (March 1, 1977), 9 (July 1, 1977), Wood Library, American Society of Anesthesiologists, Park Ridge, IL.

22. Bucklin, Hawkins, Anderson, and Ullrich, "Obstetric Anesthesia Workforce Survey," 645–53. See also Rita Rubin, "Childbirth Pain Relief Cases Triple," *USA Today,* October 12, 1999, 1.

23. Rita Rubin, "Epidurals, Other Approaches Help Manage Labor Pain," *USA Today,* August 13, 2002, available at http://www.usatoday.com/news/health/2002-08-13-labor_x.htm.

24. Practicing obstetrician, interview by author, tape recording, October 31, 2005, Highland Park, IL.

25. Richard B. Clark, "Historical Perspective: How Did Lumbar Epidural Anesthesia Become the Premier Obstetric Anesthetic in the USA?" *ACOG Clinical Review* 4 (March–April 1999): 6, 10–11; Bucklin, Hawkins, Anderson, and Ullrich, "Obstetric Anesthesia Workforce Survey." Donald Caton, professor emeritus in the departments of anesthesiology and obstetrics and gynecology at the University of Florida College of Medicine, confirmed in an e-mail exchange with the author on May 24, 2006, that epidurals solved the low-insurance-reimbursement problem.

26. Eagan, "Drugs Limiting Childbirth Pain," 14.

27. Carolyn Y. Johnson, "Childbirth Study Finds Lesser Risk in Epidurals," *Boston Globe,* February 17, 2005; quotes in Eagan, "Drugs Limiting Childbirth Pain"; Marta Poore and Joyce Cameron Foster, "Epidural and No Epidural Anesthesia: Differences between Mothers and Their Experience of Birth," *Birth* 12 (Winter 1985): 205–12.

28. Observers noticed this change in attitude immediately with the rise in popularity of epidural anesthesia. See, for example, Poore and Foster, "Epidural and No Epidural Anesthesia"; Penny Simkin, "Epidural Update," *Birth Gazette* 15 (Fall 1999): 12–16.

29. Raleigh Mayer, "Pay on Delivery," *New York Times Magazine,* November 21, 1999, 22; Rubin, "Epidurals, Other Approaches Help Manage Labor Pain."

30. Committee on Obstetrics: Maternal and Fetal Medicine, "Pain Relief during Labor," *ACOG Committee Opinion,* no. 118 (January 1993); ACOG Committee on Obstetric Practice, "Analgesia and Cesarean Delivery Rates," *ACOG Committee Opinion,* no. 269 (February 2002). Some of the studies linking epidural anesthesia with dystocia and an increase in cesarean sections include James A. Thorp, Jay D. McNitt, and Phyllis C. Leppert, "Effects of Epidural Analgesia: Some Questions and Answers," *Birth* 17 (September 1990): 157–62; and James A. Thorp, Daniel H. Hu, Rene M. Albin, Jay McNitt, Bruce A. Meyer, Gary R. Cohen, and John D. Yeast, "The Effect of Intrapartum Epidural Analgesia on Nulliparous Labor: A Randomized, Controlled, Prospective Trial," *American Journal of Obstetrics and Gynecology* 169 (October 1993): 851–58. In 2006 ACOG announced that recent studies indicated that epidural analgesia did not increase the risks of cesarean delivery. This announcement strengthened the organization's defense of epidural on demand. See ACOG Committee on Obstetric Practice, "Analgesia and Cesarean Delivery Rates," *ACOG Committee Opinion,* no.

339 (June 2006). The studies cited by ACOG include C. A. Wong, B. M. Scavone, A. M. Peaceman, R. J. McCarthy, J. T. Sullivan, N. T. Diaz, et al., "The Risk of Cesarean Delivery with Neuraxial Analgesia Given Early versus Late in Labor," *New England Journal of Medicine* 352 (2005): 655–65; and S. K. Sharma, J. M. Alexander, G. Messick, S. L. Bloom, D. D. McIntire, J. Wiley, et al., "Cesarean Delivery: A Randomized Trial of Epidural Analgesia versus Intravenous Meperidine Analgesia during Labor in Nulliparous Women," *Anesthesiology* 96 (2002): 546–51.

31. See Linda Gordon, *Woman's Body, Woman's Right: Birth Control in America* (Penguin Books, 1990), 93–113.

32. A professor in the departments of anesthesiology and obstetrics and gynecology at a southern medical school made the observation about the rising C-section rate and the need for anesthesiologists dedicated to labor and delivery. Private e-mail communication with the author on July 10, 2007.

33. Cesarean section rate statistics from 1965 to the present were compiled from Lester David and Irene David, "One in Five," *Health* (May 1984): 73–81; Paul J. Placek and Selma M. Taffel, "Recent Patterns in Cesarean Delivery in the United States," *Obstetrics and Gynecology Clinics of North America* 15 (December 1988): 607–27; Richard P. Porreco and James A. Thorp, "The Cesarean Birth Epidemic: Trends, Causes, and Solutions," *American Journal of Obstetrics and Gynecology* 175 (August 1996): 369–74; Benjamin P. Sachs, "Vaginal Birth after Cesarean: Contemporary Issues," *Clinical Obstetrics and Gynecology* 44 (September 2001): 552; Fay Manacker and Sally C. Curtin, "Trends in Cesarean Birth and Vaginal Birth after Previous Cesarean, 1991–99," *National Vital Statistics Reports* 49 (December 27, 2001): 1–16; "HealthGrades Quality Study: First-Time Preplanned and 'Patient Choice' Cesarean Section Rates in the United States," *Health Grades*, July 2003, www.healthgrades.com/media/english/pdf/Patient_Choice_Csection_Study_July_2003.pdf; "Total and Primary Cesarean Rate and Vaginal Birth after Previous Cesarean Rate—United States, 1989–2003," *Morbidity and Mortality Weekly Report*, Centers for Disease Control, January 21, 2005, http://www.cdc.gov/mmwR/preview/mmwrhtml/mm5402a5.htm (accessed June 18, 2008); Brady E. Hamilton, Joyce A. Martin, and Stephanie J. Ventura, "Births: Preliminary Data for 2005," *National Center for Health Statistics*, www.cdc.gov/nchs/products/pubs/pubd/hestats/prelimbirths05/prelimbirths05.htm (accessed October 4, 2007); Brady E. Hamilton, Joyce A. Martin, and Stephanie J. Ventura, "Births: Preliminary Data for 2006," *National Vital Statistics Reports* 56 (December 5, 2007), available at http://www.cdc.gov/nchs/data/nvsr/nvsr56/nvsr56_07.pdf. The authors of a study that demonstrates larger reimbursements by Medicaid for cesarean (as opposed to vaginal) birth argue that this practice contributed to higher cesarean delivery rates in the Medicaid population. See Jon Gruber, John Kim, and Dina Mayzlin, "Physician Fees and Procedure Intensity: The Case of Cesarean Delivery," *Journal of Health Economics* 18 (1999): 473–90.

34. In 1932 a typical doctor observed: "It is a well known fact that the better trained in obstetrics a physician is, the fewer cesarean sections he finds it necessary to perform." Arthur H. Bill, "The Newer Obstetrics," *American Journal of Obstetrics and Gynecology* 23 (February 1932): 155–64.

35. Retired obstetrician, interview by author, tape recording, July 12, 1996; Winnetka, IL; Presidential Address, Obstetrical Society of Philadelphia, February 12, 1981, J. Robert Willson, MD, presidential guest speaker, typed transcript, J. Robert Willson Papers, National Library of Medicine, History of Medicine Division.

36. Edwin B. Cragin, "Conservatism in Obstetrics," *New York Medical Journal* 114 (July 1, 1916): 1–3. Cases of rickets were exceedingly common; cows' milk had not yet been supplemented with vitamin D, and many children grew up in dangerous, heavily polluted, sun-blocked cities, where parents reared them in windowless tenements. The contribution of the diagnosis of dystocia to the high section rate is discussed in Helen I. Marieskind, *An Evaluation of Caesarean Section in the United States* (U.S. Department of Health, Education, and Welfare, June 1979), 9–10, 113–18, quotes at 9 and 10. Critics of the high cesarean section rate today continue to complain that dystocia is overdiagnosed. See M. Dabbas and A. Al-Sumadi, "Cesarean Section Rate: Much Room for Reduction," *Clinical and Experimental Obstetrics and Gynecology* 34 (2007): 146–48.

37. Joseph B. DeLee, *The Principles and Practice of Obstetrics* (W. B. Saunders, 1929), 1060–62; J. P. Greenhill, *Principles and Practice of Obstetrics* (W. B. Saunders, 1951), 924–27.

38. Retired obstetrician, interview by author, tape recording, Glenview, IL, June 29, 2006; retired family physician who attended births throughout his years of practice, interview by author, tape recording, October 11, 1999, River Forest, IL.

39. John R. Evrard, "Cesarean Section and Maternal Mortality in Rhode Island: Incidence and Risk Factors, 1965–1975," *Obstetrics and Gynecology* 50 (November 1977): 594–97; Diana Petitti, Robert O. Olson, and Ronald L. Williams, "Cesarean Section in California—1960 through 1975," *American Journal of Obstetrics and Gynecology* 133 (February 15, 1979): 391–97, "the proper level" at 395.

40. Marieskind, *An Evaluation of Caesarean Section*. For historic detail of the maternal death rate in the United States, see Irvine Loudon, *Death in Childbirth: An International Study of Maternal Care and Maternal Mortality, 1800–1950* (Oxford University Press, 1992), 365–97. For specific data on the 1920s and 1970s, respectively, see Robert Morse Woodbury, *Infant Mortality and Its Causes, with an Appendix on the Trend of Maternal Mortality Rates in the United States* (Williams and Wilkins, 1926), 181; and Jack C. Smith, Joyce M. Hughes, Penelope S. Pekow, and Roger W. Rochat, "An Assessment of the Incidence of Maternal Mortality in the United States," *American Journal of Public Health* 74 (August 1984): 780–83.

41. Evrard, "Cesarean Section and Maternal Mortality." The study showed there had been 6.95 deaths per 10,000 sectioned deliveries versus .27 deaths per 10,000 vaginal deliveries.

42. Marieskind, *An Evaluation of Caesarean Section;* NIH Task Force, "NIH Consensus Development Task Force Statement on Cesarean Childbirth," *American Journal of Obstetrics and Gynecology* 139 (April 15, 1981): 902–9.

43. Marieskind, *An Evaluation of Caesarean Section.*

44. Kenneth E. Thorpe, "The Medical Malpractice 'Crisis': Recent Trends and the Impact of State Tort Reforms," *Health Affairs* (January 21, 2004).

45. A. Dale Tussing and Martha A. Wojtowycz, "The Cesarean Decision in New York State, 1986," *Medical Care* 30 (June 1992): 529–40; Steven M. Rock, "Malpractice Premiums and Primary Cesarean Section Rates in New York and Illinois," *Public Health Reports* 103 (September–October 1988): 459–63; A. Russell Localio, Ann G. Lawthers, Joan M. Bengtson, Liesi E. Hebert, Susan L. Weaver, Troyen A. Brennan, and J. Richard Landis, "Relationship between Malpractice Claims and Cesarean Delivery," *Journal of the American Medical Association* 269 (January 20, 1993): 366–73; Laura-Mae Baldwin, Gary Hart, Michael Lloyd, Meredith Fordyce, and Roger A. Fosenblatt, "Defensive Medicine and Obstetrics," *Journal of the American Medical Association* 274 (November 22–29, 1995): 1606–10; Kristi Ryan, Peter Schnatz, John Greene, and Stephen Curry, "Change in Cesarean Section Rate as a Reflection of the Present Malpractice Crisis," *Connecticut Medicine* 69 (March 2005): 139–41. In the first national study (released in 1999) of the impact of malpractice claims risk on the cesarean section rate, investigators found negligible impact, affecting mainly low-income women. Researchers found no evidence of defensive medicine practiced on married women with a college education, although a few of the studies listed above belie this conclusion. Lisa Dubay, Robert Kaestner, and Timothy Waidmann, "The Impact of Malpractice Fears on Cesarean Section Rates," *Journal of Health Economics* 18 (1999): 491–522.

46. Marieskind, *An Evaluation of Caesarean Section*, 3–4, 82–87; Dubay, Kaestner, and Waidmann, "The Impact of Malpractice Fears on Cesarean Section Rates."

47. Marieskind, *An Evaluation of Caesarean Section*, 5–7, 29–30, 95–107.

48. Practicing obstetrician, interview by author, tape recording, June 28, 2006, Chicago. The second factor listed in the HEW report was the universal policy in the United States of not allowing a vaginal birth after a cesarean section (VBAC). In 1974 repeat cesareans represented about one-third of all cesareans; fewer than 2% of American women with a prior section delivered vaginally in a subsequent birth, and if they did, it was almost always an accident: they went into labor before their scheduled cesarean. Marieskind, *An Evaluation of Caesarean Section*, 3–4, 82–87. In 1982 ACOG agreed with the recommendation in the HEW report that women with one previous cesarean not have an automatic repeat cesarean. American College of Obstetricians and Gynecologists (ACOG), "Guidelines for Vaginal Delivery after a Previous Cesarean Birth," *ACOG Committee Statement State-of-the Art Opinion in Obstetrics and Gynecology* (ACOG, January 1982, rev. November 1984). In 1988 ACOG issued an even stronger statement favoring VBAC, observing that maternal and perinatal mortality rates for vaginal delivery after a previous cesarean were lower than for repeat cesareans. ACOG, "Guidelines for Vaginal Delivery after a Previous Cesarean Birth," *ACOG Committee Opinion*, no. 64 (October 1988). In 1994 ACOG confirmed this position with even stronger language: women "should be counseled and encouraged to undergo a trial of labor" after one previous cesarean. ACOG, "Vaginal Delivery after a Previous Cesarean Birth," *ACOG Committee Opinion*, no. 143 (October 1994). In 1998, however, ACOG became more circumspect: "Because uterine rupture may be catastrophic, VBAC should be attempted in institutions . . . with physicians readily available to provide emergency care." ACOG, "Vaginal Delivery after Previous

Cesarean Delivery," *ACOG Practice Bulletin,* no. 2 (October 1998). Then, less than a year after sounding that cautious note, a single word change in another ACOG advisory effectively dissuaded all but the largest, best staffed, urban hospitals from permitting VBACs. An *ACOG Practice Bulletin* advised, "VBAC should be attempted in institutions . . . with physicians immediately available to provide emergency care." ACOG, "Vaginal Delivery after Previous Cesarean Birth," *ACOG Practice Bulletin,* no. 5 (July 1999). Advising that doctors be "immediately" rather than "readily" available dissuaded most American hospitals and doctors from allowing VBACs. More recently, studies have supported the view that VBAC candidates who have had a prior vaginal delivery have a decreased risk for major maternal morbidities when compared with like women who do not attempt a VBAC trial. See Alison G. Cahill, David M. Stamilio, Anthony O. Odibo, Jeffrey F. Peipert, Sarah J. Ratcliffe, Erika J. Stevens, Mary D. Sammel, and George A. Macones, "Is Vaginal Birth after Cesarean (VBAC) or Elective Repeat Cesarean Safer in Women with a Prior Vaginal Delivery?" *Obstetrics and Gynecology* 195 (2006): 1143–47. ACOG has not revisited its 1999 recommendation, however. Although studies note that women not allowed to go into labor spontaneously were the ones at significant risk for uterine rupture during a VBAC, the onus for uterine rupture after a previous cesarean continues to be on VBAC rather than labor induction.

49. NIH Task Force, "NIH Consensus Development Task Force Statement on Cesarean Childbirth," 902–9. After the HEW and NIH reports, researchers across the country conducted additional studies that ultimately supported the hypothesis that rising section rates and falling neonatal death rates were unrelated. See Richard P. Porreco, "High Cesarean Section Rate: A New Perspective," *Obstetrics and Gynecology* 65 (March 1985): 307–11; Robert K. DeMott and Herbert F. Sandmire, "The Green Bay Cesarean Section Study: The Physician Factor as a Determinant of Cesarean Birth Rates," *American Journal of Obstetrics and Gynecology* 162 (June 1990): 1593–1600; Stephen A. Myers and Norbert Gleicher, "A Successful Program to Lower Cesarean-Section Rates," *New England Journal of Medicine* 319 (1988): 1511–16. Other studies arguing that there is no connection between more cesarean sections and better outcomes include Thorkild F. Nielsen, Petra Otterblad Olausson, and Ingemar Ingernarsson, "The Cesarean Section Rate in Sweden: The End of the Rise," *Birth* 21 (March 1994): 34–38; and Saed M. Ziadeh and Elias I. Sunna, "Decreased Cesarean Birth Rates and Improved Perinatal Outcome: A Seven-Year Study," *Birth* 22 (September 1995): 144–47.

50. "Monitoring Childbirth," *Newsweek,* February 6, 1967, 84.

51. "'Watching' the Unborn Inside the Womb," *Life,* July 25, 1969, 63–65.

52. "Labor-Saving Devices," *Newsweek,* April 23, 1979, 85; retired obstetrician, interview by author, tape recording, Glenview, IL, June 29, 2006; Presidential Address, Obstetrical Society of Philadelphia, February 12, 1981, J. Robert Willson, MD, presidential guest speaker, typed transcript, J. Robert Willson Papers, National Library of Medicine, History of Medicine Division.

53. ACOG, *Standards for Obstetric-Gynecologic Services,* 6th ed. (ACOG, 1985), 33–35. Since 1989 ACOG has consistently advised in every one of its *Standard Practice*

advisories that intermittent auscultation with a fetal stethoscope is as effective a tool as electronic fetal monitoring when used on low-risk women. ACOG Committee on Professional Standards, *Standards for Obstetric-Gynecologic Services* (ACOG, 1989), 36; American Academy of Pediatrics, ACOG, *Guidelines for Perinatal Care* (American Academy of Pediatrics; ACOG, 2002),133. Hon quoted in Mary Lee Grisanti, "The Cesarean Epidemic," *New York Magazine,* February 20, 1989, 56–61, quote at 58. Several studies have warned that the monitoring of low-risk patients yielded a high false-positive rate for fetal hypoxia, prompting many unnecessary cesarean sections. See, for example, Gino Tutera and Robert L. Newman, "Fetal Monitoring: Its Effect on the Perinatal Mortality and Cesarean Section Rates and Its Complications," *American Journal of Obstetrics and Gynecology* 122 (1972): 750–54; Petitti, Olson, and Williams, "Cesarean Section in California," 391–97; Michael Newton, "Why So Many Cesareans?" *Family Health,* September 1979, 18–19; Kirkwood K. Shy, David A. Luthy, Forrest C. Bennett, Michael Whitfield, Eric B. Larson, Gerald van Belle, James P. Hughes, Judith A. Wilson, and Morton A. Stenchever, "Effects of Electronic Fetal-Heart-Rate Monitoring, as Compared with Periodic Auscultation, on the Neurologic Development of Premature Infants," *New England Journal of Medicine* 322 (March 1, 1990): 588–93; Thorp, McNitt, and Leppert, "Effects of Epidural Analgesia," 157–62; Karin B. Nelson, James M. Dambrosia, Tricia Y. Ting, and Judith B. Grether, "Uncertain Value of Electronic Fetal Monitoring in Predicting Cerebral Palsy," *New England Journal of Medicine* 334 (March 7, 1996): 613–18; Margaret Lent, "The Medical and Legal Risks of the Electronic Fetal Monitor," *Stanford Law Review* 51 (April 1999): 807–37.

54. ACOG did not begin to collect nationwide data on the extent of fetal monitoring until 1990. By then, 73% of births were electronically monitored. The rate had risen to 85% by 2003. These figures were collected from the following sources by the ACOG Resource Center: 2003: *National Vital Statistics Reports (NVSR)* 54, no. 2, table 27; 2002: *NVSR* 52, no. 10, table 27; 2001: *NVSR* 51, no. 2, table 27; 2000: *NVSR* 50, no. 5, table 27; 1999: *NVSR* 49, no. 1, table 27; 1998: *NVSR* 48, no. 3, table 36; 1997: *NVSR* 47, no. 18, table 36; 1996: *Monthly Vital Statistics Reports (MVSR)* 46, no. 1 supp., table 36; 1995: *MVSR* 45, no. 11 supp., table 36; 1994: *MVSR* 44, no. 11 supp., table 36; 1993: *MVSR* 44, no. 3 supp., table 36; 1990–92: *Vital Statistics of the United States,* table 151. Obstetricians quoted in Marieskind, *An Evaluation of Caesarean Section,* 195.

55. Grisanti, "The Cesarean Epidemic."

56. Christine Coleman Wilson and Wendy Roe Hovey, "Cesareans," *Glamour,* July 1980,171–74; Matt Clark and Mary Lord, "Too Many Caesareans?" *Newsweek,* October 6,1980,105.

57. U.S. Public Health Service, *Healthy People 2000: National Health Promotion and Disease Prevention Objectives* (United States Public Health Service, 1992), Publication no. 93-1212-1, www.cdc.gov/nchs/products/pubs/pubd/hp2k/review/review.htm (accessed October 18, 2006). Benjamin Sachs, Cindy Kobelin, Mary Ames Castro, and Fredric Frigoletto, "The Risks of Lowering the Cesarean-Delivery Rate," *New England Journal of Medicine* 340 (January 7, 1999): 54–57.

58. W. Benson Harer, "Patient Choice Cesarean," *ACOG Clinical Review* 5 (March–April 2000): 1, 13–16; Deborah L. Shelton, "C-Sections Increasing as Doctors, Patients

Re-Evaluate the Risks," *American Medical News,* October 9, 2000; Ralph W. Hale and W. Benson Harer, "Editorial: Elective Prophylactic Cesarean Delivery," *ACOG Clinical Review* 10 (March–April 2005): 1, 15–16.

59. Andrea Tone notes the same phenomenon surrounding the often dangerous and deceptive advertisements for contraceptive devices in the 1930s, endorsed not by male but by female physicians "whose innate understanding of the female condition permitted them to share their birth control expertise 'woman to woman.'" Lysol disinfectant was the most heavily endorsed product for contraceptive douching. Andrea Tone, "Contraceptive Consumers: Gender and the Political Economy of Birth Control in the 1930s," in *Women and Health in America,* ed. Judith Walzer Leavitt (University of Wisconsin Press, 1999), 306–25, quote at 316. ACOG has compiled gender statistics for its members since 1990. In 1990, 20.9% of ACOG's total membership was female (6,361 women vs. 24,064 men); in 2005, 44.2% was female (21,931 women versus 27,633 men). ACOG, "ACOG Membership Statistics," available at the ACOG Library, Washington, DC.

60. Rob Stein, "Caesarean Births Hit High Mark," *Washington Post,* December 16, 2002, A1; Rita Rubin, "More Moms Opt to Undergo C-Section Births, Study Finds Concern about Labor's Toll on Their Bodies a Factor in Planned Cesareans," *USA Today,* July 22, 2003; *Good Morning America,* ABC, October 17, 2002.

61. R. Al-Mufti, A. McCarthy, and N. M. Fisk, "Survey of Obstetricians' Personal Preference and Discretionary Practice," *European Journal of Obstetric and Gynaecologic Reproductive Biology* 73 (1997): 1–4. A similar study of physicians' attitudes toward cesarean section for themselves is G. S. Gabbe and G. B. Holzman, "Obstetricians' Choice of Delivery," *Lancet* 357 (2001): 722. Another study showed that urogynecologists were significantly more likely to support elective sections than obstetricians (80.4% versus 55.4%). Jennifer M. Wu, Andrew F. Hundley, and Anthony G. Visco, "Elective Primary Cesarean Delivery: Attitudes of Urogynecology and Maternal-Fetal Medicine Specialists," *Obstetrics and Gynecology* 105 (February 2005): 301–6. The following study indicates that the percentage of obstetricians who prefer vaginal delivery and external cephalic version is higher than other studies reported without significant gender differences: Janet B. Wright, Alison L. Wright, Nigel A. B. Simpson, and Fiona C. Bryce, "A Survey of Trainee Obstetricians' Preferences for Childbirth," *Obstetrics and Gynecology* 97 (2001): 23–25. The study indicating that physicians shape their patients' birth preferences is Gregory L. Goyert, Sidney F. Bottoms, Marjorie C. Treadwell, and Paul C. Nehra, "The Physician Factor in Cesarean Birth Rates," *New England Journal of Medicine* 320 (March 16, 1989): 706–9. See also David A. Luthy, Judith A. Malmgren, Rosalee W. Zingheim, and Christopher J. Leininger, "Physician Contribution to a Cesarean Delivery Risk Model," *American Journal of Obstetrics and Gynecology* 188 (June 2003): 1579–87.

62. Wendy Mitchinson discusses this pairing of specialties with contradictory underlying premises in *Giving Birth in Canada, 1900–1950* (University of Toronto Press, 2002), 57–58. Although the physicians who advocate cesarean delivery on maternal request contend that vaginal birth prompts pathological conditions (particularly urinary incontinence), studies linking vaginal birth and incontinence have not

been conclusive. Heredity might play a greater role in the development of incontinence than either parity or mode of birth. See, for example, G. M. Buchsbaum, E. E. Duecy, L. A. Kerr, and L. S. Huang, "Urinary Incontinence in Nulliparous Women and Their Parous Sisters," *Obstetrics and Gynecology* 106 (2005): 1253–58; Gunhilde M. Buchsbaum, Michelle Chin, Chris Glantz, and David Guzick, "Prevalence of Urinary Incontinence and Associated Risk Factors in a Cohort of Nuns," *Obstetrics and Gynecology* 100 (August 2002): 226–29; and Guri Rortveit, Anne Kjersti Dalveit, Yngvild S. Hannestad, and Steinar Hunskaar, "Urinary Incontinence after Vaginal Delivery or Cesarean Section," *New England Journal of Medicine* 348 (March 6, 2003): 900–907.

63. Sanghavi, "The Mother Lode of Pain," 18.

64. Laurel Graeber, "How Do You Spell Relief? E-P-I-D-U-R-A-L," *Parents' Magazine*, July 1998, 77–78.

65. Christopher Snowbeck, "Is Elective C-Section Delivery a Good Idea?" *Pittsburgh Post-Gazette*, March 18, 2003. See also Alice Park, "Choosy Mothers Choose Caesareans," *Time in Partnership with CNN*, April 17, 2008, article at http://www.time.com/time/magazine/article/0,9171,1731904,00.html.

66. ACOG Committee Opinion, "Surgery and Patient Choice: The Ethics of Decision Making," *Obstetrics and Gynecology* 102 (2003): 1101–6; "Non-Medically Indicated C-Sections Ethical, ACOG Ethics Committee Says," *Kaiser Daily Reproductive Health Report*, November 3, 2003; Rob Stein, "Elective Caesareans Judged Ethical," *Washington Post*, October 31, 2003, A2. For recent studies that indicate elective cesareans result in higher infant and maternal morbidity and mortality than low-risk vaginal births, see Anne Kirkeby Hansen, Kirsten Wisborg, Niels Uldbjerg, and Tine Brink Henriksen, "Elective Cesarean Section and Respiratory Morbidity in the Term and Near-Term Neonate, *Acta Obstetrica et Gynecologica Scandinavica* 86 (2007): 389–94; Marian F. MacDorman, Eugene Declercq, Fay Menacker, and Michael H. Malloy, "Infant and Neonatal Mortality for Primary Cesarean and Vaginal Births to Women with 'No Indicated Risk,' United States, 1998–2001 Birth Cohorts," *Birth* 33 (September 2006): 175–82; and Catherine Deneux-Tharaux, Elodie Carmona, Marie-Hélene Bouvier-Colle, and Gérard Bréart, "Postpartum Maternal Mortality and Cesarean Delivery," *Obstetrics and Gynecology* 108 (September 2006): 541–48. Studies of the safety and efficacy of VBAC versus elective cesarean remain contradictory; some indicate a higher maternal and infant death rate in low-risk, elective cesareans versus low-risk vaginal births. See, for example, Cahill, Stamilio, Odibo, Peipert, Ratcliffe, Stevens, Sammel, and Macones, "Is Vaginal Birth after Cesarean (VBAC) or Elective Repeat Cesarean Safer in Women with a Prior Vaginal Delivery?" 1143–47; and Oscar Sadan, Moshe Leshno, Ahuva Gottreich, Abraham Golan, and Samuel Lurie, "Once a Cesarean Always a Cesarean? A Computer-Assisted Decision Analysis," *Archives of Gynecology and Obstetrics* 276 (2007): 517–21. Other studies indicate a significant percentage of placental anomalies in subsequent births after only one cesarean. See, for example, Carolyn Zelop and Linda J. Heffner, "The Downside of Cesarean Delivery: Short- and Long-Term Complications," *Clinical Obstetrics and Gynecology* 47 (June 2004): 386–93; and Q. Yang, S. W. Wan, L. Oppenheimer, X. K. Chen, D. Black, J. Gao,

and M. C. Walker, "Association of Caesarean Delivery for First Birth with Placenta Previa and Placental Abruption in Second Pregnancy," *British Journal of Obstetrics and Gynaecology* 114 (May 2007); 609–13. One article that attempts to present a balanced view of CDMR is Jane E. Brody, "With Childbirth, Now It's What the Mother Orders," *New York Times*, December 9, 2003, F7. For a discussion of the limiting of patient choice in birth even as physicians and women invoke choice, see Lawrence M. Leeman and Lauren A. Plante, "Patient-Choice Vaginal Delivery?" *Annals of Family Medicine* 4 (May–June 2006): 265–68. For a recent analysis of the safety of vaginal breech births, see H. Whyte, M. E. Hannah, S. Saigal, et al., "Outcomes of Children at 2 Years after Planned Cesarean Birth versus Planned Vaginal Birth for Breech Presentation at Term: The International Randomized Term Breech Trial," *American Journal of Obstetrics and Gynecology* 191 (2004): 864–71.

67. Grisanti, "The Cesarean Epidemic," 59, 61.

68. Nancy Wainer Cohen and Lois J. Estner, "Silent Knife: Cesarean Section in the United States," *Society* 21 (November–December 1983): 95–111. For a comprehensive list of articles discussing the risks of cesarean section, see note 66.

69. Obstetrician, interview by author, tape recording, November 1, 2005, Chicago area. One study indicates that 25% of mothers who have had cesareans feel they were pressed to have the surgery. Eugene R. Declercq, Carol Sakala, Maureen P. Corry, and Sandra Applebaum, *Listening to Mothers. II: Report of the Second National U.S. Survey of Women's Childbearing Experiences* (Childbirth Connection, 2006).

70. Obstetrician, interview by author, tape recording, June 29, 2006, Evanston, IL.

71. Presidential Address, Obstetrical Society of Philadelphia, February 12, 1981, J. Robert Willson, MD, presidential guest speaker, typed transcript, J. Robert Willson Papers, National Library of Medicine, History of Medicine Division; Thorp, McNitt, and Leppert, "Effects of Epidural Analgesia," 157–62, quote at 158. In 1990, 86.7% of ACOG fellows were men; only 13.3% were women. In 2005, 62.4% were men, and 37.6% were women. Yet among ACOG's younger members, women were the vast majority by 2005. In 1990, 55.6% of ACOG's junior fellows were men, and 44.4% were women. In 2005, only 27.8% were men, and 72.2% were women. "Manpower Statistics," compiled by ACOG, available from the ACOG Library, Washington, DC.

72. Katherine Shaver, "Birth Centers' Closures Limit Delivery Options," *Washington Post*, May 18, 2007, B1.

73. Ibid.; Dennis Thompson, "Spat with Hospital Heads to Court," *Salem (OR) Statesman Journal*, May 18, 2007; Erin Allday, "Fewer Options for Those Who Seek Natural Births. Midwives Becoming Less Popular as Cesarean Sections Gain Ground," *San Francisco Chronicle*, May 29, 2007.

74. Maria V. Gibson and William J. Hueston, "Recruiting Faculty to Perform Deliveries in Family Medicine Residencies: Results of a Residency Program Survey," *Family Medicine* 39 (March 2007): 178–83; Frederick M. Chen, Jane Huntington, Sara Kim, William R. Phillips, Nancy G. Stevens, "Prepared but Not Practicing: Declining Pregnancy Care among Recent Family Medicine Residency Graduates," *Family Medicine* 38 (June 2006): 423–26. In 1970, family physicians attended 31% of hospital births. Committee on Maternal Health, ACOG, *National Study of Maternity Care Sur-*

vey of Obstetric Practice and Associated Services in Hospitals in the United States (ACOG, 1970), 9.

75. Sandra Steingraber, *Having Faith: An Ecologist's Journey to Motherhood* (Perseus, 2001), 154–61, 175–76, 193–200, quote at 154.

76. Ibid.; a mother, interview by author, tape recording, November 2, 2005, Lombard, IL. For analyses of childbirth education classes today, see Barbara Katz Rothman, *In Labor: Women and Power in the Birthplace* (W. W. Norton, 1991), 31, 170–78; and Robbie E. Davis-Floyd, *Birth as an American Rite of Passage* (University of California Press, 2003), 32.

77. Steingraber, *Having Faith*, 154–60.

78. Ibid., 161.

79. Ibid., 175–76.

80. Ibid., 194–95.

81. For discussions of changing attitudes toward feminism and changing definitions of female empowerment (from defining social activism and antimaterialism as empowering in the 1970s to defining upscale women's achievement and self-improvement as empowering in the 1990s, for example), see Susan J. Douglas, *Where the Girls Are: Growing Up Female with the Mass Media* (Times Books, 1994), 245–94; and Joan Jacobs Brumberg, *The Body Project: An Intimate History of American Girls* (Random House, 1997), xvii–xxxiii, 195–201. See also Johanna Brenner, "U.S. Feminism in the Nineties," *New Left Review* (July–August 1993): 101–59; and Wendy Kaminer, "Feminism's Identity Crisis," *Atlantic*, October 1993, 51–53, 56, 58–59, 62, 64, 66–68.

bougie, 122; definition of, 197

Bradley, Katherine Shedd, 122

Bradley, Robert A.: obstetric anesthesia and, 4–5; theory of, 157. *See also* Bradley Method

Bradley Method: description of, 197–98, 206n9; Lamaze vs., 157

breastfeeding, hospital policies and, 160

breech birth: cesarean section and, 181; choice and, 190; obstetricians' skill at, 180

Brown, Nellie, 18

Brumberg, Joan Jacobs, 208n5, 208n6

Carmody, Francis, 55

Carmody, Mrs. Francis: death of, 68–69; Twilight Sleep Association and, 55–56

Carstens, J. H., on chloroform, 96

castor oil: inducing labor with, 105, 120, 134. *See also* elective induction of labor; induction of labor

Catholic Church, birth practices and, 139

Caton, Donald, on Dick-Read, 153

caudal anesthesia, 87; definition of, 198; development of, 89–90; side effects of, 90, 159. *See also* obstetric anesthesia

CDMR. *See* cesarean delivery by maternal request

Central Free Dispensary (Chicago): obstetric anesthesia use and, 100; twilight sleep and, 58

cervical dilation: definition of, 198; epidural anesthesia and, 177; forcible, 122. *See also* Friedman curve

cervical effacement, definition of, 198

cesarean delivery by maternal request, 178; ACOG policy on, 190; definition of, 198; female empowerment and, 195; female physicians' and, 187–88; infant morbidity and mortality and, 190; low-risk vaginal birth vs., 188; maternal mortality and, 190; mothers' attitude toward, 189–90; paternalism and, 191; perception of risk and, 190. *See also* cesarean section

cesarean section: choice and, 187–91, 196; class and, 257n33; definition of, 198; electronic fetal monitor and, 178, 185–86; epidural anesthesia and, 177, 178, 185–86, 191; female physicians and, 188, 189–91; fetal outcome and, 182; indications for, 180–81; malpractice liability fears and, 183, 259n45; maternal mortality and, 182; NICU and, 184; normalization of, 178–79, 187, 193; obstetricians' attitudes toward, 179–80, 181–82, 187,

257n34; placental anomalies and, 181, 190; rates, 166, 178, 179, 180, 181, 182, 186, 187, 196; repeat, 180; rickets and, 180, 258n36; rise in, 178–84; risk and, 179–81, 182, 183, 190–91; techniques, 180; vaginal birth vs., 182, 190. *See also* cesarean delivery by maternal request

Channing, Walter: ether and, 24, 28–29; Charles Meigs and, 28; views of birth of, 23–24, 42

Charity Hospital (New Orleans): obstetric residents at, 91; saddle block anesthesia at, 100–101, 110

Chicago Lying-in Dispensary: chloroform use at, 95; founding of, 22; maternal morbidity at, 76, 95

childbed fever. *See* postpartum infection

childbirth. *See* birth

childbirth education: attitudes toward, 168; in hospitals, 140, 246n7; hospital takeover of, 167, 193–94; physician-offered, 158–59; rivalry among methods of, 157–58; women's movement and, 146. *See also* Lamaze method; Bradley method; HypnoBirthing

Childbirth without Fear (Dick-Read), women's discovery of, 82

chloral: definition of, 198; by rectum, 34. *See also* obstetric anesthesia

chloroform: administration of, 37, 39–40, 92; class and, 33–34; debate about, 29–30; definition of, 198; discovery of, 14, 24–25; effect of, on birth practices, 42–43; ether vs., 95, 96; home birth and, 100; hospital birth and, 34; introduction of, 1; mothers' views of, 31, 37–38, 42, 113, 152; in rural areas, 41, 80–81, 96; in Scotland, 1, 27, 86; side effects, 27, 29, 70, 95–96, 102, 113, 214n52, 227n10; James Young Simpson and, 24–25; social concerns and, 14–20, 54; therapeutic uses of, 28, 54; twilight sleep vs., 51, 59; use of, to attract patients, 41. *See also* obstetric anesthesia

Christian Family Movement, 139

civil rights movement, birth reform and, 139

Cold War, obstetric anesthesia and, 109

consumers' movement, birth reform and, 138

contraception. *See* birth control

Cook County Hospital: birth at, 85; cesarean section rate, 181

Cragin, Edwin B., on cesarean sections, 180

cyclopropane: definition of, 198; physicians' preference for, 86; side effects of, 96. *See also* obstetric anesthesia

definition of, 199; side effects of, 96. *See also* obstetric anesthesia

eugenics movement: birthrate and, 53–54; maternal mortality and, 75

failure to progress. *See* dystocia

family physicians: effect of, malpractice premiums on, 193; fight of, to attend births, 230n35; low-risk births and, 193; number of attending births, 193. *See also* general practitioners

Farm, the: birth statistics, 247n20; Midwifery Center, 138–39

fathers, in delivery rooms, 146, 150–51, 179. *See also* birth: fathers' views of; induction of labor: fathers' views of

Feminine Mystique (Friedan), 170

feminism: birth reform and, 9, 11, 138, 139, 148–49, 160–61, 171; cesarean section rate and, 187; effect of, on anesthesiology, 174–75; effect of, on birth practices, 60, 149–50, 194–95; natural childbirth and, 146, 158, 165; in Reagan era, 170, 265n81; reproductive rights and, 177–78

Finney, Roy P., 79

first stage labor: without anesthesia, 42; analgesia during, 129; anesthesia during, 39, 40, 84, 114, 119, 129; definition of, 199; physicians' views of, 25–26, 39–40, 213n42; physiology of, 4. *See also* labor; transition

Flexner, Abraham, Flexner Report, 62–63

forceps: anesthesia and, 34, 38, 59, 68, 76, 94, 98, 133, 159, 195, 227n10; definition of, 199; in lieu of cesarean section, 180; maternal mortality and, 76–77; mothers' views of, 137; physicians' views of, 76–77, 134; postpartum infection and, 75–76; prophylactic use of, 120, 123; protest against, 147, 158; rates, 77; as routine, 110, 114, 119, 135; training, 75–76

Freiburg Frauenklinik: American mothers' visits to, 44–46, 47, 51, 55–56, 63–64; American physicians' visits to, 49, 57, 58, 59, 60; class and, 49–50, 56, 63

Friedan, Betty, 170

Friedman curve, 117; critique of, 241n31; definition of, 199

Gaskin, Ina May: activism of, 138–39; 147, 148–49, 151; births of, 136–38; midwifery center of, 144

Gaskin, Stephen, 137–38

Gauss, C. J.: twilight sleep and, 44, 48, 49, 51, 54–55, 57, 63; Mrs. Cecil Stewart and, 45

general practitioners, 84; low-risk birth and, 83; obstetrics and, 21–22, threat of, to obstetricians, 83, 230n35

Gerber, Michele, 188

Gilbreth, Frank Bunker, 118

Gilbreth, Lillian Moller: births of, 65–66; theory of, 118

Greenhill, J. P., 175

Greenwood, Esther, 71

Guernsey, Henry N., on birth, 26

Gwathmey, James Tayloe: American Association of Anesthetists and, 87–88; rectal anesthesia and, 69, 87, 88; synergistic method of, 87–88

gynecology, obstetrics and, 82, 84, 188–89

halothane: definition of, 199; side effects of, 86. *See also* obstetric anesthesia

Harer, Benson, on cesarean delivery by maternal request, 187

Harland, Marion: on the birthrate, 17; on obstetric anesthesia, 29

Hawkins, Joy, 175

Hawks, Graham G., on natural childbirth, 165

health insurance. *See* insurance

Heardman, Helen, Dick-Read and, 155

Hellman, Alfred, on twilight sleep, 58–59

hemorrhage. *See* postpartum hemorrhage

Henderson, Yandell, on barbiturates and labor, 94

Hendricks, Cecilia Hennel, births of, 80

heroin, as obstetric analgesic, 129

HEW. *See* Department of Health, Education, and Welfare

Heywood, Neal, on birth, 80

Hingson, Robert: on anesthesiologists, 93; on birth practices, 131; caudal anesthesia and, 87, 89–90; on fear of labor, 79, 81; on side effects of obstetric anesthesia, 96

Hirst, Barton Cooke: on anesthesia and class, 81; on marijuana, 85–86; twilight sleep and, 49

Hoffman-La Roche Chemical Company: Nisentil and, 116; scopolamine and, 56

Holt, William, twilight sleep and, 48, 71

home birth: anesthesia and, 33, 35–36, 38, 81, 100; birth reform and, 138, 143, 144, 146, 147; class and, 100; maternal mortality and, 77; medical charities and, 22–23, 32–33, 34, 100; mothers' experience of, 19, 32–33, 35–36, 66, 146, 192; physicians' views of, 64, 66, 165; race and, 145; rates, 77,

natural childbirth *(continued)*
and, 139–40; women's magazines and, 133,
161–63; women's movement and, 146, 158, 165.
See also birth; Bradley method; HypnoBirthing;
labor; Lamaze
Natural Childbirth (Dick-Read), 154
Natural Childbirth and the Christian Family (Wessel), 140
Nembutal: paraldehyde and, 87, 126; Pitocin and,
124. *See also* barbiturate; obstetric anesthesia;
pentobarbital
neonatal intensive care unit, effect of, on cesarean
section rate, 184, 186
neurasthenia, symptoms of, 15
Newell, Franklin, S., 48, 67
Newman, George, on infant mortality, 225n3
New York Academy of Medicine, report of, on maternal mortality, 76
NICU. *See* neonatal intensive care unit
NIH. *See* National Institutes of Health
Nisentil: advertisement for, 116; definition of, 201;
physicians' view of, 115. *See also* obstetric anesthesia; opioid
nitrous oxide: definition of, 201; mothers' view
of, 122; in rural areas, 80–81; in second stage
labor, 7, 126; side effects, 102. *See also* obstetric
anesthesia
Nuland, Sherwin, on Lamaze classes, 156–57
nurse-anesthetists: anesthesiologists and, 90,
174–75, 255n15; obstetricians and, 173, 174

obstetric anesthesia: advertising for, 56, 61, 65, 116,
127, 128; advice literature on, 29–30; backlash
against, 130–33, 141–51, 160–61; birth practices
and, 42–43, 108–9, 196; birthrate and, 17–18,
53–54; breastfeeding and, 94; charting, 35; class
and, 6, 33–35, 47, 47, 48–50, 56, 79, 81, 99–102,
222n52; choice and, 11, 176–78, 190–91, 196; convenience of, 10, 119; cost of, 244n66; culture and,
8; debate among physicians about, 1, 2, 10, 18,
23–30, 42–43; development of, 78, 85–90; in first
stage labor, 39, 40, 84, 114, 119, 129; forceps and,
76, 133, 227n10; home birth and, 33, 35–36, 38, 65,
81, 100; hospital birth and, 33–35, 81, 104; indications for, 33–34, 38–39, 177, 216n81; induction of
labor and, 121–24, 126, 133, 196; insurance reimbursement for, 244n66; maternal mortality and,
75–78, 103, 226n8, 254n13; medical school train-

ing and, 23; mothers' views of, 9, 10, 38, 61–62, 79,
81, 85, 88, 89–90, 94, 103–4, 108–10, 121, 141–51,
160–61, 176; multiple drugs, 7, 34, 84, 85, 87, 93,
94, 101, 103, 114–15, 126–30, 133, 174; newborns
and, 94, 102–3, 129, 131, 133; physicians' preference
for types of, 86–87; physicians' views of, 18,
23–30, 37–41, 58, 59–60, 67, 78–79, 86–87, 93,
94–95, 99, 102, 109, 114–15, 121, 130–31, 134, 216n81;
Pitocin and, 121–24; race and, 96, 100–102,
236n87; regional variation in use of, 27, 38,
86–87, 175; religion and, 28, 139–40; risk and,
11–12, 27–28, 69, 95, 96, 97–98, 130, 146; in rural
areas, 41, 80–81, 129–30; safety of, 10, 93–103; in
second stage labor, 5–6, 9, 35–36, 39–40, 81, 84,
89, 114, 120; side effects of, 85, 93–103; social birth
and, 100; social concerns and, 8, 14–20, 53–54, 55,
107–10, 143–51, 160–63, 169–72, 176–77, 196; techniques for administration of, 38–40, 49–50,
63–64, 92–93, 97–98, 127; therapeutic uses of, 28,
54, 59, 60; timing of, 5–6, 9, 42; women's magazines and, 78, 88, 89–90, 104, 109–10. *See also*
analgesia; anesthesia; anesthetic; caudal anesthesia; chloral; chloroform; cyclopropane; Demerol;
dilaudid; epidural anesthesia; ether; ethylene;
halothane; heroin; Nembutal; Nisentil; nitrous
oxide; paraldehyde; Penthrane; phenazocine;
pudendal block; rectal anesthesia; saddle block;
secobarbital; Seconal; sodium amytal; spinal
anesthesia; Thorazine; trichloroethylene; twilight sleep
obstetricians: anesthesiologists and, 172–73; as
anesthetists, 173–76; baby boom and, 119; board
certification of, 82–85; cesarean section and,
179–80; effect of feminists on practice of, 149–50;
effect of malpractice threat on, 183; family physicians and, 193; fees of, 61–62; female, 187–88; general practitioners and, 21–22, 83; medical technology and, 191–92; mothers' views of, 61–62,
110–13; natural childbirth and, 165–66; numbers
of, 262n59, 264n71; pathologizing birth, 2, 6, 28,
83–85, 120, 189, 193, 262n62; prenatal care and,
110–14; as solo practitioners, 119; status of, 10,
20–23, 61–66, 70–71
obstetric residencies, 82–85; effect of, on hospital
birth, 104, 229n33; growth in, 83
obstetric residents: training of, 85, 183–84; training
of, in anesthesiology, 91, 173
obstetrics: certifying board for, 82–85; effect of